Children's Services: Working Together

Children's Services: Working Together

Malcolm Hill, George Head, Andrew Lockyer, Barbara Reid, Raymond Taylor

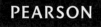

Harlow, England • London • New York • Boston • San Francisco • Toronto • Sydney • Auckland • Singapore • Hong Kong
Tokyo • Seoul • Taipei • New Delhi • Cape Town • São Paulo • Mexico City • Madrid • Amsterdam • Munich • Paris • Milan

Pearson Education Limited
Edinburgh Gate
Harlow
Essex CM20 2JE
England

and Associated Companies throughout the world

Visit us on the World Wide Web at:
www.pearson.com/uk

First published 2012

ISBN 978-1-4082-3725-0

British Library Cataloguing-in-Publication Data
A catalogue record for this book is available from the British Library

Library of Congress Cataloguing-in-Publication Data
Children's services : working together / Malcolm Hill . . . [et al.] -- 1st ed.
     p. cm.
  ISBN 978-1-4082-3725-0 (pbk.)
  1. Children--Services for.   2. Child welfare.   I. Hill, Malcolm.
  HV713.C3966 2012
  362.7--dc23
                                        2011041566

10 9 8 7 6 5 4 3 2 1
15 14 13 12 11

Typeset in 10/12.5pt Sabon by 35
Printed by Ashford Colour Press Ltd., Gosport

We would like to dedicate this book to Professor Frederick Hope Stone – our esteemed and much-missed colleague who died in 2009. Known to most people modestly as Fred Stone, he had a distinguished career in child and adolescent psychiatry and played a unique part in the creation and development of the Scottish Children's Hearings System. He was awarded an OBE for his services to children. Fred combined academic and clinical knowledge of children with intuitive sympathy for them. He was committed to inter-agency collaboration and always showed respect for the contribution of professionals from disciplines other than his own. He also had high regard for those who freely devoted their public service to the well-being of children. His spirit is reflected in themes that are core to this book.

Brief contents

Detailed contents

Chapter 24
Collaborating to improve the health of looked-after children

301

Jackie Dougall

Chapter 25
Issues in interprofessional education

314

Sally Kuenssberg, Barbara Reid and Raymond Taylor

Chapter 26
Working together in children's services: constants and changes

328

Malcolm Hill, George Head, Andrew Lockyer, Barbara Reid and Raymond Taylor

List of contributors

Bill Alexander, NHS Highland and Highland Council
Graham Bryce, University of Glasgow
John Carnochan, Strathclyde Police
Harry Daniels, University of Bath
Jackie Dougall, Glasgow Caledonian University
Alan Dyson, University of Manchester
Anne Edwards, University of Oxford
Silvia Fargion, Free University of Bozen-Bolzano, Italy
Joan Forbes, University of Aberdeen
Robbie Gilligan, Trinity College, Dublin
Lynn Jamieson, University of Edinburgh
Sally Kuenssberg, University of Glasgow
Eva Lloyd, University of East London
Walter Lorenz, Free University of Bozen-Bolzano, Italy
Gillian MacIntyre, University of Strathclyde
Kathleen Marshall, University of Strathclyde
Elspeth McCartney, University of Strathclyde
Helen Minnis, University of Glasgow
Andrea Mooney, Cornell Law School, USA
Colin Morrison, TASC Agency/The Children's Parliament
Christine Puckering, Royal Hospital for Sick Children, Glasgow
Helen Roberts, UCL Institute of Child Health
Bob Stradling, University of Edinburgh
E. Kay M. Tisdall, University of Edinburgh
Bill Whyte, University of Edinburgh
Jane Williams, University of Swansea

Acknowledgements

Author's acknowledgements

Our greatest debt is to the contributors. They responded with goodwill and patience to requests from the publishers and ourselves to make accessible their individual expertise and viewpoints, while adhering to some standardisation of format to help produce a coherent volume. Andrew Taylor of Pearson Education has been highly supportive throughout a lengthy process and made helpful suggestions to improve the book. Our thanks go to other staff at Pearson, including Lauren Hayward and Jane Hawes, for their help with the final stages of production. We are grateful for encouraging comments on plans for the book made by Sandy Jamieson of Eastwood High School, Marion MacAulay and Deirdre O'Hara of North Lanarkshire Council and Richard Hosking, organisational consultant. We'd also like to thank Sir Paul Ennals, Chair of the Children's Workforce Development Council and Chief Executive of the NCB, Anna Fowlie, Chief Executive of the SSSC and Professor Andrew Cooper at the Tavistock, London for their valued input.

We received constructive feedback from anonymous reviewers on both the outline contents for the book and a late draft, which has assisted us to make the book as relevant to multiple perspectives as we can.

Publisher's acknowledgements

We are grateful to the following for permission to reproduce copyright material:

Figures

Figure 5.1 adapted from Getting it Right for Every Child: Guidance on the Child's or Young Person's Plan, http://www.scotland.gov.uk/Publications/2007/01/22142141/3, The Scottish Government, © Crown Copyright 2007

Text

Example 11.2 adapted from Evaluation of the full service extended schools initiative: Final Report. Research report RR852, *Report for DfES*, pp.52–53 (2007), London, Crown Copyright material is reproduced with permission under the terms of the Click-Use License; Examples 15.1 and 15.2 from Highet, G. and Jamieson, L.

(2007) Cool with change: Young people and family change. Final Report, http://www.crfr.ac.uk/reports/CWC%20final%20report%202007.pdf; Example 16.1 from Fair Society, Healthy Lives: A Strategic Review of Health Inequalities in England Post-2010, http://www.ucl.ac.uk/gheg/marmotreview

In some instances we have been unable to trace the owners of copyright material, and we would appreciate any information that would enable us to do so.

Chapter 1

Introduction

Malcolm Hill, George Head, Andrew Lockyer, Barbara Reid and Raymond Taylor

Few individuals who work with children do so in isolation from other professions and organisations. For most, successful performance of their particular role requires cooperation with others. In recent years, children's policies in the UK have emphasised the need for a shared commitment by everyone to promoting children's health, welfare, learning and their ability to contribute responsibly to society. Various terms have been deployed to express this vision, from working together to integrated services.

This book is intended to provide knowledge about policy, theory, research and practice relevant to all professionals who work with children and those training to join such professions. A volume of this size cannot attempt to cover comprehensively the detailed understanding required in any particular profession. Rather, it complements more specialist texts by concentrating on topics of common interest related to children and their lives, and to ways in which interprofessional collaboration can be enhanced. It provides some core knowledge, ideas and values relevant to anyone working with children and offers critical awareness of the issues that arise when people of different training, experience and organisational settings collaborate.

Several broad themes permeate the book:

- an emphasis on situations when different types of profession and agency work together for the sake of the children and families they are seeking to help;
- an holistic approach to children, which requires understanding multiple dimensions of their lives and the key people and circumstances with which they interact;
- the importance of approaches that involve working with children, their families and other community members as active participants;
- the need for reflective practitioners, aware of the influences and assumptions shaping their own training and everyday work, and empathic towards the values and knowledge bases of different professionals;
- the importance of understanding organisational and interpersonal influences on the work of professionals and especially on interprofessional cooperation;
- recognition of a wide range of relevant clusters of theories, e.g. related to children, families, organisations and groups;

- critical awareness of key concepts shared by a number of professions, but open to varying interpretation and application, e.g. rights, risk, needs, agency, learning, social capital, attachment and resilience;
- recognition that there are different perspectives within and between professional and academic disciplines, which involve complementarity, differences in emphasis and, at times, tension or conflict.

The key principle underpinning these themes and the book is that all professionals working with children should pay close attention to connectedness – of different elements of children's lives; between children and their family, friends and communities; among agencies and professionals. Naturally the salience of connectedness will vary according to the particular functions of an individual practitioner and the circumstances they are dealing with. At times, specialist roles and skills will be applicable and predominate, as when children are in a maths class or a young person attends accident and emergency services with a serious injury. Even then the situation is not entirely one of learning or medical treatment, because the children's experiences and responses will be affected by such matters as their home backgrounds, the meanings they attribute to what is happening to them, peer relationships, availability of educational or emotional support and so on.

The rest of this chapter briefly reviews different ways of understanding children and childhood, and then considers the service, legal and policy context for working with children.

What is a child?

The answer to this question may seem obvious, but ideas about children and childhood have varied greatly across time and culture (Zwozdiak-Myers 2007; Pressler 2010). During the Middle Ages, children engaged in work and play alongside adults soon after infancy, and were usually dressed the same as adults. In traditional farming or herding societies across the world children from 6 or 7 years upwards have usually taken responsibility for care of animals, fields and younger siblings and cousins. By contrast, nowadays we tend to think of children as depending on adults materially and emotionally for a substantial number of years. They are rarely seen in adult work and leisure places, but spend much time in locations devoted largely or exclusively to children (early years centres, schools, clubs etc.) Nevertheless, considerable cultural and individual variations occur in beliefs and values about children, including different emphases on individual fulfilment or extended family commitments, the influence of nature and nurture, appropriate forms of behaviour and punishment etc.

It can be tempting to consider children largely in terms of what they lack. In other words, they do not have the competence, power, status, knowledge, experience and understanding that adults possess. It is only a short step to regarding childhood as simply a period for making good deficiencies and preparing to be adult. Much recent academic thinking, however, highlights the need to consider children's current activities, perspectives and pre-occupations as important in their own right, of inherent worth 'for now' and not only for possible future benefits. This is linked to recognition that children have 'agency', i.e. capacities to shape their own lives. This is obviously within limitations arising from immediate and wider circumstances, but children are not merely the products of influential adults around them (Mayall 2002).

The boundaries of childhood are fluid. Debates about abortion highlight that, for some people and in certain respects, a foetus in the womb can be seen as already a child. At the other end of childhood, the extension of education over the past two centuries or so has increased the length of time that children may be financially dependent. Associated with this has been a growing view that children have distinct needs and rights until well into their teens. The UN Convention on the Rights of the Child, introduced in 1989 and subsequently ratified by nearly every nation state, indicates that the 18th birthday should normally be the upper limit for the special rights attributed to children (see below). This is the practice accepted in the UK, although a wide range of age thresholds exists for such matters as criminal responsibility, school-leaving, driving, marrying and voting.

Although teenagers are legally still 'children' in the above sense, most would not describe themselves as such and many of them would be insulted to be called a child. It is, therefore, common to use the phrase 'young people' for older children.[1] Similarly, when reference is made to children in school, use of 'pupil' is increasingly restricted to primary school, and 'student' preferred in secondary, as well as in further and higher education. The term 'adolescent' is widely employed by psychologists, psychiatrists and others as representing the period of (literally) becoming adult, but is disliked by some people for having negative connotations (immature, troublesome). Young people collectively are sometimes referred to as 'youth', with distinct cultures and activities, although in North America youth can include younger children too. Matters to do with crime committed by young people are generally described under the umbrella of *youth* justice.

Diverse and changing childhoods in the UK

In many ways family life has become more diverse over the past half century. Lower rates of marriage and increases in separation and divorce have resulted in more lone-parent households (nearly one quarter of children), a larger proportion of reconstituted families with step- and half-siblings and greater numbers of children growing up with couples who live together on a long-term basis but are not married, including gay couples (Hill 2009a; Maplethorpe et al. 2009). The percentage of mothers who work has grown markedly. Some commentators have seen these trends as an unfortunate erosion of traditional family patterns; others as representing greater choice, with fewer adults and children trapped in unhappy or abusive relationships.

Ethnic diversity has become commonplace, particularly in cities and towns. The great majority of black and ethnic minority children are born and brought up in

---

[1] In this book, 'children' should be taken to denote 'children and young people' unless otherwise stated.

Britain, though usually with some degree of dual or multiple identities, reflecting the customs and religion of their families' countries of origin (Modood 2007). Early years services, schools and other agencies nowadays make considerable efforts to value the cultures present in their catchment areas and to attend where necessary to language issues. However, even well-meaning professionals from a different ethnic background to a given child may fail to understand the significance of language, family communication and attitudes – for example, in relation to eating disorders or mental health problems (Jackson et al. 2008).

Rates of child poverty in the UK diminished in the first decade of the new millennium, but still remain higher than in some other countries in western Europe (Bradshaw and Mayhew 2005; Hamilton 2011). Lone-parent households and certain minority ethnic groups are over-represented among the poor (Hansen et al. 2010a). Economic and social disparities are closely linked to inequalities in child health and educational performance (Marmot 2010).

'Childhood . . . is increasingly saturated by technology' (Hutchby and Moran-Ellis 2001, p. 1). Rapid changes have exposed children to a wider range of information and influence beyond the family and school, resulting in myriad effects on their communication, activities and culture. Patterns of computer use tend to vary with gender, ethnicity and family income (Hansen et al. 2010a). Opportunities and risks abound, which professionals need to keep up with (Livingstone 2009).

How do and should we envisage childhood?

Many specialist theories and concepts have been used to aid understanding of children, of which a few are considered in Part III of the book. Here we consider three broad frameworks that emphasise respectively:

1. how children change as they grow older;
2. how children can shape what happens to them, in the context of socially produced assumptions;
3. environment influences and settings.

Developmental approaches

Academic thinking about children in the twentieth century was largely dominated by child psychology and applications of psychological analysis in fields such as education and child psychiatry. Child psychology textbooks and journals remain valuable compendia of knowledge about children, usually organised on different broad age groupings and/or dimensions like physical, cognitive and social (e.g. Lindon 2005).

For the most part, child psychology and associated disciplines have taken a developmental perspective, i.e. seeing children as evolving and improving in various ways as they grow older, building on earlier achievements. This clearly links to the commonsense observation that, with increasing age, children typically get bigger, move more adeptly and quickly, learn to speak, extend their intellectual skills, and so on. Several key theorists have presented such progressions in terms of stages occurring at roughly similar times for most children, e.g. Freud (psycho-sexual development), Piaget (changes in ways of thinking), Erikson (psycho-social development) and Kohlberg (moral reasoning). A related concept is that of developmental milestones, a level of functioning achieved by most children at roughly the same age in a given culture, such as standing, walking and talking. It can be helpful to identify children who achieve such milestones late, or maybe not all, so that they can be given appropriate treatment or extra help. This has been the purpose of the Sheridan charts used in public health and early years services for several decades. There are, though, dangers of exaggerating the significance of natural variations and of stigmatising those who differ from the norm.

Other important conceptualisations of development have not been stage-based, or only loosely so. These include attachment theory dealing with care-giving and children's intimate relationships, and approaches derived from the Russian theorist Vygotsky concerning children's active engagement with their environments and interpretations using language and signs, both discussed later in the book.

The social construction approach to childhood

During the 1990s a growing critique of developmental psychology occurred, leading to the creation of an alternative paradigm in the social studies of childhood (James and Prout 1998). The key idea is that both lay and expert expectations and understandings of children are socially constructed. This does not mean that all ideas about children are socially determined, since the biological basis of some phenomena is accepted (Prout 2005), but the precise ways in which childhood is regarded and experienced are crucially shaped by interaction with the cultural and historical context and prevailing assumptions (Zwozdiak-Myers 2007).

The social constructionist approach to childhood was initiated in sociology, anthropology and history, but has extended to other subject areas such as geography, as well as influencing applied disciplines. It challenged what it saw as the main tenets in developmental psychology:

- childhood is largely biologically driven and comprises relatively fixed stages;
- children are lacking in adult competence, and childhood is primarily about developing knowledge and skills as a preparation for adulthood;
- children are largely moulded by adult socialisation;
- variations in childhood experience are typically treated in terms of factors like age, gender and ethnicity whose influence is best examined by means of statistical analysis.

This portrayal exaggerated the uniformity of developmental psychology and disregarded some of its more subtle and qualified accounts, which often include a very active role for the child in, for instance, learning about their worlds and developing relationships. Woodhead (2008) offers a more nuanced critique of what he called a 'crude developmental model' and highlights valuable aspects of child psychology that recognise children's agency and the fluidity and diversity of childhood.

In any case, the social studies of childhood have largely moved on to provide a range of new understandings, based particularly on children's own perspectives and priorities about their active engagement with different aspects of everyday life (e.g. Holloway and Valentine 2000; Markström and Hallden 2009). Children's experiences and accounts are valued in their own right, rather than as steps en route to adulthood. Emphasis has also been placed on the analysis of children's status as a social group, lacking power, and with distinctive experiences and characteristics as a 'generational unit' (Qvortrup 2008). Another strand has classified and questioned representations of children made by adults (in academe, policy, the media), for instance, seeing them as typically innocent, vulnerable, threatening or incompetent.

Ecological frameworks

Holistic approaches to understanding children's worlds take into account how the child interacts with the local and wider environment. Much evidence indicates that the foundations of children's well-being, learning and behaviour are laid by the families and neighbourhoods within which they grow up. Probably the best-known example of an environmental framework is the ecological model of Bronfenbrenner (1979), which he introduced as a corrective to narrow concentration on the individual and family in developmental child psychology. Bronfenbrenner portrayed a child's world as comprising four concentric circles of relationships and influences. The four systems are of different scales, ranging from the immediate situation of a child (microsystem) via family, neighbourhood and parental work (meso- and exosystems) to beliefs, attitudes and policies present in wider society and culture (macrosystem). This approach is largely descriptive, but provides a useful framework for organising information about different levels in a child's environment and how they interact.

The influence of such thinking can be seen in the assessment triangle used in government policies, which directs attention to environmental influences on parents and children from societal and policy processes, communities and schools (Aldgate et al. 2006). A further implication is that interventions often need to act with or on people other than the child in order to achieve their agreed goals. The Munro review of child protection services (2011) argued that a shift is required from 'atomistic' thinking, which concentrates on individual problems of children and families, to a 'holistic' approach that relates all aspects to each other and takes account of long chains of causality and consequences. This requires understanding not only of the socio-spatial environments of children but of the way service systems operate and interact with each other and with children and their families.

What is a children's service? Agencies and professionals that work with children

Axford (2010) highlights how the word 'service' has multiple meanings, so it is important to be clear which sense is being used at any one time:

- Professional activities aimed at assisting children and families;
- The legal status of the activities;
- The organisation in which those activities take place (the service provider).

Defining what is meant by a children's service is a far from easy task. Families, friends and neighbours often perform services for children, but that is not the sense intended here. Policy documents about children's services typically focus on more formal services that are publicly provided or 'commissioned', with the core functions falling within health, education, care and protection, policing and youth justice.

Many children's services are provided directly by public agencies, but there have always been contributions from voluntary and private organisations: for example, with respect to day and residential care. Health services for children are part of a national service based largely in primary care and hospitals, with children's nurses, paediatricians, midwives, health visitors and child and adolescent psychiatrists as the main roles specialising in children's physical and mental health. Local authorities in England, Scotland and Wales have broad responsibilities for education, child and family social work, leisure and others services for children. In Northern Ireland children's social services were traditionally part of health services, currently in joint Departments for Health, Social Services and Public Safety (DHSSPS). The police are organised into regional forces, some with units and roles that focus wholly or in part on child abuse or young people who offend.

Lawyers in private practice and in law centres provide advice and advocacy services for children and parents, while some are employed by local authorities with a remit to assist with legal matters related to children, such as contested child abuse or adoption cases. Certain bodies provide services linked to legal decision-making, such as the Child and Family Court Advisory and Support Services (CAFCASS) in England and CAFCASS CYMRU in Wales. CAFCASS handles both public law cases (court proceedings where children may need local government involvement in their care and protection) and private law cases (mainly situations where separating parents cannot agree on contact or residence arrangements for children). CAFCASS staff are mainly social workers, whereas in Scotland safeguarders (appointed to protect and advise on children's best interests in difficult cases) may be either lawyers or social workers. This is also true for children's reporters in Scotland, who act as gatekeepers to the hearings system that makes decisions about compulsory measures that may be needed for a child's care or protection, or in response to their behaviour. Northern Ireland has its own Guardian Ad Litem Agency. This body recruits and organises a panel of independent officers, experienced in working with children and families, who are appointed to safeguard children's interests in care and adoption proceedings.

It is valuable to take a flexible rather than exclusive approach to considering children's services. Certain financial transfers through the social security system and employment measures by government, such as child benefit and maternity/parental leave, can have a major impact on children's well-being, although these are not usually depicted as services. A research study that asked children themselves about what they understood to be local services found that the three types of facility mentioned most commonly included only one of the conventional list, i.e. health. The other two were shops and leisure (Wager et al. 2007). On the whole, sales of food and goods are seen as commercial activities, but the children were right in understanding that that they do indeed perform a vital service, even if the treatment of child customers by some was rated as poor. Recreation services provide opportunities not only for fun, but also for learning vital life and social skills, developing social relationships and pursuing healthy lifestyles.

Relevant services are sometimes devoted solely to children, as in the case of schools and many charitable organisations. Others cater for people of all generations. They include GPs, the police, swimming pools and libraries. Many professional groups as a whole cover most or all stages of life, but usually contain age-related specialisms such as paediatricians, schoolteachers, child and family social workers and child psychotherapists. A number of voluntary children's organisations operate nationally at UK or devolved levels, while there are many local and regional agencies. Some non-age-related charitable bodies make an important contribution to children, notably in the disability field.

Certain services are universal in that they are used by or available to all families and children, as in the case of midwives, GPs and schools. Others are targeted. This is often on the basis of particular needs or problems, e.g. child and family social services, speech and language therapy. The word 'specialist' is commonly attached to such services, though this is sometimes reserved for work with small, particular groups, for example, adoption and fostering (DfES 2003). Periodically policies and services have been targeted on certain geographical areas, normally ones with high levels of deprivation and need. Examples are Health Action Zones and Sure Start.

Within the early years context, it has been suggested by Moss and Petrie (2002) that the phrase 'children's services' is unhelpful, because it is bound up with adult-organised forms of provision and adult-defined objectives. They put forward as an alternative the concept of 'children's spaces', which they suggested allows for more flexibility and negotiation between children and adults about the purpose and use of facilities. Moss (2006) proposes that such a reconceptualisation would not only lead to more productive and ethical forms of care and education, but also contribute to democratic renewal and inclusive politics. This argument has been developed largely in relation to services in places where children spend long periods of time like nurseries, schools and youth clubs. It is less straightforward to apply to services where a professional meets a child or family on occasions in the home or at an office or clinic. Nevertheless, it highlights the importance of taking account of how children experience the spaces where their encounters with professionals take place and adapting these accordingly.

It should not be forgotten that some adult services also have relevance to children, for two reasons in particular. First, drug and alcohol agencies, adult mental health services and prisons need to be aware that many people using their services are parents and to be mindful of the consequences for their children of actions they take. Second, young people in their teens who require a continuing service as adults will be helped if communication and continuity between children's and adult's services are good.

During recent years all professional groups whether working with children, adults or both have witnessed a shift in orientation towards greater participation by the people they work with. Most commonly this has been seen at the level of involvement with individual children and family members. In the past it was not uncommon for doctors, teachers, dentists and others to talk at or down to patients and children, not necessarily with malign intentions or consequences, but simply because that was how they thought they should deploy their knowledge to teach, cure etc. This may be termed the 'expert approach'. Now it is usual for professionals and indeed decision-makers to seek to engage with the expectations and wishes of people using their service, so that expert knowledge is imparted or deployed to help someone with a problem in a way that is likely to be more acceptable and accessible. This trend has been described variously as being more subject-focused, child-centred or person-centred. Some professionals and agencies have gone further and sought dialogue with service users more collectively (e.g. through surveys or meetings). Both in the cases of individuals and groups, the aim is to be more inclusive and/or empowering. We shall return to this issue when considering policy later in this chapter and also in the concluding chapter. (The principles and nature of children's services are covered in detail in Part I of the book.)

The legal basis for work with children

The nature and role of the law

To varying degrees everyone who works with children is affected by the law. Those working in the statutory sector (local authorities, NHS, police) are expected to implement legal requirements placed on the agencies they work for. It is common to distinguish between legal *duties* given to statutory organisations, which they are obliged to carry out, and legal *powers*, which they can deploy if and when they deem it appropriate or affordable.

Those working outside the statutory sector will generally be less bound by legal considerations, but voluntary organisations must comply with charity law, while they, together with private enterprises, are also generally subject to regulation and, if they provide centre-based or residential services, to registration. In recent years it has become mandatory for any individual who has access to children not related to them to have a police check to see if they have previously committed an offence against children.

The law not only gives authority for certain official actions, it also provides supervision of how duties and powers are carried out through such means as complaints procedures and judicial review (Williams 2008). The legal system, mainly through the courts, also makes key decisions in individual cases where it is alleged that a law has been broken. Some professionals such as legal representatives and the police also need to be aware of relevant *case law*, i.e. precedents from past legal decisions relevant to the case in hand.

The influence of international law

Until recently virtually all domestic law was enacted by the UK Parliament. However, as a result of membership of the European Union and also of devolution, it has become increasingly to consider legislation from multiple levels. Membership of the

European Union has meant that a wide range of matters is subject to European law. Though many of these relate to commercial activities and trade, certain matters do affect children, notably those concerned with movement from one country to another (e.g. entitlements to healthcare, education and financial benefits). EU funding made possible a cross-border project between Northern Ireland and the Republic of Ireland, which resulted in a common framework for planning in relation to children and families (Canavan et al. 2009).

The Human Rights Act (HRA) 1998 embodied the European Convention on Human Rights (ECHR) in UK law. The ECHR was formulated not by the European Union but by the Council of Europe – a looser association of European countries. The HRA 1998 requires all public bodies to ensure that their acts and decisions are compatible with the rights and freedoms of the ECHR (e.g. the right to life, not to be tortured etc.). The HRA makes little specific reference to children, but has wide relevance to them. For instance, it affects the kinds of circumstance in which children can be deprived of their liberty and the principles for information-sharing between agencies about children and other members of their families (Goldthorpe 2004; Marshall 2006). British courts are expected to uphold the ECHR, but individuals are also entitled to bring a complaint against a public authority to the European Court of Human Rights in Strasbourg (see Williams 2008 for examples of UK cases involving children that have been considered). For the most part, the HRA has not had a major impact on the curriculum or everyday running of schools, but it has acted as a restraint on certain disciplinary measures and discrimination. It also supports involvement of children in key decisions (Whitburn 2003). In relation to youth justice, Council of Europe rules apply to the UK.

Another major international influence is the UN Convention on the Rights of the Child (UNCRC). This has been ratified by nearly all the world's nation states including the UK, which is therefore committed to implementing its provisions. The UNCRC comprises 54 Articles, which place duties on 'state parties' (i.e. national governments). A few apply to particular circumstances, such as refugee children and those 'without families'. Among the universal provisions are the rights to survival and good health; protection from ill-treatment; provision of appropriate services; and the right to have their views taken into account in decisions affecting them. All rights should apply without discrimination on the basis of gender, ethnicity, religion or ability. Contrary to some common misconceptions, the UNCRC does not undermine family unity or the authority of parents. It asserts parental rights and responsibilities and, like the ECHR, stresses children's rights to family life (Williams 2008). Moreover, Article 29 states that education should be directed, first, to the child's own talents and potential, and should also cover respect for parents, as well as human rights in general and respect for one's own and others' cultures (Osler 2010).

Children's legislation in the four UK jurisdictions

Since the late 1990s devolution has also had an important impact on social legislation, including that related to children. Pre-devolution, England and Wales were bound by the same legislation. The Children Act 1989 mainly covered England and

Wales (except for certain early years provisions in Scotland) and remains the statutory basis for the care and protection of children, post-divorce arrangements and youth offending. The 1989 Act sought to integrate private law (e.g. divorce) with public law (mainly to do with the role of local authorities and courts with regard to care, protection and crime). Subsequent statutes with more specific foci have modified and extended the law with regard to offending, antisocial behaviour and early years provision, and have updated the law on adoption (Williams 2008).

After the creation of the Welsh Assembly in 1999, the Children Act 1989 and Adoption Act 1976 remained applicable across both England and Wales. Subsequent primary legislation extends across both countries, but sometimes with separate parts referring to services in each country, as in the Children Act 2004 (see below). The Assembly is now responsible for secondary legislation in Wales, i.e. regulations and standards, for instance, as regards residential homes and private fostering (Williams 2008). Wales was the first of the four jurisdictions to establish a Children's Commissioner. The Welsh Assembly Government has developed distinctive policies in relation to such matters as child and adolescent mental health services, where all children's agencies are seen as having a part to play (Jackson et al. 2008). The Welsh approach to children's services has more explicit linking of policies to the UNCRC than elsewhere in the UK. The young people's organisation Funky Dragon, substantially funded by the Assembly, has made important contributions to policy development (Butler and Drakeford 2010).

The Children Act 2004 reformed services for children in England, leading to the creation of multi-organisational Children's Trusts, while in Wales separation between education and social work services was retained, though with a duty to cooperate (Waterman and Fowler 2004). Following the example of Wales, then Scotland and Northern Ireland, the 2004 Act created the position of Children's Commissioner in England, though with more limited powers than in the other three jurisdictions. Local authorities were required to establish Local Safeguarding Children Boards to provide strategic coordination at local levels in line with guidance from the Secretary of State (England) and Welsh Assembly (Wales). These Boards replaced the previous non-statutory Area Child Protection Committees. The Act also introduced Children and Young People's Plans (CYPPs) in both England and Wales. However, the Act transferred the functions of CAFCASS CYMRU to the Welsh Assembly, with Welsh family-proceedings officers appointed to carry out the work, some having transferred from CAFCASS. As well as carrying out case functions as in England, it also has a role in policy development (Rees 2008).

Before devolution, distinct Scottish legislation was passed at Westminster, giving Scotland among other things a different school examination system and methods for dealing with children's care and protection (children's hearings). Since the re-establishment of a Scottish Parliament at Holyrood in 1999, the responsibility for most areas of social law directly affecting children has been devolved (Tisdall and Hill 2010). However, certain matters like social security, immigration and asylum remain 'reserved', i.e. they are still dealt with at Westminster, as are economic, foreign and defence policies.

The Children (Scotland) Act 1995 is, at the time of writing, the key Scottish statute relating to children. It includes a number of elements borrowed from the 1989 Act, but has several distinctive features. In particular, except in emergency situations, compulsory measures affecting children are normally decided not by courts but by children's hearings, introduced in 1971. A panel of three lay people from the local area makes decisions following discussion with family members, social workers and sometimes other professionals (Lockyer and Stone 1998; Kearney 2000). Sheriffs (Scottish judges) only become involved if the ground for referral to the hearing is denied, or for very serious cases and appeals. The child's welfare should be the main consideration in decisions, even when the young person has committed an offence. The 1995 Act has wider interpretations for children in need and looked-after children than the 1989 Act, though the duties of local authorities towards these groups is similar. Scotland has Integrated Children's Services Plans, prepared together by education, child health, children's social work, youth justice and police services.

Northern Ireland also has separate legislation for social matters, including children's issues. The Children (NI) Order of 1995 followed the English and Welsh Children Act 1989 very closely and enabled the country to 'catch up', as it had not been included in legislative changes on the mainland for 30 years or more (Kelly and Pinkerton 1996). One key hope was to reduce use of court orders, but in fact they have increased and the time taken over applications has lengthened (Donaldson and Harbison 2006).

Throughout the UK, the key acts stipulated three key principles in decision-making:

1. The child's welfare is to be the primary consideration.

2. A compulsory order should be made only when other measures were inadequate (the minimum necessary intervention principle).

3. The child's views must be taken into account (according to the child's age and understanding).

Thus, the welfare and participation principles of the UNCRC were included, along with restraint on the use of intrusive measures, such as compulsory sentences or supervision. Although the law stipulates that children's interests should be primary considerations in legal decisions and professional actions, 'Law – like politics – has no way of knowing what is good or bad for children' (Piper 2008, p. 135). Hence, knowledge must be brought to bear about children's needs and well-being from a range of theoretical and empirical sources. [Some of these are considered in Part III of the book.]

By contrast with children's law, education legislation has been 'very much centred on the rights, entitlements and preferences of parents' (Whitburn 2003, p. 153). They have choices about which school their child will attend, for instance. Until recently the obligation of parents to ensure their children receive schooling was not accompanied by a statutory right to education for children themselves, although this has been gradually introduced.

Policy guidance and frameworks

Besides legislation, both UK and devolved governments may issue statutory guidance. Local authorities and others are not obliged to follow statutory guidance in the way

Table 1.1 Guidance for children services in the UK

Every Child Matters England	10-year Strategy for Children and Young People Northern Ireland	Getting it Right for Every Child Scotland	Core aims for children and young people Wales
Healthy	Healthy	Safe	Parenting and childcare
Safe	Enjoying, learning and achieving	Healthy	Learning and working
Enjoying and achieving	Living in safety and with stability	Achieving	Health, child protection and care
Making a positive contribution	Economic and environmental well-being	Nurtured	Play and leisure
Economic well-being	Contributing to community and society	Active	Participation and equality
	Living in a society which respects their rights	Respected	Safe home and community
		Responsible	Child poverty
		Included	

that they have a duty to implement laws, but it carries force because courts will expect them to follow it unless they have good reason not to. The main policy framework for children's services developed in England during the first decade of this century is *Every Child Matters*. The other three parts of the UK have different overarching frameworks, which vary in emphasis but embody broadly similar values and aspirations (see Table 1.1). One central thrust of these policies has been to unify objectives and actions affecting the minority of children who require intensive or specialist help with those relating to the well-being of all children – in other words, to integrate universal and targeted services. Each document has a list of desirable outcomes for children, which are similar but with slight differences in wording and order.

As the document titles indicate, these broad aims apply to every child, so each country has introduced guidance to promote 'working together' by all children's services. Aldgate (2011) describes the frameworks for assessment intended to guide the practice of everyone working with children. For instance, Northern Ireland has a very detailed framework based on thresholds and levels of interventions, whereas Scotland took a flexible approach with more scope for professional discretion. [Policies and practice with respect to interprofessional and inter-agency cooperation are considered in detail in Part IV of this book.]

Recent government policies with respect to children, education and health have placed emphasis on the overlapping concepts of prevention and early intervention. Both entail acting to nip problems in the bud. *Prevention* has been present in child welfare policy for at least 50 years, though given renewed impetus in several policy areas (Churchill 2007). Originally, preventive services and resources were meant to avert major state intervention, i.e. reduce the need for children to appear before courts or be received into care. Later the concept was broadened to encompass a range of actions to tackle child and family problems as soon as they were apparent, in order to stop them getting worse. It was a short step to seeing the need to try to prevent difficulties arising in the first place. Eventually this range of measures and stages was subsumed in the phrase 'family support'.

In the health field, the notion of prevention has long been recognised as having a similar spread. It is common to recognise three or four levels of prevention.

- primary – dealing with long-term risks in large populations;
- secondary;
- tertiary;
- quaternary – focused on a small number of individuals or families at high risk.

These correspond approximately to four tiers of service ranging from Tier 1 (universal, e.g. GPs, health visitors) to Tier 4 (highly specialised, e.g. in-patient units). A child or family may progress from one level or tier to another, but this is not necessary. A combination of services may be required, or a rapid move to Tier 3 or 4 in severe or emergency cases (Lavis 2008).

Early intervention is slightly different. It refers to action taken early in a child's life with the aim of avoiding later difficulties. This notion has been part of the rationale for early years services for many years, fortified by the evidence from American programmes that intensive educational and family support input before children started school had a range of long-term benefits for children, especially those from poorer backgrounds. The Sure Start programmes introduced in 2001–2 drew inspiration from this tradition. Some parenting programmes and intensive health visitor support to young mothers also aim to give help at a stage when difficulties are yet to have become entrenched.

Within youth justice a related concept is that of *diversion*. The basic idea is that involvement in formal procedures and alternative care and education options tends to reinforce offending behaviour as a result of the negative peer associations, alienation effects and confirmation of a criminal identity. Therefore, it is preferable to divert young people whenever possible into a less formal process such as a police caution or into sport, leisure and outdoor activities aiming to enhance social skills and esteem (Hayden 2007).

Broader policy trends

Children's services are affected not only by their specific remits and legal frameworks, but also by more general policies. Of course, some of these very much reflect the party political priorities of the government, but it is also possible to see longer-term threads in policy that have persisted across changes in government. Developments in globalisation, information technology, economic and social organisation and democratic expectations during the past 20–30 years have been characterised as post-modern or late modern, resulting in pressures on all organisations to become more flexible, responsible, accountable and efficient (Frost and Stein 2009a).

Political and media criticisms of public services for not achieving their aims or not providing value for money have persisted over the decades, sometimes linked with beliefs that professionals may sometimes act more in their own interests than those of the people they serve (Exworthy and Halford 1999). Such views have led governments in two contrasting directions, often at the same time – namely, to increase central control and to espouse localism with greater participation by ordinary citizens.

A raft of measures was developed by central government from the 1980s onwards in efforts to improve the quality and consistency of services (Kirkpatrick et al. 2005). Some were deliberately imported from private business with the aim of improving public-sector efficiency and promoting 'modernisation'. They include:

- targets and performance indicators (such as school league tables, appointment and waiting times);
- stricter registration criteria and inspections of schools and care services;
- standards of care;
- growth in documentation required to demonstrate accountability;
- management training and orientation based on generic principles often derived from commercial organisations.

Collectively these trends have been discussed by academics as 'managerialism' (Kirton 2009). One consequence of this has been that growing numbers of professionals have gained management assets (experience, qualifications) to cope with the changed environment and improve their own career prospects.

While managerialism has led to gains in service quality, many negative consequences have been identified. These include reducing the scope for local and individual initiative (Milbourne 2009). Within child protection services, particularly social work and police, the need to meet requirements about record-keeping, inspections and so on has detracted from the time available for direct work with children and families and for professional supervision (Kirkpatrick et al. 2005; Munro 2011). In some contexts, including certain primary schools, it has been found that the sense of collegiality has diminished as a result of managerial measures (Exworthy and Halford 1999). Sometimes practice has been distorted in order to improve agency figures. For instance, some schools became reluctant to admit or retain students with learning difficulties or challenging behaviour. The police in certain areas prosecuted young people for minor misdemeanours in order to increase the clear-up and conviction rates by which they were judged. Partly in response to these problems, the government has expressed a commitment to a 'lighter touch' as regards accountability procedures.

The Conservative government of the late twentieth century, the New Labour government from 1997 and the Conservative–Liberal Democrat government from 2010 have all supported the role of the market and pluralism of providers, although in different ways. Of course, private services for children have long existed in such forms as independent schools, for-profit nurseries and residential homes, and private healthcare. During the 1980s and 1990s market mechanisms were introduced into the NHS, including a purchaser–provider split, which led to new roles and bureaucratic mechanisms within the public sector for commissioning services externally and managing relationships with the independent sector (Dickens 2010). The voluntary sector was encouraged to take on a larger role in children's services. The 'New' Labour government introduced the concept of 'best value', whereby local authorities were expected to provide services themselves or commission from voluntary or private organisations depending on which offered the best outcomes at a reasonable cost. It also promoted the public–private finance initiative to fund new schools and hospitals. The aspiration of the Conservative–Liberal government after 2010 has been to enhance the contribution of private and voluntary bodies in service provision against a background of cuts in funds to the public sector.

Localism has taken various forms. It may entail a shift from a large organisation (usually a local authority department) to a constituent unit, giving local managers and professionals more influence and responsibility. In the 1990s budgets were devolved from local authorities to schools, and GPs were enabled to become fund holding if they wished. In 2011 plans were introduced to replace Primary Care Trusts in the NHS with GP consortia to commission health services. Further diffusion of power entails involving members of the community – for instance, in school management and local health partnerships. The 'New' Labour government enabled some schools to opt out of local authority control and still receive central government funding as academies. The Conservative–Liberal Democrat government has extended the right of publicly funded schools to be 'free' from local government and seeks to enable local people to manage schools in order to promote innovation and choice. In all these moves towards decentralisation from local authorities, questions arise about representativeness, self-selection and the role of profit-making agencies. Also the ability of authorities to plan for their populations is diminished.

Governments of all political persuasions have for different reasons promoted the idea of greater involvement of 'users', 'consumers', 'recipients' or 'customers' of services – each term carrying somewhat different expectations. User participation was part of both Conservative and New Labour policies based on a consumerist rights and choices and a belief that this would improve the quality of services. There are, however, dangers that only certain kinds of service user are willing and able to participate. Also, some citizens may come to feel more marginalised than before as they encounter an imbalance of power and expertise in their contacts with professionals and officials (Bochel et al. 2008).

User participation has at times arisen as much from pressures and movements by service users themselves, as from 'top-down' processes. In some ways this fits well with the commitment of many professionals to participatory practice, but others have been anxious that their expertise may be challenged or overridden. User involvement also chimes with children's participatory rights, though until recently it was common for parents rather than children to be seen as the main 'customer' to have more choice and involvement in schools and others services (Tisdall et al. 2006). Personalisation has been a key aim of policy-makers seeking to modify bureaucratic practices in public agencies and also of practitioners in the fields of disability and mental health.

A different approach is 'bottom-up' where citizens themselves develop services. This was how playgroups first developed, for example. Holman (2001) has argued passionately for resources to be given to local people and self-help organisations, particularly as a means of tackling poverty and its consequences, such as youth crime.

Working with 'the community'

Participative approaches may be largely or solely confined to engaging with individuals and families referred to services, but it is also possible to take on a wider role in relation to the whole population or a significant part of it in the catchment area or relevant neighbourhood(s) of the service you work for. Indeed, this is an explicit expectation of those involved in, for example, public health or community policing. It is supported by the ecological framework for childhood discussed earlier.

The community may be looked at in various ways – as a unit of belonging; a local environment with protective and risk factors; an activity space for social functions; or a network of relationships. It is important to recognise that such communities are multiple, may not act collectively and can produce conflict, exclusion and problems, as well as provide care, support and resources (Chaskin 2008). A different use of the word 'community' refers to a community of interest, when a selection of people from different areas are linked by a common issue. Some become organised as activity or self-help groups. Thus, looked-after children can be seen as a community of interest with their own representative organisations at devolved levels (Who Cares? and Young People in Care). Parents of children with autism spectrum disorders form another example.

The notion of partnership with the community normally refers to those living locally. Such work involves at a minimum consulting with key stakeholders locally about need or the nature of services. It can extend to involving community members in service planning and delivery, though only in recent years have children been taken seriously in such developments. Since at least Victorian times, certain agencies in both public and non-government sectors have sought to work closely with people in small neighbourhoods, especially in deprived areas, to help them organise, articulate their views to those in power and seek to change their social, economic and political circumstances. Professionals with community work or community development training and orientations have been present in education, youth work, social work and health services deploying a set of knowledge and skills with respect to neighbourhood assessment, group work, organisation building, negotiation and advocacy (Henderson and Thomas 2002). During the past 10 to 15 years, community social work and, to a smaller extent, community education and youth work have declined, but new opportunities for community development have opened up in relation to training, anti-poverty measures, youth employment and housing, mostly in the voluntary sector and often in multi-agency partnerships (Henderson and Glen 2005).

For several decades government policies have sought to promote the contribution of community providers to welfare services. According to Henderson and Glen (2005) the governments of the 1980s and 1990s favoured volunteering, voluntary organisation and self-help, but were suspicious of local campaigning. The 'New' Labour government sought to engage more with community groups in its social inclusion and locality regeneration projects. Sure Start projects were intended to be developed in negotiation with local communities. Schools were expected to act as a resource for the whole community – for instance, by offering family learning opportunities (Anning et al. 2010). Since 2010 the Conservative–Liberal Democrat government has reasserted policies intended to shift power and responsibility from the 'state' to citizens under the umbrella term of the 'Big Society', based on beliefs about the importance of contributions by local people and scepticism about bureaucratic public services. This can be viewed as involving greater democratic involvement (as with appointment of Police Chief Constables) or taking over services from local authorities, notably through free schools. Critics argue that this model can act as a rationale for cuts in services, may overestimate the capacities and willingness of lay people and may give undue influence to those with more resources and confidence. It remains to be seen whether these policies will be open to bottom-up pressures for change as opposed to top-down handing over of responsibilities. Also, history suggests than some community-based movements and organisations may lobby for improvements and expansions of publicly provided services rather than to take them over.

[Issues of participation and community are discussed in Part II of the book.]

Evidence-based policy and practice

During the first decade of the new millennium it was common for politicians, policy-makers and professionals to espouse a commitment to 'evidence-based' policy and practice (EBPP). However, this could mean different things. Some wished evidence to be a guide, while others argued more strongly that evidence should determine actions, i.e. interventions should only happen if evidence demonstrated their effectiveness or if they were being formally tested. One broad definition is 'putting the best available evidence at the heart of policy development and implementation' (Nutley et al. 2010, p. 133).

The extent to which direct or clinical practice can or should be evidence-based, and in what ways, remain contested. On the one hand, researchers have been urged to make their findings more accessible, and practitioners to be more open to evidence and its implications. By contrast some have claimed that the EBPP movement stultifies critical thinking and seeks to impose simple conclusions onto complex situations (Midgley 2010). Views vary, too, about what counts as relevant evidence (see Part III). Should it comprise only systematic research, or even be confined to experimental studies? Some argue that more qualitative research is also relevant, while strong arguments have been put forward that the findings of research must be integrated with clinical expertise arising from work with individuals (Black 1998). Both proponents and opponents have supported the need for more evidence to be produced directly from practice. Indeed, some have advocated an approach to research and theory that is grounded in everyday practice and in practitioner reflections (see e.g. McNiff and Whitehead 2006).

It appears that politicians may attend to research evidence that fits with their own values and preconceptions, supported by tales they hear from constituents. Having reviewed the relationship between research and youth justice policy in Scotland, McNeill (2010) concluded that 'policy is driven by evidence of popular appeal and electoral success'.

Policy makers have emphasised that services should be 'outcome-led'. Use of the word 'outcome' serves several purposes, such as to identify what are seen as commonly accepted broad aspirations for children (child-centred outcomes) and to encourage all professionals to work towards the same set of goals rather than pursue solely their own. Another reason for referring to outcomes is that they are seen as lending themselves to measurement and accountability, so that agencies and partnerships can be judged. A structured approach using outcome grids has become common. This involves first identifying what desired results are wished for as a basis for planning change. Assessment is then based on the quantity and quality of effort put in (the scale of services and how well they performed) and in particular the effects on children and/or families (Chamberlain et al. 2010).

However, application of the concept of outcome is not straightforward (Frost and Stein 2009b). Once a move is made from very broad 'apple-pie' aspirations that virtually everyone would agree with (e.g. positive well-being) to more precise indicators, questions arise as to who decides what the key dimensions are and then how they are measured. In clinical practice and research, it is common for professionals, young people, parents and others to reach different conclusions about levels and significance of symptoms and behaviour (Worrall-Davies and Cottrell 2009). How are differences between national, regional and local priorities to be reconciled?

Furthermore, the word 'outcome' suggests that whatever is being measured (e.g. educational achievements, rates of obesity) results from (comes out of) the policies or interventions under consideration. In practice, it is difficult to disentangle a complex set of environmental and interpersonal factors at play. The evaluation of children's trust pathfinders showed improvements in a range of indicators ranging from teenage pregnancies and child protection referrals to school absences and school-leaving qualifications, but the researchers admitted that the gains were due to multi-causal and multi-level mechanisms. Hence, it was possible to conclude only that 'expenditure and service-level professional practice probably play some part in the process of change' (O'Brien et al. 2009, p. 330). As the debates about school league tables showed, judgements cannot rest purely on what follows from a service, since these depend as much on prior capacities and circumstances, if not more so. A school in a very deprived area may help its pupils to make great progress, yet they may still perform less well in exams than those living in a more favoured area.

It is important not to focus entirely on the 'products' of a service to the neglect of how it is delivered and experienced. Children themselves place great emphasis on the manner in which they are treated, as well as having their expectations fulfilled (Wager et al. 2007).

The rest of the book

After this introductory chapter, the book has four sections dealing with the following broad elements:

- the organisational, legal and policy context of services for children within the UK;

- ways in which professionals engage with members of the community – as 'service users/clients/patients', pupils and students, parents and carers, supporters, volunteers, citizens etc.;
- principles, concepts and research findings concerning children and families that are valuable for collaborative assessment and joint work;
- factors and processes that promote and hinder cooperation among professionals.

Many of the chapters relate to more than one of these themes, since they are interconnected, and have been allocated to the part that provides the best fit. It is impossible to include detailed consideration of every possible relevant topic, so we have tried to concentrate on issues that are significant beyond any single professional area. The book also includes contributions from a range of professional and academic disciplines, with many of the chapter writers being former or current practitioners.

Part I

CHILDREN'S SERVICES

'The level of civilisation attained by any society will be determined by the attention it has paid to the welfare of its children.'

Billy F. Andrews M. D. 1968 (Huth and Murray 2006 p. 59)

If as societies we are to achieve the best for all children and particularly for those who are in need, it will require providing them with the best possible services. It also means listening to the users of the services, overcoming policy and professional barriers that can get in the way, and a willingness to change. In this part contributors cover these issues.

Even before birth, children are involved with universal services through antenatal and neonatal care. Thereafter, a variety of provision has an impact on their lives – mainly through health and education. For most children the interface with services is not problematic – they visit doctors and dentists when required – and move from being cared for within the home to nursery care and then on to school and, in many cases, further and higher education. When children and young people encounter problems, they will seek informal help through family and friends.

However, some children – usually through no fault of their own – face difficulties which bring them to the attention of a wide range of both universal and specialist services. As noted in the Introduction, recent policies have emphasised the importance of taking a holistic approach, so that any additional support needs are seen in the context of other aspects of a child's life. Similarly, a commitment to social inclusion has meant that only in extreme cases should children with behaviour problems, physical impairments or learning difficulties be separated from mainstream facilities (Head 2007). This means that generalist services for all children, such as schools and health centres, should work closely with those having a more targeted role – for example, psychologists and psychiatrists. The law requires that children's best interests should be the main consideration for professionals and decision-makers (Williams 2008). In addition, children's views must be taken seriously. Normally their perspectives will also be a good guide to what is in their interests, but when a judgement is made that an action is best for the child but contrary to their wishes, then careful explanation and sensitive support is necessary. These welfare and participatory rights of children take on particular significance when the 'state' intervenes in their lives through formal processes and, in some cases, legal compulsion.

In policy-making and in service provision for children and young people in the UK, attempts are increasingly being made to seek the views of children and young people, not only about decisions taken about them, but also about the services provided. Therefore, we thought it was vital to begin with an overview by Hill and Morrison of the ways in which children seek help and from whom. This suggests that experiences of formal services are very much affected by informal help-seeking that often precedes or accompanies contact with professionals. Differing approaches and strategies for seeking the views of children are explored in the chapter, along with evidence about children's perceptions of what is good or deficient in services. Professionals and agencies need to be aware of such experiences and address concerns.

The importance of seeking children's views and protecting rights is further developed by Marshall and Williams, writing on the role of the Children's Commissioners. They note the participation of children in the appointments process. In Scotland the importance of children playing a part in areas which affect them has been further enhanced by the role that children will have in the appointment of the National Convenor of Children's Hearings, Scotland and in the selection and training of children's panel members (Children Hearings (Scotland) Act 2011). The chapter explores the role and remits of commissioners in the context of their commitment to the UNCHR. Marshall and Williams describe not only how commissioners consult with children, but also their cooperation and collaboration with other relevant organisations and with commissioners in other jurisdictions.

The next two chapters move on to consider service delivery within the context of national and agency policies encouraging inter-disciplinary cooperation. Both review research evidence about the impact of such policies at local levels. Daniels and Edwards consider the issues facing professionals in universal and specialist services as they all seek to promote children's welfare while pursuing various particular aims in their work. Drawing on their own research in England, the authors reinforce the need to build a common base of knowledge and understanding. They highlight the importance of learning from, and recognising, the expertise of others – including the views of children and families – in order to develop integrated responses and services for children. The chapter gives details of concepts and methodologies to support inter-professional learning and collaboration.

The impact of the recurring child abuse inquiries into failures in protecting vulnerable children (Corby 2006; Munro 2011) has led to major policy, organisational and practice shifts to enable and ensure cooperation and collaboration between all the agencies involved in the life of a child. The need for coordinated work among many agencies at national and local levels was also highlighted by the Marmot Review (2010), which detailed the close relationship between health, education, income, employment and housing. Stradling and Alexander outline the policies developed in England and Scotland with the goal of integrating universal and targeted services. They share the findings and experiences of the Highland Pathfinder project whose aim is to develop 'a seamless network' to support children and families. They stress the interconnectedness of changes in professional cultures, organisational arrangements and workforce development, along with adherence to clear, shared principles and careful preparation, training and support.

Further insights into how services can be provided may come from international comparison. Lorenz and Fargion note common demographic trends in western Europe, then examine the differing welfare models that have been developed, especially in relation to vulnerable children. The chapter illustrates how different views about children, the family and the state help shape policy (see also Harding 1996; Thomas 2000; Jones et al. 2008). Social pedagogy is discussed as a common professional tradition on the continent, which blends features of education, social work and health promotion in a holistic way, as some agencies in the UK are striving to do.

These three chapters just summarised deal with issues relating to a cross-section of children's universal services and their relationships with more specialist services dealing with children who are in need on account of inadequate family care. Another vital part of the field comprises the services and decision-making mechanisms that respond to children whose behaviour is challenging. In most cases they have also experienced problematic care and poverty. Whyte's chapter highlights the wide variations in attitudes and approach to youth offending within the United Kingdom and in the rest of Europe. Whyte discusses the impact on rights of these differences, as in relation to the age of criminal responsibility. International treaties require that youth justice systems integrate welfare and justice considerations. This means that a collaborative approach is necessary so that services address the needs and deeds of the young person.

REFLECTIVE EXERCISE

The issues raised in this section range from seeking and taking account of the views of children and young people, putting children's legal rights into operation and the importance of integrating services in ways that recognise the complexity of the lives of children and families.

- How can professionals gather the views of children appropriately?
- How can agencies better protect the rights of children receiving their service?
- What challenges do you face in seeking to address the interconnectedness of children's needs, e.g. as regards health, learning, behaviour and social care?

Chapter 2

Children's help-seeking and views of services

Malcolm Hill and Colin Morrison

Summary points

- Children's concerns and views about matters that require professional attention often differ in nature and emphasis from adults expectations.
- It is vital to understand the informal processes and pathways that precede professionals' contacts with a child. Children are likely to seek help from their family and friends first. These will usually continue to exert influence during contacts with formal agencies.
- Professionals should offer children clear explanations of their own roles and, when referring elsewhere, inform them about who will do what and why.
- Children's appraisals of what they want from professionals include qualities that apply to all encounters – friendliness, respect, informality; confidentiality and having promises kept.

Introduction

The core argument of this chapter is that it is vital for professionals working with children to understand and respond sensitively to the expectations and views of children using the service.

This is important for legal and ethical reasons. Legislation in the UK and the UN Convention on the Rights of the Child require that children's views are taken into consideration when decisions are made affecting them. Similarly, government guidelines in most policy areas state that service recipients, clients or patients should be 'listened to and properly informed' (Day 2008: 4). There is also a pragmatic rationale for knowing and responding to children's perspectives. They are much more likely to accept and cooperate with a service when they feel respected and listened to.

One consequence of a commitment to attending to children's thoughts and feelings is that agencies and their staff should engage in dialogue with service recipients about their expectations and experiences of the service, including providing information they require to make sense of an intervention. Many methods have been developed to ascertain children's views on services, ranging from traditional questionnaires, one-to-one interviews and group exercises to online and texting surveys (McLeod 2008). Expertise is also available on approaches to communication with very young children and those with serious impairments and learning difficulties or complex health care needs (Clark and Moss 2001; Watson et al. 2006). It is important to be aware that children vary in the modes of communication they prefer, and efforts to obtain views can be counterproductive unless professionals make a genuine effort to respond (Hill 2006; Lewis 2010). Increasingly, schools and other agencies involve children themselves in carrying out evaluations (Kellett 2010).

While there is no substitute for knowing the perspectives of the particular children you work with, it is also helpful to draw on wider information about how children think and feel about different kinds of service. In this chapter we shall summarise key lessons that we have derived from our own experience in practice, consultation and research and from an extensive literature review.[1]

Children's concerns and worries

Most children in the UK who are old enough to take part in surveys report being fairly satisfied with their lives most of the time, though a significant minority (between 10 and 20 per cent) feel unhappy, helpless or lonely. The main sources of distress are:

1. Experiences or fears about loss, separation and ill-health of others, especially close relatives.
2. Tensions and conflicts with peers.
3. Parental behaviour including arguments and violence (Borland et al. 1998).

As would be expected, anxieties among children vary with age. Among pre-school children, common fears relate to separation, getting lost, imaginary beings, scary dreams and certain animals like snakes (Muris et al. 2009). The intensity of both fears and worries tend to decline during middle childhood, but rates of depression rise during the teens, especially among girls. As children grow older, worries related to social relationships become more prominent, as do concerns about not meeting social expectations. Teenagers express anxiety about their appearances, school work and educational or employment futures, or about national and world issues (Menna and Ruck 2004). Children living in poor neighbourhoods often voice concerns about the quality of their schools and local environments. Fears of dangerous objects and buildings, aggressive individuals or groups restrict where they can go and what they do (Turner et al. 2006; Osler 2010). Cheap, frequent and reliable public transport is a critical consideration in accessing services, especially for those in rural areas or lacking an adult with a car available to assist (Wager et al. 2007).

While the issues and areas highlighted above may seem obvious, it seems that children's concerns or worries differ somewhat from matters that parents, policy makers or media might regard as the main risks of childhood – abduction, drug misuse, early sexual experience (Borland et al. 1998).

---

[1] In order not to clutter the writing, only some of the references used will be given.

Children's help-seeking

The most common response for children to a worry or concern is to tell someone. Among the purposes this can serve are sharing and offloading (catharsis), feeling less alone with the problem, obtaining information, advice or action which can help with a problem, gaining comfort or reassurance about one's self-worth or identity or learning from the experience of others.

Help-seeking for personal and interpersonal problems

Help-seeking by children has been examined in relation to several distinct types of help including personal or emotional issues, practical problems and academic learning. Most children are selective about the kinds of issue they want assistance with. They are more likely to seek help when the cause of the problem is attributed to other people or external circumstances. Issues with internal origins are regarded as a reflection of personal inadequacy and so are often kept private (Fallon and Bowles 2001; Menna and Ruck 2004).

American and Australian studies show that about half of young people in their teens seek help for a distressing problem during the course of a year and mainly from family or peers. Girls ask for help more often than boys, and this gender difference is apparent from an early age. Females are more likely to admit to emotional issues, while males tend to acknowledge school-related problems more (Hallett et al. 2003; Menna and Ruck 2004).

Coping alone

It is not uncommon for both boys and girls to cope with a worry or problem alone. For some children dealing with a problem on their own is a matter of pride and avoids the danger of 'interference'. Others do not confide out of embarrassment or fear of stigma. In one study nearly one in ten said they had nobody to share their feelings with (Gordon and Grant 1997). When children lack trusted and supportive resources, their isolation may compound the original difficulties. They may suffer silently, so adults only become aware there is an issue if they detect unusual behaviour or demeanour.

A constructive but indirect way children deal with worries is to engage in activities that take their minds off the troubles at hand. Children report sometimes coping with negative feelings by being with friends, not as a means of sharing the problem but as a distraction from their problems (Hallett et al. 2003). Teenagers who self-harm sometimes engage in alternative activities to counter an impulse to hurt themselves – for instance, playing sport or taking a shower. Diversionary measures can involve positive coping strategies, such as listening to music, watching TV, going for a cycle ride or writing in a diary. These actions support reflection and perhaps putting the matter in perspective. Another response to stress is to compensate for negative emotions by 'treating oneself' by eating, shopping etc.

Coping with the help and support of others

From children's point of view the significant people and world around them comprise a range of *resources*, of which formal services are only a part and often a small part. A helpful distinction may be made between *resources at hand*, discussed here, and resources which are *out there*, described in later sections (Weirenga 2009).

Resources at hand are easy to access and include relatives, friends, neighbours or other informal contacts. Many children feel they get adequate and appropriate assistance informally, so do not need to approach professionals (Sullivan et al. 2002), particularly when communication with professionals is experienced as negative (Catan et al. 1997; Drury 2003). Even children who are in public care and have more problematic access to trusted family resources prefer familiar people to help with their difficulties rather than be referred to unknown specialists (Hill 1999).

As they grow older, children increasingly see their friends as their first or main source of advice and assistance (Sullivan et al. 2002). This applies particularly to matters that can cause embarrassment or shame. Children may also feel that adults lack the understanding to intervene effectively, and may make matters worse. This applies particularly to peer disputes including bullying (Craig et al. 2007). Studies in Sweden and the USA of young people who had been sexually abused found that most had confided in a friend of their own age but few had told professionals. Sometimes the friend acted as a bridge to seeking formal help (Priebe and Svedin 2008; Ungar et al. 2009).

Children do not necessarily use the word *trust* when accounting for their willingness to seek or accept help from their resource networks, but that is implicit in three crucial ingredients they highlight – children prefer to have people dealing with their problems whom they know well, think will react supportively and believe will respect privacy (TASC 2005a). These characteristics of trust are based on previously established and positive experiences, and are difficult for an unfamiliar person to achieve quickly.

Often children will have a tight circle of trusted individuals with whom they are prepared to discuss a problem. This applies also to revelations of identity or status that the child perceives as shameful or stigmatised, such as being 'in care', 'poor' or having a parent with a mental health problem or addiction. Research on attachment has shown that children who have experienced seriously defective parenting or care-giving tend to generalise the resulting mistrust to other adults. They may then behave in challenging ways that make professional sympathy or empathy more difficult (see Chapter 18).

Experiences and views of professionals and services

From children's perspectives, most professionals except some teachers are *resources out there* – less familiar and difficult for children to know how to reach. Hence, when more formal help is needed, this will usually follow attempts to resolve the issue informally, and it is important for professionals to understand what has already been done before they get involved.

Freake et al. (2007: 640) remind us that it is when we are young that 'patterns of service use are developed which tend to continue through adult life – if young people have positive early experiences of accessing help from professionals they are more likely to continue seeking help when they need it throughout their lives'. Thus, it is vital that initial contacts with a service involve comfort, attractiveness and (as discussed above) trust-building. Very few children lack contact with at least one professional they like and trust, though quite often this is not a specialist in relation to their 'main' problem(s) (Hill 1999). Indeed, a minority of children's lives are heavily influenced by or even dominated by professionals; for example, those in residential care or unaccompanied asylum seekers, or with very high needs for educational and/or medical support. A key need of this minority may be for help in developing informal relationships and the skills to sustain these.

Of course, views about professionals vary considerably depending on the child, the service and the context. Nevertheless, it is possible to identify themes which apply across most or all services. These are summarised in the following sections.

When professionals/services get it wrong

Individual professionals, teams or a service can behave in ways, or have features, that impede children's meaningful or constructive engagement. Children often make clear distinctions between an agency and an individual staff member, so that they may feel negatively about an organisation but like one or more of the staff, and vice versa. On the other hand, repeated negative experiences will colour attitudes to the whole service.

Before the child develops a view from direct experience of a professional or service, they may have prior fears that inhibit approaching professionals or speaking freely. They may feel ashamed or worry they will lose control of the situation (Hallett et al. 2003). Children also bring expectations shaped by views acquired in various ways, including family, peers and the media. Some will be inhibited or unresponsive on account of personality, the power imbalance which typifies adult–child relations or more transient features such as mood. Some children also think they will be judged on account of their age or behaviour, others because of their sexuality or sexual activity (Freake et al. 2007). A further barrier to initial engagement is that some professionals, including GPs, school nurses and guidance teachers, are seen as too busy or difficult to access (Hallett et al. 2003).

At referral, time needs to be spent clarifying both the child's and the professional's understandings of the service and its purpose. Not uncommonly, children do not understand why they have been referred. Some want help with issues *other* than those seen as important by professionals. This may lead them to resist attempts by professionals to shift attention to what the latter see as underlying or causal issues (Coleman et al. 2004; Davies and Wright 2008). On the other hand, some children think that formal responses are too superficial. This applies, for instance, to some children who self-harm or have mental health problems (Buston 2003).

Once engaged with a professional or service, several issues can impact negatively on the development of effective relationships. A key issue is that of communication.

Studies of police, doctors and others have shown that they often find older children difficult to communicate with and tend to interpret the unforthcoming child as sullen and poorly motivated, when in fact this may reflect the power imbalance and failure of the professional to put the child at ease (Drury 2003). Children resent being 'talked down' to or patronised (Freake et al. 2007). Many children welcome parental support and may like their parent to speak for them, but they also resent being treated as an appendage of their parents. In consultations with doctors children are normally seen with a parent or other relative – they often take little part in the communication and feel marginalised from discussions between the adults (e.g. Watson et al. 2006).

When several agencies are involved, children commonly report a lack of explanation about who they are seeing and why. Some resent being excluded from decision-making meetings or case conference on matters affecting them and about which they have expertise. Equally, it can be puzzling and intimidating to attend discussions with adults present who are unfamiliar and whose role is not known (Children's Parliament 2010b; Osler 2010).

Confidentiality and privacy are central considerations in children's evaluations of services. If they suspect or have experienced that this is not respected, they will often not engage or withdraw from contact. Many children doubt that professionals, including teachers and GPs, will keep confidences, which makes them disinclined to discuss personal matters. A significant factor for many professionals in considering information-sharing without the child's permission is when they see a conflict between the child's right to confidentiality and anxieties over child protection – for example, when a 14 or 15 year old engages in consensual sexual activity. This can result in the professional/service erring on the side of what they perceive as a requirement to share information despite their obligation to the child's confidentiality (TASC 2006).

One of the most complex set of relationships between a child and a professional/service occurs in response to abuse. Children report that, when official agencies become aware of abuse, their early contacts with these agencies are often experienced as intrusive and insensitive. Furthermore, an initial absence of belief on the part of police or other professionals, whether genuine or conveyed by the need to check evidence, tends to discourage children from taking further action. For some children there are risks in discussing a concern and seeking help – for example, in relation to bullying where there is a common fear that 'telling' can result in the adult taking over and making things worse (TASC 2004).

When professionals/services get it right

We do not wish to suggest that interaction between professionals and children is inevitably, or even usually, fraught. For example, the majority of children say they like (most of) their teachers (Keys 2006). Similarly, most young people are positive about their GP, though may not want to communicate with them about sensitive matters (Bundle 2002).

Across these and other professional groupings, research findings are consistent about a number of approaches or characteristics that children value. An overarching theme is that children want to be seen as individuals and that professionals and services must provide them with enough time to deal with an issue fully (Freake et al. 2007).

While underscoring that children are a heterogeneous population, research suggests that they give their trust to *individual professionals*, especially when they show a genuine interest and respect (Catan et al. 1997). This requires time to build up trust before difficult issues are tackled, as well as continuity of staff input (Children's Parliament 2007). The professional should display a caring and helpful attitude, empathy and be non-judgemental. As well as likeability, competence and effectiveness are also important. That includes involving the child in the discussion of options, carrying out the necessary action, reliability, keeping promises and punctuality (Buston 2003; Freake et al. 2007). Questions should normally be sensitive and open-ended, but at times directness is required. For example, when clinicians ask children straight out if abuse has occurred, this considerably increases the likelihood of disclosure (Ungar et al. 2009).

Example 2.1

Children like professionals to explain who they are and what they will do. Explicit interest in their views and welfare is valued. Jenny aged 13 spoke warmly about her dentist, who gave her explanations about treatment and, unlike previous experiences, sought her consent: 'She asks you before she does it'. David, 10, reported that hospital staff showed concern for his general well-being, not just his illness: 'asking me if I was hungry and getting me a video'.

(Wager et al. 2007, p. 116)

Children often have little idea about the roles and functions of specialist professionals such as psychologists, psychiatrists, social workers and counsellors, perhaps because they do not encounter them routinely or see their role represented in soap operas. Therefore, it is especially important that careful explanations are given when referrals are made or received. Likewise, avoidance of jargon, careful listening and responsiveness are particularly wanted from these less familiar services (Hallett et al. 2003; Morgan 2006).

The majority of children tend to prefer professionals who are young adults and seem more on the same wavelength, although some do like older people. A wish to be helped by someone of the same gender can be important; this is more often true for girls and where sexual health issues are involved (Hallett et al. 2003; Freake et al. 2007). However, it is important to check assumptions about what children might want in relation to the individual traits of the professional; one group of Black/Minority ethnic young people said that they normally would *not* want staff at a sexual health clinic to be of the same ethnicity because they would then feel judged or fear a breach of confidentiality (TASC 2005).

With regard to the characteristics of *whole* services, these are considered more positively when they adopt a consultative or participative approach, display skills and creativity in their communication and avoid stereotyping children as uncommunicative

(Drury 2003; Hallett et al. 2003). In practical terms the service should be easy to access, though when dealing with sensitive issues, it needs to be discreet (TASC 2003). Furthermore, the role and functions of the service should be explained clearly, with agency policy on confidentiality clarified.

Views on specific professionals or services

In addition to these general themes, it is possible to identify some key messages for specific professional groups. Space allows us to provide just a sample of potential lessons.

Key messages

Teachers (e.g. Keys 2006; Osler 2010)

Most children would like to have more of a say about what is taught in school and how it is taught. Many want a personalised, stimulating and respectful approach from teachers if they are to commit themselves to academic work or be open about non-academic issues. Many students want a more reciprocal relationship and feel teachers should listen better. This applies particularly to those from disadvantaged homes or who lack self-esteem. Children are often reluctant to share personal issues at school out of embarrassment or fear of others finding out, so respect for confidentiality is crucial. Children who experience difficulties in school tend to resent being singled out and shouted at, but value time for dialogue in private.

Health professionals (e.g. Birch et al. 2007; Davies and Wright 2008)

Children like staff who treat them with respect and consideration. They prefer continuity of contact with people they know. They usually want active involvement in discussions and decisions about their treatment. Confidentiality and effectiveness are also important. Many are reluctant to talk about emotional or sexual matters with their GP. Young people tend to think that a nurse or doctor is less likely to keep confidences in a school setting than in a clinic or surgery setting. Children tend to see hospitals as an adult-dominated space which does not take account of their needs. They would like staff to know and respond to their wishes, e.g. about who visits and when. Some think accident and emergency services lack understanding or sympathy in relation to self-harm and mental health issues. Children can find mental health professionals' language and style off-putting.

Police (e.g. Norman 2009; Children's Parliament 2010a)

Many children see the police as fair, honest, reassuring and helpful, but dissatisfaction tends to be higher in the teens. Being stopped or followed is often experienced as harassment, and many children from black and minority ethnic communities see the police as treating them in a negative, discriminatory way. Children suggest police officers should engage with them more positively in public spaces – talk to them informally, get involved in activities and listen to their perspectives.

Social workers (e.g. Morgan 2006; McLeod 2010)

Children who have little contact with social workers are mostly puzzled about what they do. Young people who see social workers frequently value those who combine practical and emotional support, give clear explanations and respond to the wishes and interests of the children. Children in care criticise some social workers for not listening, being unreliable in carrying out promised actions, talking inappropriately to others about confidential or sensitive matters and not speaking up for them.

Material and organisational factors affecting service use

A number of factors other than staff qualities impact on views and access to services.

Cost of services

Children from diverse economic backgrounds and across the urban–rural spectrum highlight the importance of having free access to services, since otherwise the cost would be a disincentive to use. This applies to such services as libraries (including internet access) and recreation, as well as health and education. Affordability of services is also strongly affected by indirect costs such as travel and clothing or equipment required (e.g. for swimming, uniformed organisations, trips). Many children in low-income families and/or living in 'deprived' neighbourhoods think that formal leisure facilities and organised clubs are either lacking locally or too expensive to use, so they rely more than others on informal spaces (Ridge 2002; Wager et al. 2007).

Location

Some professionals, including health visitors and social workers, have a tradition of seeing people in their own homes, whereas others typically see children at school, clinics or offices. Office appointments save time and money for professionals, while home visits reduce time and financial costs for service users. Home visits can help busy or stressed families who may simply not turn up after an invitation to attend an office. Further, home contact can facilitate informal communication and helpful observations of children and families in more natural settings. In serious child abuse cases, indeed, seeing the child at home may be essential. For some purposes it is useful to consider contact on 'neutral territory' like a community centre, especially if home contact might be regarded as intrusive.

When it comes to children accessing services several issues can arise. Distance from home may make the costs of travel difficult or prohibitive and the journey may be stressful (Wager et al. 2007). Children may be reluctant or unable to attend certain locations; situations where attendance is highly visible may elicit fears about being seen, especially if the issue is perceived as private or stigmatising (e.g. abuse, contraception). Routes to a service can involve exposure to safety risks – for instance, passing through the territory of a hostile gang. For some children, particularly those with disabilities, travel to a service can be prohibitive because of physical/environmental barriers or lack of autonomy.

Premises

Students have strong and sometimes very critical views about the layout, resources and quality of school buildings and play areas, and how these impact on their learning and behaviour (Osler 2010). Primary school pupils want bright colours, natural light, adequate space and a friendly atmosphere (Ghaziani 2010). Children like colourful surroundings and play equipment in waiting areas, as at the dentist and in hospitals. However, commonly these are designed for young children, so older ones feel belittled and would like games or reading material more suited to their age (Birch et al. 2007; Children's Parliament 2010b). For some services, having a non-specific name on signs and correspondence is helpful to avoid possible embarrassment when a young person is seen entering. Reception staff are not always experienced as welcoming or informative (Taylor and Dogra 2002). Cleanliness and safety are important considerations, as is privacy.

Children who stay in hospital would like more choice about a range of matters, such as being placed close to others of the same age. They would like access to space to be alone, or private discussions with visitors. The ability to communicate with friends by text and internet is also important (Birch et al. 2007).

Opening hours and appointments

As with adults, children like to interact with services at times that suit their availability and fit with other priorities (Wager et al. 2007). Some prefer drop-in arrangements on account of the flexibility. Travel delays and forgetting may lead to lateness or non-attendance for appointments so that some children with 'chaotic lifestyles' may only cooperate if supported and accompanied. However, some young people prefer to have a fixed time (TASC 2003).

Telephone and online help

Telephone helplines for children have become common across the world and more recently forms of internet-based support have been developed (Fukkink and Hermans 2009). In the UK, ChildLine is well known and widely seen by children as a good first port of call for dealing with a wide range of worries. Scottish children expressed concerns about talking to a stranger on the phone and the dangers of being overheard, but also recognised the positive attraction of helplines as anonymous and confidential (Children's Parliament 2007).

Increasingly young people see the internet as a means of gaining information and advice. A Dutch study showed that children were more likely to raise emotional problems during more anonymous online chat conversations than using the telephone helpline (Fukkink and Hermans 2009). However, most still prefer face-to-face contact for serious mental health or interpersonal matters (Burns and Rapee 2006).

Example 2.2

An evaluation of a service concerned with the sexual health of young people yielded conclusions about information, access and staff approaches that could apply to many services (TASC Agency 2003). For instance:

■ Positive word of mouth is the best way of helping young people find out about services, especially if attractive elements of the service are promoted.

■ All staff, including reception, should be respectful, polite and non-judgemental.

■ Long opening hours and a mix of drop-in and appointments are helpful.

■ Confidentiality is vital.

Conclusions and implications

Professionals working with children must understand how the specific reason and nature of their contacts mesh with the priorities, expectations and informal resources of children's lives. Pathways to seeking formal help usually entail prior stages of coping alone, informal confiding and/or external assistance. Peers are often the first people to know about problems and advise what to do. Children want contacts with formal services to be based on dialogue and respect, information-giving and understanding of the child's pathway to the service. Research on children's appraisals of what they want from professionals indicates a high degree of common ground, including friendliness, continuity, respect, confidentiality and action in response to their wishes.

Professionals and other adults can help promote a sense that having a problem and seeking help are not shameful. Peer helpers should be made aware of how and where they can link a victim of harm or worry to a professional helper. Where possible, professionals should be flexible about the timing and location of contacts to suit young people's wishes and needs. On occasions it may be helpful to use or share another agency's premises.

Both initial reception and ongoing contacts need to be prompt, welcoming and accepting. Clear explanations are needed of an individual's own role with a child and that of other relevant agencies, with checks that the child has understood. Clarity is necessary about confidentiality, and time must be taken to engage before tackling sensitive matters. Listening seriously and empathy are vital. Children also want to see action – or explanations if their wishes cannot be fulfilled. They especially value individuals who combine professional competence with friendliness and informality. Continuity of contact is desirable, ideally with a single individual. This builds trust and minimises confusion in the child's mind about who does what and why. The increasingly common practice of having a lead professional or named person taking on a primary role when several professionals are involved is a helpful trend, but it is vital that children have a say in the choice of key person. In such ways will agencies become more rights- and relationship-based, and also more effective.

Exercise

1. Describe the nature of the **relationships** you want to build with children in your current or professional future role.
2. What **rights** do children have in their interactions with services?
3. What considerations should inform the timing and nature of professionals' discussions with children about **confidentiality** and **trust**?

Recommended reading

Hallett et al. (2003) examine young people's worries and coping strategies, along with their help-seeking behaviour and negotiation of pathways to access services.

Newman (2000) reviews evidence about how, when and why children seek help with school work from peers, parents and teachers.

Wager et al. (2007) describe the views of children from both disadvantaged and more affluent backgrounds about services that are salient in their lives.

Weiringa (2009) conceptualises children's use of informal and formal supports and resources in their communities in the light of views expressed by a sample of Australian children.

Chapter 3

Children's commissioners: representing children's interests and views

Kathleen Marshall and Jane Williams

Summary points

- Children's commissioners are independent offices established by law to undertake functions with regard to the rights, interests, and views of children.
- There are separate commissioners for Wales, Northern Ireland, Scotland and England.
- They all must have regard to the 1989 UN Convention on the Rights of the Child (UNCRC).
- They comment on law, policy and practice issues and adopt policy priorities that interested agencies and individuals can influence.
- They seek to involve children and young people in their work through listening, hearing and responding to them.
- The separate commissioners collaborate with one another and with other agencies and groups to maximise their impact.
- They can all undertake formal investigations/ inquiries with legal powers, but their ability to take on individual cases varies.

Introduction

This chapter describes the role and status of the four Children's Commissioners in the UK and explains the differences in their remits. There is potential for confusion arising from these differences, but this has been mitigated by the close working relationships established by the four offices. The commissioners' processes and policy priorities are a rich resource for those with an interest in children's issues who would like to help shape the policy agenda. The common focus for the four offices is the UNCRC, which covers the whole spectrum of children's rights and is an essential reference point for everyone working with children.

The emergence of children's commissioners

On 20 October, 2008 the Children's Commissioners for Wales, Northern Ireland, Scotland and England gathered in the Palais Wilson in Geneva to hear the UN's assessment of the state of children's rights in the UK. The commissioners and staff had prepared a report for the UN Committee on the Rights of the Child to use as a critique of the Government's report to them. Now it was time for the verdict.

In its usual, balanced way, the committee commented on positive developments since their previous scrutiny, before launching into criticisms and recommendations about what remained to be done. When it had first scrutinised the UK in 1995, there had been no children's commissioners and the committee had commented on the lack of an independent, coordinating and implementation mechanism focusing on the rights of the child (UNCRC 1995). In its second scrutiny in 2002, the committee was able to welcome the establishment of a Children's Commissioner for Wales, and moves towards similar offices in Northern Ireland and Scotland, but regretted the lack of plans for England (UNCRC 2002a.). By 2008 it was able to welcome the establishment of commissioners in all four countries and their initiatives to promote and protect the rights of children, while recommending that the powers and independence of the commissioners be enhanced (UNCRC 2008). The committee views Children's commissioners as critical tools in entrenching the UNCRC in societies across the world (for the committee's understanding of this role, see UNCRC, 2002b).

The UNCRC

Time and place condition how we view our children. It was therefore little short of a miracle when, in 1989, the United Nations General Assembly adopted the UNCRC. It had taken ten years to produce a draft acceptable to member states with their varied cultures and family systems. There had been earlier international statements – starting with the Geneva Declaration of the Rights of the Child passed by the League of Nations in 1924 – but these were merely exhortations. The difference with the Convention was that it was a treaty – a piece of international law, with a monitoring mechanism attached to it. The Convention has been ratified by all states across the world with the exception of the USA and Somalia. Two years after ratification, states have to submit an initial report to the UN Committee on the Rights of the Child, which scrutinises it, receives alternative reports from independent agencies working in the country, discusses the situation with government representatives, and then produces 'Concluding Observations and Recommendations'. These form the starting point for the next scrutiny five years down the line, and every five years thereafter. The committee reports and policy documents provide a fascinating and valuable resource for anyone interested in children's rights. Children's commissioners have a particular interest in monitoring government compliance with the committee's recommendations.

The Convention looks at children as whole persons with a range of indivisible rights. But there are four basic principles that are said to permeate all other articles of the Convention:

- Article 2 guarantees all rights to all children without discrimination of any kind.

- Article 3 says that the best interests of the child should be at least 'a primary consideration' in all decisions by institutions, courts, administrative bodies or parliaments.

- Article 6 is about the right to life and to survival and development 'to the maximum extent possible'.

- Article 12 is about the child's right to express views on all matters affecting the child. The views of the child must be given due weight in accordance with the child's age and maturity. It includes the right to be heard, either directly or through a representative, in all relevant proceedings.

The central articles for the purpose of this chapter are therefore articles 3 (interests) and 12 (views), but it is important to bear in mind the whole scope of the Convention and the connections between all of the articles.

By ratifying the Convention, the UK Government has agreed to ensure that these rights are extended to children within its borders, that children and adults are made aware of them and that agencies of the state actually implement them. Children's commissioners sometimes identify themselves as the independent guardians of the promises made to children by the government.

Rights, interests, welfare and views

While each of the four children's commissioners in the UK has some reference to 'rights' in their founding legislation, there is also varying emphasis on 'interests', 'welfare' and 'views' of children. This is how these concepts appear in the legislation, set out in chronological order according to the time of the offices' establishment (and with emphasis added):

- Wales
  'The principal aim of the Commissioner in exercising his functions is to *safeguard and promote the rights and welfare* of children' (Section 72A of the Care Standards Act 2000 (as amended by the Children's Commissioner for Wales Act 2001).

- Northern Ireland
  'The principal aim of the Commissioner in exercising his functions under this Order is to *safeguard and promote the rights and best interests* of children and young persons' (Article 6 of the Commissioner for Children and Young People (Northern Ireland) Order 2003).

- Scotland
  'The general function of the Commissioner is to *promote and safeguard the rights* of children and young people' (Section 4(1) of the Commissioner for Children and Young People (Scotland) Act 2003).

■ England

'The Children's Commissioner has the function of *promoting awareness of the views and interests* of children in England' (Section 2(1) of the Children Act 2004).

In each case the legislation also refers to UNCRC. The Welsh, Northern Ireland and Scottish Commissioners are all under a duty to have regard to the UNCRC in exercising their functions. However, the English Commissioner, whose general function does not encompass 'rights', is required only to have regard to the Convention when considering what the 'interests' of children might be.

Nevertheless, in practice all four commissioners have made children's rights prominent in their work and have advocated for effective implementation of the UNCRC. Each commissioner has actively sought children's views on various issues and has sought to promote awareness of their rights. This is obvious from even a cursory glance at each of the commissioners' websites. As indicated above, the four commissioners have also collaborated to engage in the UNCRC monitoring process.

Political debates (with a small 'p') have shaped the focus of the founding legislation. There are some who would contest the notion of 'children's rights', arguing that they have needs rather than rights, and that interests or welfare are more important than views. At the other end of the debate, the Scottish legislation reflects a view that the rights of the child (including the right to express a view and have it taken into account) encompass respect for the child's interests or welfare; therefore, there is no need to refer explicitly to interests or welfare in the basic function, although interests are given prominence elsewhere in the Act.[1]

Certainly, there is a close relationship between interests and views. Earlier drafts of the Convention were clearer about this than the final version where a tidying-up exercise consigned interests and views to separate articles. The earlier drafts manifested the thinking of the drafters that taking account of a child's views (where the child wished to express them) was an integral part of identifying a child's interests (Detrick, 1991; Marshall, 1997); and, indeed, it is pertinent to ask how a decision-maker can claim to be acting in a child's best interests if the child has views on the matter under discussion and the adult does not know what they are.

History of commissioners/ombudsmen

The first ever children's ombudsman was appointed in Norway in 1981. The European Network of Ombudspersons for Children (ENOC) now boasts 24 members.

---

[1] Section 4 of the Commissioner for Children and Young People (Scotland) Act 2003 sets out the general function of the commissioner which refers solely to 'rights'. Section 5 continues that, in carrying out this function, the commissioner must have regard to the UNCRC and in particular must regard, and encourage others to regard, the interests and views of children and young people.

There are similar offices across the world, some of which have their own networks. ENOC was formed in 1997 to promote implementation of the UNCRC and the establishment and mutual support of such offices. Some are called 'ombudspersons' and some are called 'commissioners' and their remits and status are quite varied. Some focus on individual casework, while others have a more strategic role at the level of law and policy. Some have elements of both. ENOC membership criteria require independence from government, but the actual mode of appointment, accountability and status of its members show significant variations. ENOC's website, hosted by CRIN (Children's Rights Information Network), contains a wealth of information about its constituent offices and their work. ENOC also produces some agreed statements on behalf of its members.

Within the UK, the four children's commissioners joined together with the Republic of Ireland to form BINOCC – the British and Irish Network of Ombudsmen and Commissioners for Children. The commissioners/ombudsman and their staff meet regularly to share knowledge, experiences and ideas.

Although there are many similarities between them, the UK's four commissioners were set up in different ways and in the context of different policy agendas. As well as differences in their overall aim (noted above), there are differences in their specific powers. The Welsh Commissioner has the power to 'review, comment and make representations' on any matter affecting children in Wales,[2] as well as specific reviewing, monitoring and investigative functions in relation to children provided with care services by Welsh public bodies. The Northern Ireland Commissioner has similar reviewing, monitoring and investigative functions accompanied by powers and duties which focus on promotion of awareness of the rights of children and young people and on influencing policy and legislation. Both the Welsh and the Northern Ireland Commissioners have powers to provide advice and assistance and to investigate individual cases. The Northern Ireland Commissioner is the only one with explicit powers to bring legal proceedings and is the only commissioner who has brought a legal action against government. The Scottish Commissioner has no powers to carry out investigations in relation to a particular child, but can investigate 'whether, and by what means and to what extent, a service provider has regard to the rights, interests and views of children in making decisions or taking actions that affect those children and young people'.[3] The term 'service provider' is meant to include individuals and agencies in the public, private or voluntary sector.[4] The English Commissioner's remit is yet another variation on the theme – he or she can investigate individual cases only where the case raises 'issues of public policy of relevance to other children'.[5]

The four commissioners each have slightly different relationships with the devolved governments. The English, Northern Ireland and Welsh Commissioners are appointed by their respective government ministers, whereas the Scottish

[2] Section 75A Care Standards Act 2000, as amended by the Children's Commissioner for Wales Act 2000.

[3] Section 7 of the Commissioner for Children and Young People (Scotland) Act 2003.

[4] See the explanatory note referring to Section 7 of the Commissioner for Children and Young People (Scotland) Act 2003, available on the OPSI website – www.opsi.gov.uk.

[5] Section 3 of the 2004 Act.

Commissioner is appointed by the Queen on the nomination of the Scottish Parliament. Each is formally separate from government (neither they nor their staff are to be regarded as 'a servant or agent of the Crown'). However, the English Commissioner must consult the Secretary of State (UK Government) before initiating an inquiry into the case of a particular child and may be directed by the Secretary of State to conduct an inquiry, whereas the other three cannot be directed by their respective governments as to the exercise of any of their functions. The Northern Ireland Commissioner, who, as stated above, has explicit powers to bring legal proceedings, has twice brought legal challenges alleging children's rights violations against the government.

Independence from government is important in the context of the UNCRC and human rights implementation generally; the UN's 1993 'Paris Principles' on the status of national human rights institutions emphasise this (UNCRC 2002 b.). The power for the Secretary of State to direct the English Commissioner is a limitation on such status and contributed to the English Commissioner only being admitted to ENOC with associate rather than full member status. Having said that, none of the commissioners' offices complies fully with the characteristics of national human rights institutions set out in the Paris Principles and recommended by the UN Committee on the Rights of the Child. For example, when it comes to funding, only the Scottish Commissioner is clearly independent of government, being funded by the Scottish Parliament. The other three, whose budgets are allocated by government departments, are vulnerable to indirect control via the imposition of conditions about financial management. Arguably this could undermine their independence of action even where (as in the case of the Welsh and Northern Ireland Commissioners) there is no formal power to direct them as to the exercise of their functions.

The current budgets for the offices are as follows (to nearest £100,000):

Welsh Commissioner	Northern Ireland Commissioner	Scottish Commissioner	English Commissioner
£1.8 million	£1.8 million	£1.3 million	£3 million

The impact of devolution

The existence of four separate commissioners and the variations between them are a consequence of devolution within the UK. The interface with UK Government is different for each of the three devolved countries and the Welsh, Northern Ireland and Scottish Commissioners have formal powers only in relation to matters within the remit of their devolved parliaments and assemblies. They can comment on other matters, but cannot exercise legal powers in those areas. The English Commissioner has authority in relation to all matters to do with children in England, as well as non-devolved matters in other parts of the UK, but must consult the other children's commissioners about these matters.[6]

[6] Sections 4, 5 and 6 Children Act 2004.

The variation in powers devolved to Wales, Northern Ireland and Scotland means that there is a very complicated jigsaw of responsibilities among the commissioners. Youth justice is a good example. In Scotland, that is a matter for the Scottish Parliament and therefore for the Scottish Children's Commissioner. Justice is not devolved to the Welsh Assembly, so the Welsh Commissioner has no powers to review the youth justice system. This has not stopped the two people who have held the post from taking a significant interest, and support has been provided in individual cases with no evident tension in practice. Youth justice was not initially devolved in Northern Ireland, but transferred later as part of wider policing and justice functions, in April 2010.[7] What that means is that the English Commissioner has had formal responsibility for youth justice in England, Wales and Northern Ireland (until April 2010), but not in Scotland. The matter becomes even more complex when the issue of individual casework is introduced. As explained above, the commissioners in Wales and Northern Ireland have a power and responsibility to take on individual cases, while the English and Scottish Commissioners do not. So, if a child approaches the Welsh Commissioner with a complicated life story (as is often the case), the Welsh Commissioner can formally deal with the devolved parts of the story but not any that relate to youth justice. These he could refer to the English Commissioner, but the English Commissioner does not have a remit to pursue individual cases unless they highlight 'issues of public policy of relevance to other children' – and then only after consulting the Secretary of State. The potential confusion this could cause, as well as damage to the rights of children, has been mitigated by the close working relationships established among the commissioners' offices across the UK.

Example 3.1 Working together on asylum

Asylum and immigration matters are reserved to the Westminster Parliament and therefore fall within the jurisdiction of the English Commissioner. Nevertheless, the commissioners in other parts of the UK have felt it necessary to address the issue, even if they could not exercise formal powers on it. The Scottish Commissioner explained that, while matters could be reserved to Westminster, children themselves could not. The immigration status of children affected their welfare, education and mental well-being in the face of threats of 'dawn raids' (early morning removals from home), detention and deportation. The Welsh Commissioner has responded to a number of individual contacts from children arising out of their asylum status and the commissioner's 2009 report, *Child Trafficking in Wales*, drew attention to the way in which assumptions and decisions about the immigration status of children could render them more vulnerable to exploitation by traffickers and less likely to benefit from child protection procedures. The Northern Ireland Commissioner has commented on the lack of respect for children's views and experiences in the asylum process and her inability to intervene in individual cases as a result of the restriction on her statutory remit on Westminster matters.

(UK Children's Commissioners 2008 para. 170)

The English Commissioner relentlessly highlighted asylum issues and the situation of children held at the Yarls Wood Immigration Detention Centre. The English

[7] Northern Ireland Act (Amendment of Schedule 3) Order 2010.

office's employment of a specialist in asylum and immigration provided a resource that the other commissioners' offices could draw on. In March 2007 the four commissioners issued a joint statement on children seeking asylum alone, having arrived in the UK without a supporting adult. Asylum also featured prominently in the commissioners' joint report to the UN Committee on the Rights of the Child.

Setting priorities

The children's commissioners have exceptionally wide remits, so choices have to be made about which areas of work to focus on and how resources should be allocated across the different functions of each office.

Both the UNCRC and the laws of each country emphasise consulting and involving children and young people. Real consultation and effective participation take time. If the commissioners' offices are to be true to their founding principles they have to find ways of allowing children and young people to help set their agendas. The early work of the four offices demonstrated their commitment to finding the best ways to do this.

Each office has taken pride in the inclusion of children in arrangements for setting up and recruiting senior staff, including the commissioners themselves. Each set out to develop ways of ensuring children and young people could contribute to settling the commissioners' work programmes.

In Wales a school ambassadors scheme was established mainly for primary school age children. For older children and young people there are two advisory groups which help plan the commissioner's future work programme and advise on how to engage and work with children and young people. The Welsh Commissioner engages with children and young people in a wide range of ways and regularly meets, listens and responds to individuals and groups of children and young people.

The first Northern Ireland Commissioner initiated a major research project comparing children's rights and welfare in Northern Ireland with the standards of the UNCRC. The research, conducted by Queen's University, Belfast, included canvassing the views of a wide range of children and young people, and the report contributed to the commissioner's first priorities. The commissioner also developed an advisory group from the Youth Panel that had contributed to his appointment.

In Scotland 16,000 children and young people and over 300 key stakeholders took part in the consultation exercise leading to the first set of priorities, based on the theme 'Safe, Active, Happy' (SCCYP 2009). Children and young people were consulted through a voting exercise online or using voting cards. Organisations were invited to respond to a consultation document and participated in seminars to help identify which of the three offered themes should be adopted.

The English Commissioner's remit embraces by far the largest number of children, reflected in the brand '11 Million' adopted by the first holder of that position. He established 'Assistant Commissioners for England' to devise ways of ensuring representation of views from children and young people across the English regions. An annual conference of children and young people has been used to help determine project budgets.

At the time of writing, the current Welsh Commissioner's 'goals' are to:

- increase understanding of children's rights and the commissioner;
- reduce inequality and discrimination;
- provide inspirational leadership;
- ensure effective service delivery;
- improve attitudes towards children and young people;
- build a strong, confident, inspiring and resilient organisation (CCfW 2009).

The current Northern Ireland Commissioner has five 'priority areas':

- Play and Leisure;
- Having Your Say;
- Well-being and Mental Health;
- Protection;
- Equal Treatment (NICCYP 2008).

The English Commissioner's six 'major themes' are:

- Safeguarding;
- Education;
- Health;
- Youth justice;
- Positive contribution;
- Asylum (CCfE 2010).

The new Scottish Commissioner's priorities for 2010–11 are:

- Awareness and understanding of UNCRC;
- Participation;
- Children of Prisoners;
- Asylum;
- Disability;
- Youth Justice;
- Trafficking.

A new strategic plan for Scotland will be produced for 2011–2015.

A continuing challenge for the commissioners' offices is to balance allocation of resource between proactive work (identified through consultation and prioritisation) and reactive work (responding to significant issues or cases that arise and to government proposals for law and policy development). The fact that it is not possible to fully identify the scale and demands of reactive work, combined with the high expectations of stakeholders and the commitment of the commissioners and their staff, demands careful judgement to ensure sufficient flexibility. There was a danger, especially in the early years, of being too ambitious in terms of proactive work. The Scottish Commissioner acknowledged this in her final annual report in 2009.

Working in partnership

With their relatively small budgets, working in partnership with other organisations and groups is crucial to the commissioners' ability to fulfil their aims. As well as the international cooperation referred to above, the offices have developed approaches to collaboration within their respective areas. For example, The Welsh Commissioner, in addition to working with existing groups, its schools ambassadors and youth panels, has sought to expand capacity to reach children and young people in communities by means of volunteer schemes and engagement with representative groups and networks including Funky Dragon, and the Children and Young People's Assembly for Wales.

The Northern Ireland Commissioner has established a forum for non-governmental organisations as one of four reference groups to provide advice and support in key areas (the others being the Youth Panel, the Ethics Committee and Audit and Risk Committee) and to update the NGO community on the commissioner's work.

An early concern of the Scottish Commissioner was that her office should add value and not duplicate the work of the voluntary sector. She explained this as 'adding a little lightning' to their work rather than trying to 'steal their thunder'. This could be important where there was a need to tackle sensitive issues that were difficult for voluntary agencies to raise as they might frighten off funders. Collaborative working can also enable the commissioners to voice criticism that might otherwise have remained silent. For example, the Scottish Commissioner received many concerns about the rights of young people leaving care, sometimes from staff employed by voluntary agencies that were providing under-resourced services on behalf of local authorities. The commissioner's office was able to receive those concerns and address them in an independent manner, using information from local authorities that others would have found difficult to obtain. The commissioner's legal power to lay a report before the Scottish Parliament on any matter was a hugely powerful tool in gaining the cooperation of local authorities because they did not want to be identified in a parliamentary report as having failed to provide the information requested.

Because of their unique remit, the commissioners may be in a position to encourage and inspire other public, voluntary and private sector bodies to find ways of involving and listening to children and young people. A good example is the English Commissioner's 'Takeover Day', an initiative which has resulted in around 17,000 children and some 700 organisations finding ways in which children can take over a role normally carried out by an adult for one day, with resulting gains in insights and experience for the children and organisations alike.

Involving children and young people

As well as consulting children and young people about their priorities, the commissioners' offices have explored different ways of involving children and young people in their work. These mechanisms are constantly evolving in response to feedback.

For the English Commissioner, gathering and representing the views of children and young people *is* his work, since his 'function' is to promote the views and interests of children. The commissioner supports and funds research into the effectiveness of participation methodologies across England, in collaboration with the National Participation Forum and other stakeholders. A network of 'Young Friends of 11 Million' is planned to act as key advisers. The commissioner's office has undertaken 'Listening Tours' seeking direct meetings with children and young people in various settings in different local government areas (11 Million 2009a).

The approach of the other three commissioners, servicing their differently defined functions, has been slightly different. Certainly, all have sought to gather, collate and represent the views of children and young people, to encourage communications from young people and to promote awareness of the commissioners' role. The Welsh, Northern Ireland and Scottish Commissioners have each established advisory groups comprising young people. The Welsh Commissioner has also sought to engage children and young people in a relatively early evaluation of the work of his office – the resultant report fed in to ongoing plans and priorities but also reveals some of the difficulties (not least, of scale and cost) in attempting this kind of involvement (Cook et al. 2008). In Scotland the commissioner initially set up three groups of young people: a general Reference Group of twelve young people aged 14 to 21, a Care Action Group of eight young people and a similarly sized Young Persons Health Advisory Group. Contact with younger children was effected through a partnership with the Children's Parliament, a voluntary agency operating in Scotland. The first commissioner's final annual report (2009) commented on what had been learned from these experiences.

Influencing law, policy and practice

An important role for the commissioners is to comment on proposals for law and policy reform to assess compliance with the UNCRC. This can be a very time-consuming activity and some of the commissioners have been 'taking stock' to assess the priority they should give to it and the most effective ways of doing it. The Scottish Commissioner adopted a prioritisation approach which took into account which other agencies were going to respond and the likely added value of the commissioner's response. However, it often happened that, even where the commissioner and staff felt the issue would be adequately covered by others, there was an expectation that there would be a submission from the commissioner's office with potential criticism if it was not forthcoming.

As well as addressing specific issues, the commissioners' offices can provide tools for others to tackle matters using a children's rights approach. The Children's Rights Impact Assessment is a tool developed by staff from the Scottish Commissioner's office that has obtained international recognition. The Scottish office has also produced practical guidance on consulting pupils about school closures. The Northern Ireland Commissioner's office has developed and piloted a child impact assessment tool for use internally and externally, based on the Scottish model. The English Commissioner has demonstrated the application of child rights impact assessment in scrutinising draft legislation, in relation to the Equality Bill in May 2009 (11 Million 2009b).

Individual case work

The ability to undertake individual case work is a strong affirmation of the significance of the views of the child client. Nevertheless, as indicated above, only two of the UK Commissioners (Wales and Northern Ireland) have this function. When the Scottish Parliament was shaping the legislation for a Commissioner in Scotland, it took evidence from the then Welsh Commissioner who explained that the pressure to deal with individual cases did risk inhibiting his ability to take forward more strategic issues. Nevertheless, he felt it was a valuable function if used with discrimination and it helped make his role understandable and credible to children. However, the Scottish Parliament decided against a focus on individual case work, but with an indication that they might be willing to reconsider it at another time. The UN Committee recommended in 2008 that all of the commissioners should be able to investigate individual cases.

Formal investigations/inquiries

Each of the commissioners can undertake a formal investigation/inquiry with associated legal powers to compel witnesses and the production of papers. The names and extents of these powers vary among the offices. It is a potentially powerful but resource-intensive tool. At the time of writing, it has been exercised only once – by the Welsh Commissioner, early in the first term of office. For the other commissioners, it has been important to have this power because it emphasises the importance attached to the office and helps secure the cooperation of those potentially subject to investigation.

The Welsh Commissioner's 2004 *Clywch Report* ('Clywch' means 'listen') was the result of his inquiry into allegations of sexual abuse of children by a schoolteacher who, but for his suicide on the eve of his court appearance, would have been tried for serious criminal offences. Although a local authority serious-case review was held to examine the application of child protection procedures in relation to the allegations, the commissioner's inquiry ranged much more widely and resulted in recommendations for change in teacher training, whistle-blowing policies, education and child protection procedures and for action to be taken by the Welsh Assembly Government. The inquiry, which lasted three years, attracted criticism on various grounds including one that it was an inappropriate use of the commissioner's resource and function. However, without the inquiry, the full extent of the abuse would not have been exposed and the victims and their families would not have had the opportunity to contribute to bringing about improvements that could prevent repetition of the systemic failings that were discovered (Rees 2010). The Welsh Commissioner was very generous in sharing his valuable experience, and the lessons learned, with the other UK commissioners and their staff at one of the annual BINOCC staff conferences.

Changing the culture

As indicated earlier, both the concept and substance of 'children's rights' can be controversial. Children's commissioners must be at the forefront of the battle to change our culture towards recognition of the fact that it is essential to meet the claims of children if we are to have happy and healthy individuals – and a happy and healthy society.

A child-centred approach would necessitate a willingness to examine professional cultures against the standards and values of the UNCRC. Commissioners can promote the Convention as an accepted starting point, providing a common language for exploring professional attitudes and values. It will be easier to promote culture change if we can be sure that all those working with children are pulling in the same direction.

Because of the time it takes to change culture and the way it happens, it can be difficult to identify and measure success and the contribution of different agencies and individuals. For example, a central concern of the first Scottish Commissioner's 'Safe, Active, Happy' priority was the 'over-protection' of children that leads to a sterile and unstimulating environment. This was a novel idea at the start of the commissioner's five-year term of office. It had to be explained to some partners, who were then convinced and came on board with it. Now, this insight is a part of the culture. There has been a degree of culture change even within this short period, even though much remains to be done to translate it into practice. However, new thinking – new culture – quickly becomes assumed as the norm and it is then difficult to reflect back on the challenges faced at the time when it was innovative. It can also be difficult, in a matter so ethereal, to identify exactly when, how and why change occurred and what influence any one person or agency had.

True culture change on children's rights will be effected when children's commissioners have succeeded in mainstreaming children's rights to the extent that they have done themselves out of a job. But we are still a very long way from that eventuality.

Conclusions and implications

In this chapter we have introduced you to the office of Children's Commissioner and the potential for it to shape the policy agenda in a way that is influenced by children and young people and responsive to the experiences and insights of those working for children in the statutory, voluntary or private sectors. The commissioners' offices are well placed to draw together insights from diverse sources and focus on the whole child. They can be a valuable source of information and advice for workers, as well as sensitive recipients of their professional concerns and insights.

Exercise

1. Read the 2008 Concluding Observations and Recommendations of the UN Committee on the Rights of the Child on the UK's third and fourth periodic reports under the UNCRC (available at http://www2.ohchr.org/english/bodies/crc/). Reflect on the relevance of these observations and recommendations to your own work.
   Consider:

   - how you might link into the work being undertaken by the commissioners' offices to monitor implementation of the recommendations;

   - how else you might in practice make use of and/or contribute to the activities of the commissioner for the UK country in which you are working.

2. Are there lessons for child-service agencies from the way the UK children's commissioners have collaborated among themselves and with other agencies to promote the rights of 'the whole child'?

3. Reflecting on the case study 'Working Together on Asylum' (above), what other issues do you think might benefit from collaboration across the UK, whether by the children's commissioners or other agencies?

Recommended reading

The websites of the four commissioners:
Children's Commissioner for Wales: http://www.childcom.org.uk/
NICCY: http://www.niccy.org/
SCCYP: http://www.sccyp.org.uk/
11 Million: http://www.childrenscommissioner.gov.uk/

ENOC website: http://www.crin.org/enoc/

UN Committee website: http://www2.ohchr.org/english/bodies/crc/

Williams (2005) Details in references.

Cleland, A. and Sutherland, E. E. (eds), (2009) Details in references.

Chapter 4

Integrating children's services

Harry Daniels and Anne Edwards

Summary points

- Preventing social exclusion and addressing social problems requires practitioners to identify and respond to accumulated risk in children's lives.

- This calls for a multi-faceted, interprofessional response involving collaboration across professional boundaries.

- The chapter draws on a study of inter-agency working that revealed the knowledge used by practitioners to underpin their collaborations.

- New cooperative practices revealed contradictions in local systems, which made demands on their organisations.

- Key concepts discussed include the building of common knowledge at places where the practices of different professionals overlap, and the emergence of expertise which is distributed across groups or teams.

- Integrated working calls for an enhanced form of professional practice which includes both core expertise and the capacity to work relationally with others across professional boundaries, both of which make demands on current ways of organising services.

The policy background

The 'prevention of social exclusion' has been until recently a major policy driver in welfare services in England (Bynner 2001; France and Utting 2005). Its core concept 'social inclusion' now carries with it the idea of entitlement to integration into society as both an individual right and a societal necessity. That attention to social inclusion represented a shift over the past 20 years, from seeing problems among children and young people in terms of their being disadvantaged to their now being 'at risk' of being excluded from what society both offers and requires. This move has been regarded as helpful by policy-makers as it is future-oriented and allows the State to think about how it might prevent the exclusion of children from what binds society together and from their responsibilities to society.

However, vulnerability to social exclusion is multi-faceted and may not be recognised unless one looks across a child's life. It was therefore argued that the welfare services that work with children should find ways of enabling collaboration between practitioners (Home Office 2000; OECD 1998; Daniels et al. 2007) to allow responsive interventions to give support to children who appear vulnerable. This belief lay behind a raft of measures in England which aimed at producing joined up responses to the multi-dimensional problem of social exclusion in England. These included establishing the government's Social Exclusion Unit; the Green Paper *Every Child Matters* (DfES 2003); and the subsequent Children Act (DfES 2004) which together set out an agenda for more responsive interprofessional work. Particular government initiatives included:

- Sure Start, which worked with children and their families in local centres from birth (Melhuish et al. 2005; see Chapter 8);
- The Children's Fund, which set up local partnerships to encourage interagency collaborations across services working with children aged five to thirteen (Edwards et al. 2006);
- On-Track, which focused on children and crime prevention in targeted areas (France et al. 2004);
- Local Network Funding;
- Extended schools, which offer support for families, activities for children, community access and quick access to other services (see Chapters 11 and 23).

The need for practitioners to be able to understand the totality of a child's life circumstances has also led to major reconfigurations of children's services in local authorities in England. We have seen, for example, the merging of education and social care services under single directorates in English local authorities and a short-lived reorganisation in central government to produce, in 2007, the Department for Children, Schools and Families (DCSF).[1] These mergings represented a massive change. The Policy Action Team 12, when looking at services for young people, reported that collaboration between services was not being achieved, for several reasons (Home Office 2000):

- local authority budgets for intervening in a crisis were different from those which funded preventive activities;
- priorities for services set out in policy guidance did not encourage collaboration;
- professional cultures worked against the kinds of collaborations that were needed).

Our own Learning in and for Inter-agency Work (LIW) study found many of these difficulties still in place when it completed its report in 2008 (Edwards et al. 2009).

Another element of the policy response to the problem of social exclusion reflected the link between exclusion and lack of engagement with the democratic processes of society, which marked European discussions during the 1990s. Alongside increased attention to collaboration between professionals was an expectation that citizens

[1] Following the 2010 General Election, the DCSF was restructured and named the Department for Education (DfE).

identified as vulnerable would participate in the development of the services that were to be provided for them. Sinclair and Franklin (2000: 2) summarised the reasons for involving children as: upholding children's rights; fulfilling legal responsibilities; improving services; improving decision-making; enhancing democratic processes; promoting children's protection; enhancing children's skills; empowering; and enhancing self-esteem (see also Chapter 12). The Children's Fund, for example, reflected the view in government that children should play a greater role in developing policy and practice. In 2000 its strategy document stated:

> we want to hear the voices of young people influencing and shaping local services; contributing to their local communities; feeling heard; feeling valued; being treated as responsible citizens.   (Children's and Young People's Unit 2000: 27)

This strategy required service providers to become more responsive to the needs and strengths of the groups with whom they were working. However, it was not always easy for them to adjust from being the expert who inhabited a culture of specific expertise to learn to recognise the expertise that parents and carers brought to discussions of their children and neighbourhoods (Anning et al. 2006; Edwards et al. 2006).

The systemic changes were not limited to specialist and targeted services and how they worked together and with families. There was also a role to be played by universal services such as schools. The 2007 discussion paper produced by the UK Treasury, as a result of its policy review of services for children (Treasury-DfES 2007), first outlined the need for a broad interpretation of social inclusion and a whole-system response.

> . . . the system needs to be capable of providing a continuum of support across services throughout childhood and to be able to intervene when poor outcomes do arise . . . new interventions would still be needed to deal with those who will begin to signal a higher likelihood of poor outcomes at a later age but who had not done so before . . . (p. 19)

The paper then pointed to how universal services had a part to play in the rethought system:

> The need to identify children experiencing poor outcomes, and to monitor children to identify who might be showing signs of developing poor outcomes, implies a key role for universal services. These services, such as health visitors, GPs, children's centres and especially schools – which have constant contact with children throughout their childhood – could play the primary role in identifying which children might be vulnerable.   (p. 19)

This chapter engages with the challenges that practitioners and policy-makers face as they attempt to provide joined up solutions to joined-up problems. We will discuss our own empirical work which directed attention towards the way in which professionals learn to do, what is in essence, a very new form of work.

The LIW study

The whole system approach that has been developed has marked a considerable change for children's services, which have been used to working to their own goals and their own professional standards. The LIW (Learning in and for Inter-agency Work) study was an attempt to identify what these changes meant for practitioners who worked with children and families and for local authority systems. The four-year study was designed to support practitioners and systems as they experienced these changes and:

■ focused on the changes in practice identified by practitioners from different practitioner backgrounds as they began to work across organisational boundaries with other professionals;

■ elicited the ideas they were using as they worked interprofessionally to support vulnerable children and young people; and

■ identified the implications for the organisations in which they were employed.

In achieving these aims we worked in case-study sites, selected on the basis of their strong commitment to the development of multi-agency working, in England. These were:

■ a new multi-professional team that was learning to work together;

■ a loosely coupled team working with looked-after children;

■ the boundary between an extended school and the wider children's services in the same local authority, which were reconfiguring.

The work of Vygotsky (1978, 1987) made a profound contribution in revealing for us how people were making sense of new practices (Daniels 2001; 2008). Vygotsky analysed 'consciousness' – i.e. what we would now see as how people think and make sense of the world. His argument was that people reveal their understandings in the way that they interpret a problem and use the tools available, including forms of talk, to work on it. The tools used may be material artefacts such as calculators, but also include the conceptual tools revealed in how language is employed while working on a task.

Vygotsky argued that people could be helped to reveal thinking through a method that he called 'dual stimulation'. A simple example of dual stimulation is to give a child a task and a tool, which may be an intellectual tool, and to see how they use the tool to work on the task. How they are making sense of the task and the tool will be revealed in their actions, which will, of course, include the language they use.

We present details of our methods here since they have the potential to be adapted for self-reflection by teams of professionals. Our work in the case-study sites was oriented around a series of two-hour structured sessions in each site. The methodology we used in these sessions was Developmental Work Research (DWR) (Engeström et al. 2003; Engeström 2007). DWR is based on the Vygotskian idea of dual stimulation and was used to help practitioners reveal the thinking that is embedded in their accounts of their practices and to examine the systemic tensions and contradictions they encountered when developing new ways of working. The 'second series stimuli' offered in DWR are the conceptual apparatus of activity theory such as the relationship between 'rules' both implicit and explicit in the system and how participants are interpreting the new 'object of activity', i.e. the problem space that they are working on, such as preventing social exclusion. The ideas coming from activity theory are provided as second stimuli by the research team as resources to be used by participants to analyse and make sense of their everyday practices in relation to inter-agency work.

In the DWR sessions, evidence about the practices from the research was presented by the research team or sometimes by participants with the support of the team. Participants were then helped to examine those practices using activity theory. In doing so they revealed the ideas they were using as they engaged in or hoped to develop their work (Edwards et al. 2009). The methodology enabled the LIW team to see what practitioners, such as social workers, education welfare officers, psychologists and teachers were learning in order to undertake new inter-professional collaborations and what adjustments they were making to existing practices and their own positions as professionals within those practices.

The DWR sessions focused on:

- *Present* – identifying contradictions (structural tensions) in current working practices;
- *Past* – encouraging professionals to consider the historical emergence of these working practices;
- *Future* – working with professionals to suggest new forms of practice that might effectively support innovations in multi-agency working.

In short, the aim of the workshops was to address professional learning by:

- encouraging the *recognition* of areas in which there is a need for change in working practices;
- suggesting possibilities for change through *reconceptualising* the 'objects of activity', i.e. problems that professionals are working on and the 'tools' that professionals use to work together on the problems.

The knowledge in use in interprofessional work

Our analysis of talk in the sessions (Daniels 2010, in press; Edwards et al. 2009; Middleton 2010) revealed challenges arising from contradictions in practices which were not the discrete province of any one profession, but required complementary knowledge and skills drawn from across the professions, i.e. distributed systems of expertise. We identified the following responses to the challenges of interprofessional work in the teams with which we were engaged:

1. **Focusing on the whole child in the wider context.** Practitioners found this crucial to the diagnosis of vulnerability that may not be evident unless they look across aspects of a child's life and build a picture of accumulated risk. It was also essential in their orchestration of responses.
2. **Being responsive to others – both professionals and clients.** Professionals claimed and demonstrated a growing awareness of the need to work relationally with each other and moved towards working more responsively with the strengths of their clients to build resilience.

3. **Clarifying the purpose of work and being open to alternatives.** The discursive work in constructing explicit understandings of previously tacit assumptions of the practices of others opened possibilities for alternative ways of working. These were resources for identifying how to work together.

4. **Knowing how to know who can help.** Practitioners identified the importance of knowing the people and resources distributed in their local networks. For example, established networks were not sufficient for working on the new objects of activity that co-configured multi-agency working demanded.

5. **Rule-bending and risk-taking.** Practitioners described taking risks involving rule-bending as responses to contradictions between emergent practices and systems of rules, protocols and lines of responsibility. They demonstrated the need to question the legitimacy of the existing rules in relation to their professional actions on increasingly complex objects of activity, and the necessity of making visible the ways in which they worked around the barriers to action.

6. **Creating and developing better (material and discursive) tools.** Practitioners identified the limitations of tools such as assessment protocols. They responded to the contradictions between currently available tools and new and emergent objects of multi-agency activity by developing and refining new conceptual and material tools, e.g. electronic assessment and communication devices.

7. **Developing processes for knowledge sharing and pathways for practice.** Practitioners recognised the importance of demonstrating an outward-looking stance and an awareness of what it takes to be 'in the know' as the complex landscape of multi-agency work changes. DWR sessions provided a forum for precisely this form of activity.

8. **Understanding oneself and one's professional values.** Participants recognised that articulating the particularities of their own expertise and values in order to negotiate practices with other professionals was a basis for questioning them. Enhanced forms of professional practice arose from questioning how values-driven practices might be reconfigured in relation to other professionals.

9. **Taking a pedagogic stance at work.** Participants described consciously 'teaching' others, e.g. when mediating contradictions between practitioner priorities and client demands (e.g. from a school or parent); needing to communicate across boundaries between professions; enabling operational staff to communicate the implications of emergent practices with strategic managers.

Subsequent analyses of these data (Edwards 2010; Edwards and Kinti 2010) suggest that an important process was at work in the DWR sessions. In brief, the nine ideas discussed above were ones to which all participants eventually subscribed, with the result that they constituted a form of common knowledge which had been built in the meetings and could function as a foundation for future joint problem-solving and collaborative support for children and families.

Responsive interprofessional collaborations to support children and families were mediated by new official tools such as the Common Assessment Framework (CAF). However, as we indicated earlier, the use of tools is intertwined with the knowledge of the users, how they interpret the problem being worked on and what knowledge and beliefs are informing how they use the tool. One relatively mundane way of using CAF was as a *'what tool'*, i.e. to assist descriptions of diagnoses and tracking of responses. By contrast, CAF was sometimes used as a *'where to tool'*, to help support a child's long-term progress towards social inclusion. This latter use signalled a sharing of longer-term intentions for children and families, which reflected the professional values embedded in common knowledge of the practitioners involved. Indeed the making explicit, sharing and enhancement of professional values proved to be an important element in the development of common knowledge and the practices that emerged as a result, and appeared to be important in giving direction to practitioners' engagement with each other.

Conversations at the boundaries of practice about what matters for each practice, when working with children and families, can provide the foundation for cross-boundary responsive work. An extended discussion of these ideas can be found in Edwards (2010) – the key point here is that the capacity to operate within a system of distributed expertise needs some prior work among the practitioners so that they can not only 'know how to know who' but also how to make sense to others and understand what is important for others in their specialist practices.

Challenges faced by agencies and professionals

As we have just indicated, practitioners involved in preventing children's social exclusion share a common interest in children's well-being, based on sets of professional values that can overlap. In other words, the interprofessional work we observed was more likely to be child-led than service-led.

Through examining their developing practices and practitioners' frustrations together with them, we noted that they were usually related to the old rules that still governed new practices and the barriers that existed at the organisational boundaries which were tested by the new practices. For example, existing systems of referral meant that organisations passed on 'bits of the child', as one practitioner put it, from one to the other. These rules were opened up for scrutiny and criticism of how slow the respective organisations were in enabling parallel interprofessional collaboration which was more responsive to the needs of children. Rule-bending was sometimes observed, reflecting practitioners' frustrations about the responsiveness of systems to new demands of child-centred collaborations. These were likely to be a matter of bypassing organisational hierarchies in order to make direct contact with the practitioner in another service who could help quickly.

The need to rule-bend pointed to the different timescales involved in achieving change through a systemic approach, and the different capacities of the organisations in which practices were changing to learn from and respond to these changes. This is not an uncommon problem when new practices are being developed (Schulz 2001). In the LIW study, we observed that local strategists' timescales differed from the practitioners, who were often far more aware of the organisational implications of interprofessional work, while the tools created to support practices were frequently lagging behind the practices in their development.

This disjunction highlighted for us the need for systemic approaches to change to include time for systemic learning. Time is needed for management strategy to learn from practice, and for the development of strategies that are informed by the learning that is occurring in practice as practitioners develop new ways of working. People use familiar resources in fresh ways; develop new ideas as they use those resources; question the practices that get in the way of their work; and work with different people, or the same people in new ways.

However, systems don't simply evolve – changes are stimulated by imbalances in the system which, in turn, lead to dynamic shifts of the kinds just outlined. Sometimes these shifts are barely discernable, as they arise from small tensions that occur (see Example 4.1).

Example 4.1

James was displaying problems in school, and it was decided to discuss these with his parents. It was unclear whether it was best for the approach to be made by the head of year (with good understanding of the within-school issues) or the education welfare officer (with responsibility and experience in relation to relationships beyond the school). A brief conversation between these two staff resolved the matter in this case, but they also recognised that there were wider issues, since the head of year felt his pastoral activities were constrained by the EWO's primacy in links with parents. Hence, discussion was needed about how better to apportion family contacts and when these should be made jointly.

According to Engeström's (1995) activity theory framework, changes in systems occur as a result of participants recognising and working with the contradictions in them. Contradictions are to be found everywhere because few systems are so completely bounded that new ideas, resources or expectations are prevented from entering. When people first meet a contradiction, they will feel frustrated with either the expectation or the rules. We found this occurred particularly when a new expectation that staff collaborate in parallel with other professionals to support a particular child ran up against continuing rules in their workplace based on onward referral without further cooperation.

If they are convinced, because of professional values, that parallel interprofessional collaboration is best for the child, they are likely to try to work on or round the rules in order to change them. For example, they would adopt new patterns of informal referral that 'bent' the rules. We found that rule-bending was something that practitioners had learnt to do to take forward interprofessional work (see examples 4.2 and 4.3). They also learnt to create new resources which, for example, helped to sustain interprofessional collaboration. These examples of creative responses are important, because they help us to see that changes made by individual or small numbers of practitioners can shift systems. Indeed, from our perspective, if people don't try to adapt their work systems, then development in their systems will be limited.

Examples 4.2 and 4.3 show the use of informal processes to sidestep agency policies about referral.

Example 4.2

A primary school head was frustrated by the local authority's refusal to consider two pupils for special education. The head used her informal contacts with a special school so that the pupils could spend part of the day there. After two weeks the assessments persuaded the local authority to change its mind.

Example 4.3

It was the policy of the education authority that referrals to educational psychologists should be sanctioned by the relevant school, because it was responsible for deploying the time allocated by the local authority for this service. However, as a result of working in collaboration, Mrs Wood (an attendance officer) had formed a good, trusting relationship with Ms Starkie, a psychologist. Therefore, when Mrs Wood was concerned about one of her pupils, she decided not to follow the expected process, but to have an initial informal conversation with Ms Starkie. She believed this would lead to more appropriate and timely help.

There were, therefore, frequent struggles in the DWR sessions which were reflected in subsequent interviews with, for example, teachers who were not convinced by their colleagues' resistance to interprofessional work. These non-resistant teachers found themselves experiencing significant conflicts in the motives for their work – between student attainment, prioritised by existing school practices, and student well-being, which was supported by the system of distributed expertise that was developing outside the school. Such conflicts in the motives for practice are hugely challenging. It is extraordinarily uncomfortable to be, for example, a teacher whose professional values focus on developing children's well-being working in a school where improving pupil attainment is the primary purpose.

The practices and the learning that we were examining were part of a major shift in policy for work with children and families. Practitioners had little option but to move forward, however slowly, and engage with what the new policies requested of them. Standing still and hoping that the juggernaut would pass was not an option. Yet, developments in practices were frequently out-pacing institutional responses to them. Practitioners were therefore in the vanguard of unavoidable changes and bearing the brunt of the contradictions between old rules and new responses that emerged at almost every turn. At the same time they needed to sustain their sense of themselves as responsible, functioning professionals. It was a stressful time.

We argue that the emotional or affective aspects of changing organisations and practices should not be downplayed. Vygotsky was quite clear that emotion cannot be filtered out of analyses of how we act in the world. For example, he argued that if emotion were ignored

> . . . thought must be viewed . . . as a meaningless epiphenomenon incapable of changing anything in the life or conduct of a person.　　　　(Vygotsky 1986: 10).

Coping with change is not simply a behavioural response, but also involves a relatively slow process of working through contradictions or 'crises' and gaining new forms of mental equilibrium that enable functioning. This situation was certainly the case for many children's services and schools at the time of the study. Practitioners working on the ground were constantly meeting these contradictions and developing professional responses as their practices raced ahead of the inevitably slower institutional responses of their work systems.

Conclusions and implications

Responsive collaborations by practitioners in children's services call for seeing local systems in terms of the expertise that is distributed across all of them, with practitioners both contributing to and drawing on that expertise as they work with children and families. Our focus on distributed expertise indicates the importance of core professional expertise and the professional values associated with it. However, our attention to the building of enough common knowledge to permit responsive collaborations suggests that an additional more relational form of expertise is also needed to augment specialist strengths (Edwards 2010). Recognising the distributed nature of local expertise enables practitioners to move from passing over 'bits of the child' towards parallel support for children and families (Puonti, 2004).

Before we move on to discuss the organisational implications of the LIW study, it is important to reflect on what we did not find as an aspect of interprofessional working. It seemed that the recent attention to how professionals work together to support children and families has led to an understandable focus on how practitioners make sense to each other and how they jointly interpret the needs of families. Unfortunately the outcome, at least in the early days of emergent practices that we tracked, was that the children and families became objectified as shared tasks to be worked on. Consequently the interesting developments in, for example, social work on more relational forms of engagement with clients became downplayed. We suspect that this is an outcome of the challenges of setting up interprofessional work and would expect the situation to be remedied once practices have settled.

When we turn to organisational practices, our findings echo Glissen and Hemmelgarn's (1998) view that attention should be paid to developing positive organisational climates for professional decision-making rather than a focus on more rigid forms of interprofessional coordination. There was evidence of the need for organisational adjustments. The most frequent was the rule-bending that occurred when it became apparent that existing rules of, for example, sequential referral were impeding parallel responsive work.

Our starting point was the workplace learning of practitioners as they undertook new forms of work and how that might impact on systems to ensure that learning continues. Recognising tensions and contradictions and working creatively to overcome them is a good thing, as these endeavours will help to take systems forward so that they can deal with new demands, work more effectively and make the most of new resources. We have observed examples of values-led, responsible, professional action being promoted within inter-agency working, but also of constraints where organisations had not yet adjusted to the new demands this places on them.

The capacity for interprofessional work was accelerated by the DWR sessions, which had an impact on professional learning. These sessions operated as sites of intersecting practices (Edwards 2010) where professionals could discuss values; reveal their expertise in their interpretations of problems of practice; and begin to work on extending their sense of who they were as professionals. We, therefore, suggest that interprofessional meetings are useful to enable practitioners to focus on how they might deal with concrete cases and have the time to reveal and discuss different ways in which they interpret and respond to particular problems.

These meetings are not the same as case conferences, where it is often crucial that decisions are made quickly and there are often several cases to move through fairly rapidly. Rather, we are suggesting lessons are taken from DWR to structure dedicated professional development sessions so that practitioners can focus on a problem and reflect, for example, on how current rules or processes are helping or impeding what they see as their interpretations and responses. Two things will happen. First, the systemic contradictions that are getting in the way of their responsive work will be revealed and should then be worked on at a strategic level in local authority. Second, the practitioners themselves will be engaging in the building of the common knowledge they need to enable them to work purposefully and productively together and with families.

Our very strong message from the LIW study for organisations was that practices on the ground were racing ahead of the systems and strategies which should be supporting them, and that, therefore, local systems should develop ways of enabling what we have termed 'upstream learning'. This involves attention to processes that would allow local strategists to learn from the often groundbreaking work going on as practitioners collaborated and worked with children and families so that they could adapt systems to support these developments.

Exercise

■ Discuss the activities undertaken in collaborative work in one or more agencies you are familiar with. Consider:

    (a) intended outcomes of the activities, such as improving a child's attainment or school attendance;

    (b) the object of activity – i.e. something that needs to be engaged with and transformed if those outcomes are to be achieved, like a child's trajectory as a learner.

■ Next investigate the 'tools' available to work on those objects of activity such as learning mentors, home visiting or a specialist programme. Review how suitable the tools currently in use are and what others might be helpfully employed.

Recommended reading

Edwards, A., Daniels, H., Gallagher, T., Leadbetter, J. and Warmington, P. (2009) *Improving inter-professional collaborations: multi-agency working for children's well-being*, London: Routledge.

> This book outlines the project on which this study was based and gives more details on the approaches used and the findings.

Daniels, H. et al. (eds), (2010) *Activity Theory in Practice: promoting learning across, boundaries and agencies*, London: Routledge.

> This collection of papers explores how the activity theory framework used in the LIW can be applied in a wide range of different settings including schools, occupational health and manufacturing.

Morris, K. (ed.) (2008) *Social Work and Multi-agency Working*, Bristol: Policy Press.

> Aimed at social workers in training, the collection of papers in this collection explores interprofessional work from the perspectives of the different professionals involved.

The European Network of Ombudspersons for Children (ENOC) at http://crin.orq/enoc/

Chapter 5

Getting it right for children: promoting effective change

Bob Stradling and Bill Alexander

Summary points

- It has been increasingly recognised across the United Kingdom that a more streamlined and better integrated approach to children's services is needed to reduce the likelihood of children being passed around the services without getting the help they need and vulnerable children being overlooked.

- Systems, structures and processes need to be rationalised to improve information sharing, reduce duplication of effort across services, make the experience more seamless for children and families and ensure that the delivery of additional help is effectively coordinated and monitored.

- In Scotland *Getting it right for every child* has developed a national practice model, including tools and training materials, to support assessment and evidence-based professional judgement.

- Professional development, mentoring and quality assurance are also needed to ensure that practitioners develop the analytical skills needed to employ these tools effectively.

- A professional culture shift is also needed if each practitioner is going to 'let go' of the old ways of working and trust the judgement and expertise of colleagues in other services. This also has implications for workforce development.

Introduction

Since 2000, beginning with the Victoria Climbié case in England and the Caleb Ness case in Scotland, a recurring theme in many Enquiries and Serious Case Reviews involving the death or abuse of children has been that agencies have often held key information about the child and family but either did not recognise its significance or failed to share this information with other services who might have been able to intervene earlier in order to prevent a tragedy. It was widely recognised that cooperation between the various services working with children and families needed to be improved and more needed to be done to improve the assessment, decision-making and planning skills of all front-line practitioners.

In England the Green Paper *Every Child Matters*, and the subsequent consultation exercise, led to a national framework for transforming services for children and young people, also called *Every Child Matters*. In Scotland a number of initiatives were introduced to improve children's services culminating in the *Getting it Right for Every Child* initiative launched in 2006. Cooperation between different services in order to provide support for children and families was not a new phenomenon, but over the last 20 years there has been a stream of national and local government initiatives designed to make joint working more effective, and from the late 1990s a number of national developments and initiatives in Scotland played an important part in setting the direction for change in children's services. The Children (Scotland) Act 1995 required local councils to consult and cooperate with other statutory and voluntary agencies in drawing up children's services plans to identify and meet children's needs. Sure Start provided support for innovative programmes to bring together early education, childcare, health and family support to strengthen the well-being, development and learning of vulnerable children. However, it was probably the publication of *For Scotland's Children* in 2001 that had the greatest impact on the development of a more integrated approach to the provision of children's services in Scotland. It offered an action plan containing a range of different ways in which local authorities, the National Health Service and the voluntary sector could work together to create a single children's service that would ensure that all children would have the necessary support when they needed it.

Since 2001 in Scotland a number of other national policy developments have impacted on children's services. These include: changes in child protection guidelines and risk-assessment procedures following a number of high-profile cases and public inquiries; the Education (Additional Support for Learning) Scotland Act (2004) which replaced the traditional concept of special educational needs with the wider notion of additional support needs and replaced the child's Record of Needs with a Coordinated Support Plan; Health for All Children (HALL 4), which reflected a move away from a wholly medical model of early screening for disease and physical and mental disorders towards a model that placed much more emphasis on health promotion, primary prevention and joint working between health professionals and professionals in other services, and, finally, *Getting it Right for Every Child* (GIRFEC) (Scottish Executive 2005a).

During this period a number of Scottish local authorities responded by merging certain services or departments; others exploited the potential for co-location of services; and a few retained their existing service and departmental structures but agreed to pool part of their budgets to support joint working. However, while structural and systemic changes can facilitate joint working they do not necessarily ensure that all of the child's needs are addressed in an integrated way.

Traditionally practice had tended to be unsystematic and variable. Cooperation tended to take the form of a sequence of referrals from one professional to another and from one service to another. Information was shared on a need-to-know basis, usually determined by the person with the information. Additional support for the child tended to be initiated by one professional who then made an informal referral to another professional in a different service, who might take on responsibility for the intervention or make a further referral to another professional or agency.

This sequential model of joint working (Edwards 2004) raises concerns about equity of provision and the importance of working to the same standards for every child, regardless of where they were being provided or by whom. It also raises concerns about the prevalence of a referrals culture within children's services where the referrer might disengage from providing any form of additional support to the child that would complement the additional support provided by other services. A referrals culture also tends to increase the demand for targeted and specialist services for children who, after assessments have been undertaken, may not meet the criteria for those additional services. This either means unnecessary delays before the child receives appropriate and proportionate support or increased caseloads for professionals working in targeted and specialist services. There was also a growing concern by the late 1990s that the sequential model was providing an unsatisfactory experience for many children and families. As they were passed from one professional to another, they found themselves participating in different assessments of their child's needs, even though these often involved answering the same questions. These separate assessments then led to different and parallel action plans and pathways through the various support services. Finally, there was also a risk with the sequential model that availability of service rather than assessment of the child's needs might determine the sequence of referrals (Stradling and MacNeil 2007).

By 2005 two additional developments were being promoted in Scotland. First, more emphasis was given to needs-led rather than service-led provision, with success and effectiveness being measured in terms of the outcomes for children and families rather than in terms of the delivery of specific inputs and outputs. Second, the Scottish Government felt it was necessary to articulate certain common goals for children's services around the concepts of well-being, welfare and child development (Scottish Executive 2005). Meanwhile, similar approaches were being developed in England, Wales and Northern Ireland.

Getting it Right for Every Child and the Highland Pathfinder

Fundamental to the *Getting it Right* programme is the idea that a seamless network of support, coordinated at the point of delivery, should be built around the child's needs, rather than that the child and family should have to adapt to the requirements of the system.

Development work began in 2006, with priority given to the development and trialling of a practice model for all services working with children and families. To support these developments, the Scottish Government initiated some pathfinder projects to help shape, develop and test practice tools and training materials and to inform the development of national guidance (Scottish Government 2008).

The Highland *Getting it Right* Pathfinder, based around Inverness, one of Scotland's fastest-growing cities, was formally launched in September 2006. It was the only pathfinder with a remit to address all aspects of children's needs, from birth through to eighteen, and encompassing all services whose work significantly affects the lives of children and their families. Over the previous ten years Highland had already made substantial moves towards integrated children's services, and this was one of the main factors influencing the Scottish Government's decision to invite them to be a GIRFEC Pathfinder. In the rest of this chapter we shall focus on the new systems, processes and practices that were implemented in Highland and their impact on children and families.

Changing systems and procedures in line with *Getting it Right*

Traditionally, services for children and families have tended to operate independently of each other, even if some level of cooperation has been necessary in individual cases. Each service has had responsibility for managing its own budget, and this has encouraged some degree of gatekeeping with each service employing its own eligibility criteria to control access to support, its own referral and assessment procedures, and its own record-keeping system. Service-specific performance indicators, statutory requirements and distinctive professional cultures have also tended to act as barriers to more effective multi-agency collaboration.

Given these variations in the systems supporting children's services it is not surprising that the implementation of *Getting it Right* was widely perceived in Scotland to be challenging. Within Highland a broadly based governance and strategic management structure was already in place before the Pathfinder phase began in order to facilitate joint planning and decision-making between the local authority, the health board, the police, the Children's Reporter's Office, the voluntary sector and other stakeholders, including groups of service users. Steps were then taken to ensure that the procedures and pathways to be followed when a concern about a child was raised would be more streamlined. Before the pathfinder phase it was not uncommon for the parents of children with a complex set of different needs to find themselves attending four or five separate meetings, yet answering the same questions and providing different professionals with the same chronological narrative. It was also possible for a child who was on the Child Protection Register, looked after away from home and experiencing severe learning difficulties, to have several different action plans, which were drawn up, implemented and reviewed by different groups of practitioners.

That situation has changed. Business process mapping was deployed to map the procedures and pathways that were being used by the universal, targeted and specialist services and this highlighted a number of areas of duplication. Now, regardless of whether a concern is raised about a child in education, health, a voluntary agency, social work or the police, professionals ask themselves the same five questions:

- What is getting in the way of this child's well-being?
- Do I have all the information I need to help this child?
- What can I do now to help them?
- What can my agency do to help this child?
- What additional help, if any, may be needed from others?

On the basis of their answers to these questions they will then follow the same sequence of procedures:

- gather evidence about the concern;
- determine if the child is at risk and requires immediate protection;
- determine if other agencies need to be involved;
- obtain consent from the child and parents to share information with other agencies;
- work together to produce, implement and monitor an agreed plan.

Systems for recording information within different services were also upgraded to ensure that professionals undertaking an assessment of the child's needs would have a comprehensive chronology of significant events that have previously impacted on the child's well-being and development, and the interventions taken in response to earlier concerns.

The planning process has also been rationalised so that each child with additional needs, even those with needs that require multi-agency support, will have just one plan rather than several parallel plans and that plan will be managed by the same group of practitioners who are working closely with that child and family.

The seamlessness of the assessment and planning process is facilitated by the allocation to every child, of a Named Person within health or in education if they are of school age. The Named Person is responsible for making sure that the child has the right help in place to support his or her development and well-being. Where that child or young person requires additional help and support from more than one agency or service, a Lead Professional is nominated to coordinate the planning process and make sure that the different services provide a network of support around the child in a seamless, timely and proportionate way.

The evaluation of the Pathfinder phase (Stradling et al. 2009) highlighted a number of ways in which these systemic changes have impacted on professional practice:

- The quality of the information being shared across services has improved significantly.
- Better inter-agency sharing of information is reducing the likelihood of children at risk 'going off the radar screen' even when their families move frequently or cease to engage with specific services.
- This is also leading to a more comprehensive picture of each child's unmet needs and this, in turn, is increasing the likelihood of the support provided being more appropriate and proportionate.
- Planning meetings for individual children are now more likely to be concerned with addressing the needs of the whole child, rather than just the needs or concerns that have been prioritised by the individual service which first raised a concern.
- Named Persons within universal services are identifying unmet needs at an earlier stage and this is enabling the necessary support to be put in place more quickly.

Changing professional practice

These systemic changes need to be accompanied by changes in practice. The new processes and procedures only deliver improved outcomes if practitioners are willing and able to exercise professional judgement. Whether a practitioner is gathering evidence to back up his or her initial concern about a child or to assess that child's needs and determine the most appropriate actions, he or she still needs to analyse that information in order to determine the impact on the child's well-being and development. This requires skill, experience, confidence, some understanding of child development and a repertoire of methods that can be used to gather and analyse the evidence and reach a considered judgement in a systematic and rigorous way.

Systematic analysis is also required to ensure that interventions will be proportionate to the level of need presented by children. Otherwise there is a real risk that the increased emphasis on identifying and responding to concerns and needs may lead to an ever-growing demand for scarce resources (Stradling and MacNeil 2010).

The national practice model for *Getting it Right* has been critically important in the development of the skills and confidence of the professionals working with children and families in Highland. The model is informed by two decades of theory and research evidence on good practice in assessment and planning for children's needs within a single-agency and multi-agency context (Scottish Government 2008).

There are three main components in the model:

1. The eight **Well-being Indicators** – safe, healthy, achieving, nurtured, active, respected, responsible and included – which are used to summarise the child's needs and to identify and monitor the intended outcomes for any planned intervention for that child.

2. The **My World Triangle** helps practitioners to examine the strengths and pressures in children's lives that may be impacting on them. As Figure 5.1 illustrates, these are organised under three headings: 'How I grow and develop', 'What I need from people who look after me' and 'My wider world'. For children with additional needs it is important to recognise that going round the triangle and simply listing the strengths and pressures is not enough – they need to be analysed in terms of how the interactions between these factors are impacting on the child's development and well-being.

3. The **Resilience Matrix** supports the analytical process by enabling the practitioner to group the strengths and pressures around the two axes shown in Figure 5.2. The vulnerability–resilience axis focuses mainly on the strengths and pressures that are intrinsic to the child's development. The adversity–protective factors axis focuses on the strengths and pressures within the child's family, school and wider community. Plotting strengths and pressures on the matrix helps to clarify what needs to be done to strengthen the child's resilience and the protective factors around the child.

'Resilience' here relates to the capacity of children and young people to arrive at positive outcomes despite adverse circumstances and can be defined as 'normal development under difficult conditions' (Fonaghy et al. 1994 p. 233; see also Chapter 19). But, as Daniel and Wassell have observed, 'the assessment of resilience

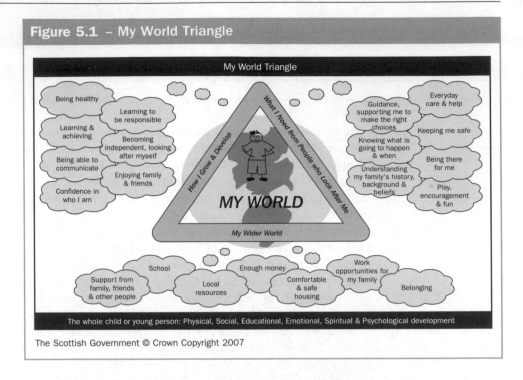

Figure 5.1 – My World Triangle

The Scottish Government © Crown Copyright 2007

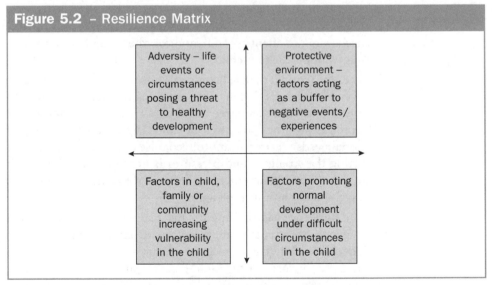

Figure 5.2 – Resilience Matrix

is not straightforward.' (2002, p. 12) Apparent coping behaviours exhibited by a young person cannot always be taken at face value. They may be internalising the symptoms. This level of interpretative analysis requires skill, sensitivity, training and experience.

Highland developed a modular training programme to support *Getting it Right* and this covered awareness-raising for all staff working with children and families, single-agency training on pathways and processes and a multi-agency training module for Lead Professionals and Named Persons (see Chapter 25).

Findings from the Pathfinder evaluation

The evaluation showed that the majority of the professionals who had participated in the training, and regularly assessed and planned for children with a diversity of additional needs, quickly gained confidence in using the My World Triangle. Health visitors and school nurses reported that they found the assessment process helpful in identifying the needs of the child, relating these to the needs of the mother and identifying a course of action which was both appropriate and proportionate. The social workers who had been using the My World Triangle to help them assess the needs of looked-after children and children in need of protection also reported that it was very helpful in organising a lot of disparate information about the child and his or her circumstances. It was also apparent that as professionals became more experienced and confident in using the assessment process, they were more likely to perceive that the initial concern raised about a child was often just a symptom of a complex of other concerns and problems. This, in turn, led to a more holistic child's plan.

Example 5.1

Chrissie is 17. She left home in her mid-teens and now has a baby, Liam, but doesn't know for sure who the father is. Recently she moved into a house with friends. Police were called to the house by a neighbour because of a disturbance. They found Liam asleep and unattended, and evidence of drugs in the house. Chrissie was not charged with any offences, but police passed on their concerns about Liam's safety to social work (see Chapter 10). Chrissie's social worker, her health visitor and a professional from Social Work Children and Families Service visited Chrissie at home and then carried out an initial assessment of the welfare and well-being of both Chrissie and Liam using the My World Triangle. This identified some evidence that Liam might be at risk if they continued to reside in the same house. Other concerns were also identified relating to Liam's low body weight and general health, the lack of a stimulating environment for him, Chrissie's health, her deficient independent living and parenting skills, and the lack of support from her family. Further information was sought from other agencies. The social worker from Children and Families Services took on the role of Liam's Lead Professional and convened a multi-agency group to draw up a Child's Plan.

Generally, then, the pathfinder training helped and professionals were learning from experience, but some further structured professional development was necessary to bring all professionals' skills up to the same level. For example, those who only used the new practice model occasionally tended to describe and summarise the needs that emerged from organising the information around the three sides of the triangle but were less likely to analyse this systematically as part of the process of drawing up a plan. It was also apparent that some professionals were confusing outputs with outcomes and therefore emphasising what each service would do, rather than what difference these actions would make for the child and family.

The evaluation also identified very few examples of the Resilience Matrix being used (see example 5.2 for an exception). The matrix is an option that Lead Professionals would probably only need to employ with cases where the child is very vulnerable or has very complex needs. However, the evaluators examined a sample of 100 different cases of children with multi-agency plans and many of these were complex. Even so, the matrix was rarely used. Without it there was a tendency to focus on the pressures and to either *exclude the strengths from the analysis* or *downplay their significance*.

Example 5.2

The multi-agency assessment process for Chrissie and baby Liam identified a wide range of concerns. On all three sides of the My World Triangle the pressures far outweighed the strengths. The analysis on the *Child Development* side of the triangle identified concerns about Liam's safety if he and his mother remained in their present accommodation, but it also indicated that he was not thriving as well as expected for his age. Signs of neglect, poor eating and sleeping patterns, irregular nappy changing and lack of learning stimuli were impacting negatively on his development. The analysis on the *People Who Can Help* side of the triangle focused mainly on Chrissie. While her love for and commitment to Liam was apparent, her capacity to nurture him effectively was impeded by physical and mental-health issues, low self-esteem, exposure to an environment where drugs were being used and poor parenting skills. On the third side of the triangle, the *Wider World*, the risks associated with her friendship group, the absence of a family support network, her financial struggles and the unsuitable accommodation were also affecting her and Liam adversely. In a situation where there were so many pressures operating on mother and baby, the Lead Professional and others in the assessment team found it helpful to use the Resilience Matrix. This assisted them to weigh the relative impact of all of these factors on the mother's resilience and vulnerability, and to identify how best to enhance the protective factors around the mother and baby when drawing up a multi-agency plan of action for them both.

The evaluation also showed that the development of skills in using the practice model is necessary but not sufficient to ensure effective planning. Practitioners also need a conceptual overview of the practice model – the linkages between recording information, assessing it, identifying intended outcomes and a timescale for measuring progress, identifying evidence-based actions and systematically reviewing whether or not any progress has been made towards improved outcomes for the children and, if not, what else needs to be done.

Consequently, while the training has been important in supporting the change process it has also been essential to reinforce this with effective quality assurance and mentoring by line managers. Highland have put into place some of the mechanisms that could support professional development here, and steps are being taken to check for consistency of practice and to establish benchmarks of good practice. However, it has also become clear that changes in practice of this scope cannot be imposed on a workforce. Hearts and minds need to be won over, and that necessitates a significant shift in professional cultures.

Changing professional cultures

Each profession tends to evolve a professional culture with distinctive elements – a specialised vocabulary, values, operating principles and a distinctive set of competencies. These determine what it is to be a professional within a particular occupation. There is an additional dimension, which is best described as a concept of professionalism and relates to how one behaves towards clients and colleagues.

However, a number of recent research studies (Cameron and Lart 2003; Edwards 2004; Sloper 2004) have highlighted how inter-agency working can challenge existing professional cultures:

- Initial professional training does not prepare practitioners for working outside established organisational practices, e.g. cross-agency responsibilities.

- Integrated planning requires each professional to think about the individual child in a holistic way rather than perceive them just as a user of their own service.

- Their expectations about who coordinates cross-agency support may not be shared by their colleagues.

- Different professions may use apparently-shared concepts, such as 'at risk', 'vulnerable' or 'additional needs' in different ways.

- Colleagues in different services may not understand each other's statutory obligations, operational priorities and constraints.

Therefore, there is a need to foster a parallel interprofessional working culture. This is partly about working collaboratively according to a set of agreed principles and values. It is also about recognising that the specialised language and the working assumptions that each profession takes for granted will not be familiar to their colleagues in other agencies. An interprofessional working culture also needs to be flexible enough to ensure that the professional expertise of each individual in an inter-agency team is recognised and valued, but at the same time those individuals do not hide behind their professional authority.

The development of a parallel integrated service culture needs to be planned. The proposed changes in practice need to be internalised by the workforce, with each individual professional being willing and prepared to adapt and 'let go' of the old ways of working and embrace the new approach. This transformation is the single most unpredictable element in the whole management of change process. Some specialist professionals in Highland, for instance, found it difficult at first to let go of the responsibility for a particular case even when progress made by the child indicated that the universal services could now take on that responsibility. The other side of the coin from 'letting go' is trusting other services to do what is best for the child. Building such trust takes time and depends on experience of multi-agency working.

In the early stages of the pathfinder process some professionals, particularly in the universal services, were reluctant to take on the role of Lead Professional responsible for coordinating the delivery of support for the child, either because of anxieties about workloads or because they associated the role of the Lead Professional with a specific service rather than with a set of responsibilities that any professional working with children might take on. In such circumstances an embedded referrals culture within universal services can be particularly difficult to erode.

Nevertheless, and in spite of these challenges, a cultural shift has been taking place across Highland:

- A common language around the Well-being Indicators and the My World Triangle is now understood and widely used across the services and agencies. Previously practitioners had assessed the needs of children and families according to whether they met the criteria for different levels of service provision.

- Each service had its own criteria and its own professional language of levels, tariffs and thresholds, which was not always understood by practitioners in other services. While the use of criteria and the language associated with it has not disappeared altogether, it is now less common in interprofessional discourse.

- There is now far more inter-agency trust, particularly between the targeted and specialist services on one hand and the universal services on the other. There is a greater willingness to share information with other agencies about the child, which was an issue initially for some health practitioners, and it is also clear that health specialists and social workers are now more willing to hand cases back to universal services when there is evidence of significant progress being made.

- More practitioners are putting the child at the centre of their joint concerns. They are also using common tools and processes.

- There is a growing perception within children's services that the effectiveness of integrated working needs to be measured in terms of the outcomes for the child rather than in terms of whether or not the specific service outputs were delivered.

Overall, the evaluation indicated that there are two parallel developments that need to take place in order to create an inter-agency professional culture. The first is when practitioners become less anxious about their professional identity. Their discourse about their work is no longer punctuated with concerns that they are being asked to do someone else's job. The fact that they no longer say this does not mean that their professional identity has become more blurred than it used to be. Rather, it means that they recognise that a central part of their professional responsibility is that they work with children and in order to do their work effectively they often need to understand the whole child. The second interrelated development is that when professionals work together to provide support for a particular child or young person, they look at the child in the round and no longer think in terms of labels such as pupil, looked-after child, young offender, child protection case or youngster with mental health problems.

This is most likely to happen where individual practitioners are not only trained to apply the new processes but also have an overview of what *Getting it Right* is seeking to achieve which drives their thinking about how best to respond to children's unmet needs.

Conclusions and implications

Implications for agencies

A more streamlined and integrated approach to children's services helps to reduce duplication and overlap. As the GIRFEC Pathfinder evaluation showed, a number of procedures and processes that existed before *Getting it Right* have either been made redundant or are only used for a small number of children now. This is providing more time for professionals to focus on the core activity of working with and for children, young people and their families. However, these are mainly non-cashable savings. They are unlikely to release resources for use elsewhere in public services but they are releasing resources for better service provision within children's services. This in turn, given the positive outcomes for children shown in the evaluation, means that streamlining has helped to ensure a more effective service.

The greater emphasis on early identification and intervention (and not just crisis intervention) has meant that in the shorter term more concerns about children are being identified. In this stage of the implementation process it is not surprising that there is an increased demand on resources and services that were only intended for a few children with higher-end needs. In the longer term it is anticipated that more systematic and comprehensive assessments, based around the *Getting it Right* practice model, will lead to more targeted support for children and bring about a longer-term saving as the needs of children are picked up before they reach crisis point and are addressed within universal services or require less input from targeted and specialist services (Stradling and MacNeil 2010).

Implications for practitioners

It is vital for practitioners to develop an integrated service culture that complements their individual professional identities. The streamlining of systems and processes to improve information sharing, reduce duplication of effort across services, and make the experience more seamless for children and families can ensure that the delivery of additional help is effectively coordinated. However, new systems will only deliver improved outcomes for children if practitioners not only gather and share information about children and families, but also analyse and interpret this information to build up a holistic picture of the child's needs and to facilitate sound, evidence-based judgement about the best course of action for the well-being and development of that child. The analysis is ecological, focusing not only on children's unmet needs and problems but also on the pressures in their immediate and wider environment that may be impacting on them. The analysis also takes account of children's strengths and resilience and the potential strengths in their environment when identifying the best course of action.

Implications for workforce development

A greater emphasis on a more analytical, ecological and holistic approach to assessment, planning and reviewing progress has implications for workforce development.

First, there are implications for higher education. The increasing emphasis on competencies in professional training has tended to introduce a false division between theory and practice. It is critically important that students understand how current theories of child development have influenced new practice models such as *Getting it Right* and how the effectiveness of their own working practice depends on their ability to apply these theories, particularly the ecological model of child development, to an analysis of the needs and concerns of the individual children they will be working with.

Second, it also has implications for local authorities, health boards and other statutory and independent bodies. The GIRFEC practice model acts as a guide to good practice, but it is not a substitute for systematic analysis and sound professional judgement. Training helps, and the more that professionals use the practice tools the more likely they are to adopt new practices. However, the evaluation of the *Getting it Right* pathfinder phase shows that continuing professional development, mentoring and feedback by line managers and experienced staff and quality-assurance processes are also essential if practitioners are going to 'let go' of old ways of working and embrace not only new methods but also the different assumptions and expectations that underpin the *Getting it Right* approach and similar policy assumptions elsewhere in the United Kingdom.

Exercise

Ian is a 9-year-old boy. Both of his parents have long histories of substance misuse and, while it is clear that both love him very much, neither has been capable of caring for him properly when they were misusing drugs and alcohol. Following a period of social work supervision, it was decided that a placement with his paternal granny would be in Ian's best interests. The parents had split up acrimoniously. The father enjoys supervised contact with Ian at the granny's house but Ian's mother only sees the boy at locations arranged by Ian's social worker. The mother is strongly opposed to the placement with the father's mother, and the granny is opposed to the mother having any access to the boy. The mother reports that she has been clean of drugs for six months and wants Ian to live with her. Ian talks about being under pressure from all three family members to support their particular positions. At a six-monthly review meeting, the parents and the granny argued vehemently about what would be best for Ian, who has said that he does not want to attend such meetings again. Some of the professionals working with Ian feel that he would be better off if he moved to foster carers, but this would mean that Ian would have to change school. The head of Ian's primary school argues that his school, friends and local community are providing a strong support network around him and a move to foster care could undermine this.

If you were Ian's Lead Professional how might an assessment using the My World Triangle and the Resilience Matrix help you to make a judgement about the goals and actions that would be best for Ian? Bear in mind that you might need to persuade a court or hearing of the wisdom of your plan.

Recommended reading

Aldgate, J., Jones, D. P. H., Rose, W. and Jeffery, C. (eds) (2006) *The Developing World of the Child*, London, Jessica Kingsley Publishing.

> This focuses on how the latest theories on child development can be applied to professionals working practice.

Cleaver, H., Walker, S. and Meadows, P. (2004) *Assessing Children's Needs and Circumstances*, London, Jessica Kingsley Publishing.

> A research study which reviews how the ecological Framework for the Assessment of Children in England and Wales impacted on professional practice and inter-agency collaboration.

Munro, E. (2008) *Effective Child Protection*, 2nd edn, Sage, London.

> This looks at the processes and the difficulties involved in assessing risk to children and reasoning skills and knowledge required for making professional judgements in complex cases.

The Scottish Government website for *Getting it Right for Every Child*.

> Provides further details about the policy initiative and research discussed in this chapter, with resources for practitioners. (For details see main bibliography)

Chapter 6

European developments in professional practice with vulnerable children

Walter Lorenz and Silvia Fargion

Summary points

- Professional practice to safeguard children is strongly connected to the diverse family patterns and social policy orientations that characterise European countries today.

- Three main models for helping vulnerable children are apparent in western Europe, with emphases on child protection, paternalistic child welfare and rights. Although the first has been most influential in the UK and Ireland and the other two on the continent, each system experiences tensions between these orientations.

- Under a child protection model, vulnerable children and their families tend to receive specialist attention depending on assessed risk levels and the potential for legal action. Elsewhere, they are more likely to be linked to universal services, while use of residential care is also more common.

- A similar set of practitioners are present in most European countries, but their roles and functions vary greatly, as do the ways they interact with each other.

- The concepts and practices of social pedagogy were developed in central Europe and cannot simply be 'copied', but they offer a comprehensive theoretical analysis as a basis for multi-dimensional intervention.

Introduction

Professional intervention to protect and promote the quality of children's life is widely recognised as among the most multi-faceted and challenging professional tasks. This is directly related to the complexity of the situations in which social and health services are called into action, particularly when dealing with vulnerable and mistreated children. Practitioners have to deal with many different problems simultaneously – low quality of life, poverty, marginalisation, alienation from learning, poor and difficult relationships, perhaps to the point of violence and abuse. This multiplicity of issues explains why a multidisciplinary approach is usually required. In all countries several professional groups are involved, albeit with considerable variations as to the type of practitioners and to the roles they are expected to perform. Hence, this chapter gives an overview of issues that concern practitioners in different professional positions from a western European perspective, with a particular emphasis on services for vulnerable children and their relationships with universal services for all children.

A wider international orientation can help practitioners to distinguish more clearly between factors that are universal and those that are culturally or legally specific. However, comparing the forms of social intervention toward children (and their families) in different countries encounters several obstacles. Many terms used in different languages to describe services can be translated, but often the local nuance is lost, while certain labels have no equivalent (Hearn et al. 2004). Policies and practices stem from national and local heritages and are set against different cultural backgrounds, which ought to be understood from the inside rather than stripped of their context (Seckinger et al. 2004). Further, what happens in practice does not necessarily correspond to official policies. Something that works well in its own context may not be readily transferable. For instance, France has children's judges (*juges des enfants*) whose specialism in children's cases combines investigatory, decision-making and case-review roles that are kept quite distinct in the UK. This reflects the French inquisitorial tradition of justice where the judge seeks the truth, which contrasts with the Anglo-Saxon adversarial model where prosecution and defence seek to convince the judge of what is true.

In most countries of Europe the set of professions involved with vulnerable children tends to be similar and includes medical doctors and health professionals, educators, social workers, psychologists, police officers and care workers. Continental countries also have a traditional role that has not been present in the UK, but is being introduced there on an experimental basis. This is the social pedagogue (and its equivalents with names like *animateur* in France or *animatore* in Italy). Hence, the chapter will also give particular attention to social pedagogy, which is receiving attention as a field of theory and practice experience that could underpin the development of the entire children's care sector. First, we review the shared and varying effects of family change, to which professional practice has to respond. Then, differences in policy traditions that shape service delivery are examined.

Professionals, children and families

We adopt a constructivist approach to the family and to child welfare, which sees the generation of social problems and the nature of helping interventions as intimately linked to each other and to a complex mix of psychological processes, economic and social changes, political orientations and societal values. In all countries, difficulties arise in seeking to gain the trust of families in crisis, but this will play out differently depending on the structures and professional staffing of agencies in touch with families.

Family patterns and child-rearing practices are subjected to broadly similar fluctuations across European countries (see Chapter 15). Common trends include:

- a general decrease in fertility rate;
- the related tendency to have children later in life than in the previous generation;
- the high frequency of two-child families;
- a decline in marriage rates and an increase in divorces, with growing numbers of children born out of wedlock;
- the increasing variety of household forms.

Compared with 50 years ago, nearly all European countries have experienced increased cultural diversity of family practices and more variation in household forms (Sobotka and Toulemon 2008). Thus, there is now more variation within countries, but less between them. Nonetheless, the same phenomenon can sometimes be attributed to different factors in different countries. For instance, the decrease of the fertility rate in western Europe at the beginning of the 1980s has been related to changes connected to economic affluence and associated culture of individualism. In eastern European countries the decline in childbirths occurred later (in the 1990s) and more in response to poverty (Frejka et al. 2008).

Countries have responded in different ways to demographic change. Nordic countries which were the first to show a decrease in fertility rates are now seeking to reverse the trend by means of proactive family-support policies. Together with France these are among the countries where support to families with children is given the greatest priority in terms of financial help, parental leave and care services for small children (Saraceno 2009). By contrast, eastern European and Mediterranean countries tend to regard fertility as a private responsibility. Here financial social investment in children is low, living arrangements create greater familial dependencies and stigma still attaches to having children out of wedlock (Flaquer 2000). Laws and social policies there have been slower to facilitate divorce or recognise same-sex couples.

Against a background of change, a common 'old' issue is poverty, particularly affecting those growing up in lone-parent families. Migration has rendered growing up a complex task for many children, and new forms of migration, such as that of non-accompanied children, require special attention. Child rearing and parenting have become more challenging as a result of the complexities of society, transformations related to electronic communications and 'time poverty'. Responsibility for dealing with these complex issues moves backwards and forwards between the public and the private spheres. The state is by turns accused of not doing enough and of interfering too much in the lives of parents, children and young people.

This difficulty in reaching a consensus on what would be the right amount and appropriate forms of intervention helps explain why child welfare measures emerged relatively late in the development of welfare states compared to measures relating to health, work and old age. A comprehensive rights perspective emerged only with the UN Convention on the Rights of the Child which has been signed by all European countries and for which a monitoring system for implementation is in place. However, its impact on actual practices has been felt more in an increase of protective measures than in general welfare improvements (Nicklett and Perron 2010).

Policy orientations towards children and families

The way different professions are involved in children services, especially those concerned with child protection or safeguarding children, the way they act, their knowledge foundations and their methods, are all strongly influenced by the welfare system and by the policy directions under which they operate.

From our constructivist perspective, both 'childhood' and 'the modern family' are seen as products of complex social, economic and political changes that culminated in the Industrial Revolution and the attempts of modern nation states to concern themselves with social integration. This led to a gradual separation of private and public spheres with, however, very different approaches to that differentiation, and subsequently to the degree to which public social policies defined the confines of social responsibility in both. Several types of approach to the welfare state have been recognised in Europe, for example:

- Nordic – a strong tradition of universal services based on high tax rates.

- Central European – with an emphasis on social solidarity founded on insurance-based entitlements and a big role for voluntary and faith-based organisations.

- UK and Ireland – a more residual role for the state (except in health) and greater exposure to American ideas.

- Mediterranean – reliance on extended family support and limited public services.

- Emergent east European – diverse patterns developing in post-Communist societies.

Within this broader framework, corresponding differences in approach to children's issues are apparent, particularly with regard to services for vulnerable children. These reflect not only differing views about the role of the state, but different versions of 'the child' and 'the family'. A particular contrast in emphasis has been whether public services should be mainly reactive or proactive. The former focus on those in crisis or with particular problems, whereas the latter envisages a broader role to promote the welfare of children at an early stage (Lorenz 1994). The *child protection approach* is centred on targeting vulnerable children in order to safeguard them against harm. It has been strong in the UK, Ireland and North America. Emphasis has been placed on the surveillance role of professionals like social workers and health visitors, and on resort to legal measures. By contrast, the *child welfare approach* to be found in continental western Europe has been concerned with securing the well-being of all children in the expectation that this will reduce risks of harm (Khoo et al. 2002; Brunnberg and Pecnik 2007). This puts more stress on family cooperation – for instance, via open access social services in Sweden or the confidential doctor services in Belgium and the Netherlands. It should be recognised, however, that these represent differences in policy emphases rather than completely opposite policies, since all countries have to balance these two main considerations.

Thus, the refocusing of policy in England and Wales in the 1990s promoted more welfare-oriented practice (Platt 2006), while child abuse scandals in Belgium caused criticisms of the reliance on voluntary measures. Financial crises and the spread in neoliberal ideology has also modified the strong tradition of well-resourced public services in Scandinavia.

The child protection tradition

The child protection perspective originates from a blend of medical and legalistic cultures. It has been defined as an approach which gives primary importance to protecting children against abuse, both in the public domain of work and other dangers of exploitation and, more hesitantly, in the private domain of the family. This political tradition necessitates and emphasises 'objective' sets of criteria and indicators where neglect and abuse occurred or are likely to occur, in order to maintain the principle of minimal interference of the public in the affairs of private individuals. While not being limited to countries with a prevailing political orientation of liberalism, this approach has been often more influential in English-speaking countries such as the UK, Ireland, the United States and Australia (Jack 1997; Healy 2010).

Historically, in the UK specialist private initiatives like the National Society for the Protection and Care of Children (NSPCC) pioneered the protection approach and subsequently lobbied for their rescue work to receive a basis in law. Similarly, the liberal, residual tradition of welfare prevalent in the UK and in the United States provided the context for a strong 'Child Guidance Movement' which emerged in the 1920s. Psychiatric competences were called on to deal more effectively first with problems of youth delinquency and later with more general crisis situations in families or in schools not covered by child protection measures. Highly trained professionals developed their role as experts in childcare who offered direct 'treatment' for problems of parenting and of child 'maladjustment'. Within this tradition the focus of interventions tends to be individually and psychologically oriented. As a civil society movement, this did not generate similar visibility and influence in other European countries. Research has shown that social services in both England and Ireland tend to concentrate on the behaviour of children and to consider the needs and circumstances of the parents as largely secondary, in contrast to a focus on the latter in Finland (Buckley 2000; Hearn et al. 2004).

Since the 1970s a series of child abuse scandals in England has led to a strong judicial emphasis, which has also been influential in other parts of the UK and Ireland. In order to gain access to the private sphere of families and children, which in liberal traditions is highly valued, professionals require clear legal reasons and authority for their intervention, based on assessment and calculation of risks and a focus on the definition of strictly legal reasons for intervention (Hutchison and Charlesworth 2000). Legal sanctions are required to overcome lack of cooperation from parents. The role of social services is defined mainly as consisting of investigations to detect potential harm in family situations. Moreover this implies operating with a 'justified suspicion' concerning a perpetrator of wrongdoing which gives the relationship between child-protection workers and parents an adversarial character, even where supportive measures are simultaneously made available. Within a child-protection orientation, the assessment becomes an inquiry. Social work and medical staff work closely with the police to increase the probability that their actions will be endorsed by the courts. This has inevitably resulted in a reduction in discretion as practice becomes increasingly procedure-driven in order to objectivise the process (Cradock 2004; Littlechild 2008).

The corresponding aim of professional training and development is to foster diagnostic and legal competences. In practice, child abuse and neglect have blurred boundaries and are not always easy to distinguish from less serious sub-optimal care, but the focus on risk assessment and obtaining evidence that will stand up in court means they have to be constructed as clear-cut phenomena that can be identified, predicted and hence prevented (Buckley 2000). Furthermore, when episodes of this kind occur, someone must be blamed and consequently punished (D'Cruz 2004).

Expertise in risk assessment and diagnosis has been developed to a higher level in the UK and Ireland than other European countries. This is undoubtedly valuable and necessary, but problems arise from the context in which such assessments are being made. Under pressure to reduce risks and satisfy public demand to 'rescue' children and punish parents, the procedures are inevitably focused on identifying problems, difficulties and incidents of abuse which can obscure the positive aspects and strengths in the situation (Hutchison and Charlesworth 2000).

Promoting children's welfare

The second tradition identified by comparative studies reveals a broader view of state and public responsibilities towards children in the context of the needs of their carers. Research by Seckinger et al. (2004) compared social workers' interventions in relation to children in seven European countries. This showed that in those countries with a broader child-welfare orientation, the focus was less on investigation of concerns and more on trying to identify and meet the welfare needs of the families more comprehensively. This perspective aims not to separate the need for protection from other needs:

> The root ethos of child welfare can be described as the desire to create those material and social conditions within which all children are given sufficient opportunity to reach their full human potential.
> (Cradock 2004, p. 318)

A child-welfare orientation, therefore, casts the protection of children as one element of a broad spectrum of interventions aimed at promoting the life quality of children and families. Moreover, by contrast with the UK and Ireland, organisationally there are no or few separate agencies and units devoted purely to child protection. The underpinning theories for practice are based on understanding acts or circumstances thought to be harmful to children in the context of psychological or social difficulties experienced by families (Davies et al. 2007). Social service interventions are characterised by rounded assessment rather than legal-actuarial inquiry, with a view to providing services and meeting the needs of families rather than taking legal action (Brunnberg and Pećnik 2007).

Not surprisingly, research on parents who have had dealings with social work applying the child welfare model in relation to concerns about childcare has shown that they regard the support they receive as extremely helpful. Parents do not feel judged and they consider that satisfactory attention is given to their circumstances, needs and other priorities, unlike the suspicion and tension often found with the child-protection approach (Platt 2006; Dumbrill 2006).

Within this framework we can identify a further distinction corresponding to fundamental social-policy orientations. One model, prevalent in central Europe, may be characterised as paternalistic, since it relies largely on expert opinion in determining need. The other, found in Nordic countries, is participative, based on the fundamental rights of children and their families to have their needs recognised.

The paternalistic model

This model operates with a taken-for-granted view of what constitutes a 'good family' as the measure for children's needs. This perception is rooted in regional or national culture (Brunnberg and Pećnik 2007). Interventions tend to be more top-down than in the rights approach. On the other hand, intrusive effects are legitimated by the privileged knowledge of experts about what is right for families and their children, rather than by legal affirmation or sanctions as in the child-protection approach.

Within the paternalistic model it is typically the professionals who, following assessment, determine the needs of children and families and who decide what action to take. Subsequent steps may range from warning and supervision of parental performance to depriving parents of their parental rights. Common measures include 're-educating' the family and the temporary institutionalisation of children (Brunnberg and Pećnik 2007). Qualitative research showed that, compared with their English counterparts, German social workers tended to have higher expectations of the family and its potential to improve if supported (Heatherington 2002). Residential and other forms of alternative care tend to be viewed more favourably than in the UK. For instance, the rate of young people per 10,000 taken into care in Germany has been much higher than in England (Janze 1999). Also, most UK children who live away from their families in public care are fostered, but in Germany and many other parts of Europe residential care is much more extensively used. Residential care institutions are very well organised in Germany with over four-fifths of staff having professional qualifications.

The paternalistic model has many variations, and traces of it can be found in practically all countries. Often, as in Italy, there is a strong orientation towards supporting the family as a whole and keeping children with their natural carers, but this can change abruptly when, as a result of 'moral panic', a narrow view of child protection takes over. In Germany and France families have more rights to refuse or accept the treatment offered than in other countries. In France all decisions regarding families and children have to be taken in the presence of the parents, which gives them considerable power (Seckinger et al. 2004).

Rights-based model

The question of rights both of children and their families is central in Nordic countries, where all interventions have to respect and promote those rights. The basic assumption is that an abusive parent is somebody who needs help and has the right to receive help. Consequently, assessment in the child-welfare approach looks for resources and strengths in families, not just for difficulties and problems as risk-assessment tools often do (Spratt 2003).

While child protection, policies tend to restrict professional discretionary power to specifically defined legal criteria, the child-welfare orientation emphasises professional autonomy, which forms the basis for the personalisation of interventions, with social workers spending much time and energy on clients. Khoo et al. (2002) compared social work interventions with respect to child maltreatment in Sweden and Canada, whose approach is similar to that of the UK and Ireland. The Swedish social workers using a child-welfare model were more likely to undertake early interventions, intervene on the basis of an individualised assessment and consider the child's best interest in broad terms, including the well-being of the family. Interventions were highly flexible and often involved the use of non-statutory resources. It implies

> . . . a greater willingness of the state to intervene in the private realm of the family – providing supporting measures such as adequate housing, decent day care, medical and dental services for children and economically viable parental leave from work.
>
> (Khoo et al. 2002, p. 467)

In Canada the central question for practitioners is 'Do we have a case here?' By contrast, Swedish workers are asked 'Are there unmet needs in this family? Is there a need for help?'

The social pedagogical paradigm

A professional identity with its own skills and training geared to a child-welfare orientation is present in most parts of continental Europe, but until very recently was absent in the UK and English-speaking world. This is the social pedagogue, who operates in a wide range of settings working with children of any age (and also adults). Pedagogues combine education in its widest sense with social care and support roles. It has been suggested that such a professional would be valuable in the UK to provide holistic support to children and families, as well as improve communication between different professionals (Glaister and Glaister 2005; Moss 2006). In the past few years some British local authorities and voluntary agencies have introduced social pedagogues in early childhood services and/or to work with older children in youth work and residential care. Pedagogues from Germany and Denmark have been recruited to work alongside British staff and help create a pedagogic culture.

However, transfer of ideas and models from one country to another may not work well unless care is taken to understand the original fully and to adapt to the new host environment. Writing from the perspectives of the Dutch–Belgian tradition of social pedagogy, Coussee et al. (2010) caution that pedagogy could become applied in the UK in too narrow a fashion. They warn that a focus on individual educational and developmental goals could sideline social development and addressing problems in the social and policy context, which they suggest is crucial to the role in continental Europe. Social pedagogy has traditionally fitted within a child-welfare rather than child-protection policy ethos. Social pedagogues offer a non-stigmatising service to meet the needs of the whole child as part of a balance between family and societal responsibilities for enabling all children to prepare broadly for life. Their role is sometimes depicted as working with the whole person – head, hands and heart, i.e. blending reflection and learning, practical activities and emotional engagement (Petrie et al. 2006). Social pedagogues have a key role in residential childcare, but also operate in a wide variety of community settings, such as after-school projects or leisure activities aimed at greater social integration. They may also assist families within their own homes.

Significantly, the movement of social pedagogy, which is so characteristic of the welfare scenario of Germany, grew as a pivotal part of the corporatist approach to welfare. The aim of German children's legislation has always been to integrate supportive and preventive measures for troublesome or troubled children with universal welfare and indeed recreational services. This was also the central intention of the Children and Young People Act (*Kinder- und Jugendhilfegesetz*) of 1989, which committed all social services working with families and children to adopt a community-oriented perspective (Lorenz 1991). The fundamental basis of social pedagogy, at least in its German version, is that 'education' is an inclusive right aimed at the full participation of children and young people in and contribution to the life of a society. While the state is supposed to create the general conditions that make this possible, it is through the efforts of individuals and associations of civil society that these goals are being reached. Moreover, socialisation of children and the general 'civilising' task of culture is regarded not as a largely private matter, but also as a public concern and as an element of care for the general welfare of the whole of society (Lorenz 2008). Similarly, social pedagogues in Denmark and other Nordic countries work closely with specialised child-welfare and protection services to ensure that any targeted actions are closely linked with the general public state system of social services.

While the 'education' element underpins direct work with an individual child, the 'social' aspect refers to a community dimension to be considered in all interventions and highlights the need to maintain or re-establish the links of all children with their social environment. When a situation arises of risk and danger for a child, remedial or compensatory measures are put into effect, which are not targeted on the child or the family alone but equally on community resources that require further development so that they can have a preventive effect. Such programmes typically involve not just social service personnel but youth workers, educators and animateurs.

This is not to say that a social pedagogy approach *per se* can tilt the balance from child protection to family welfare. Quite often social pedagogy has been practised in a restrictive and even punitive way. Therefore, the exact aims of the 'educational' orientation have to be a matter of a wider policy debate. We now turn to illustrate the connection between the policies and practices that we have discussed above through an example illustrating its complexity.

Example 6.1 Different policy frameworks, different approaches

Ms. Ramirez has three children, the youngest being a toddler, which prevents her from seeking more than casual work. Her husband abandoned her and a new partner died a year ago in a car accident. The schoolteachers refer Mrs Ramirez to social services for support during summer holidays for her two elder children. During an interview with a social worker she starts crying persistently, says that she cannot manage her life any more and expresses suicidal thoughts. From hints in the conversation, the social worker gathers that, when Mrs Ramirez loses her temper, she beats the children.

Within a child-protection framework, social workers dealing with this situation would find themselves under conflicting demands: to detect and measure possible risks of harm for the children, to avoid intruding in family life and yet encourage the mother to find a solution herself in financial and social terms. The police and doctors would probably be approached in relation to concern about harm to the children and specialist help might be sought for the mother's mental health problems.

Professionals operating within a paternalistic frame would be expected to decide what the family needed and to intervene accordingly, whether or not there was a legal basis surrounding care of the children. Social workers would seek to link the children up to an array of youth services that offer leisure and holiday activities. Often other professionals would be involved, such as clinical psychologists, to carry out a comprehensive assessment of the mother's needs and capabilities and organise a plan for meeting the family needs. In some countries such as Italy, from the beginning social pedagogues offer assessment, help and control within the household. A short-term residential placement might be arranged.

In a framework of child welfare with a focus on the rights of children and their families, Ms Ramirez would be seen as a single mother who through her unfortunate life circumstances has been prevented from giving her children the opportunities and support that children can normally expect to receive. Risk would be interpreted as connected to unmet needs and lack of opportunities. Social workers would be the lead professionals in these circumstances and are generally resourced so they can spend time to engage with the family and then work intensively with them.

Conclusions and implications

One of the impacts of globalisation on welfare states and children's services is that the tensions between protection and welfare have become sharper in most western countries. On one hand, demands increase for more preventive approaches to child welfare. This stems partly from glaring failures to reduce child poverty which remains persistently high, partly from the exposure of severe cases of child abuse that demonstrate failings in child protection measures. On the other hand, fiscal measures seek to reduce welfare support generally, to make conditions for obtaining social security more restrictive and compel social service personnel to resort more to control measures. While the child welfare approach is being advocated by experts, by welfare lobby groups and by politicians when responding to such demands and when taking a 'theoretical' position, trends in economic and social policy militate against the realisation of such measures and produce instead the effects of a residual welfare regime. This leads to a concentration on narrowly defined 'risk groups' with the effect of rendering those interventions, often against their design intentions, punitive and discriminatory. This explains the frequently contradictory tendencies in legislation and in the organisation of social services (Munro and Calder 2005). For instance, Spratt (2001) points out how in the UK the law has set principles and goals which espouse a child welfare perspective, but at the same time children's services are often under crossfire for not having detected dangers to children in time or for invading the private sphere of families. This pushes agencies and practitioners towards putting all their energies in a narrow child protection perspective. Another example of contradictory tendencies can be found in Italy, where the law and the rhetoric are all in line with child welfare social policy. Yet the scarce resources and understaffed social services force social workers to deal mostly with emergencies and with risk assessment in a manner more consistent with a child protection policy approach.

These observations imply that the development of appropriate methods and approaches to children and families needs to take cognisance of broader policy developments and indeed seek to engage with them directly. International comparisons and contacts can be a valuable source of inspiration and encouragement for all professionals, even though the direct transfer of methods is not advisable. Ultimately child and family care in all fields is very closely related to issues of cultural and ethnic identity and – with all due respect to psychological constants and universal human rights – can never be separated from the concrete historical and political context in which it is being practised.

Exercise

Consider the ways in which the activities of social pedagogues can be seen as enhancing or duplicating what other professionals aim to do in their work with children.

Recommended reading

Cameron, G. and Freymond, N. (2005) *Towards Positive Systems of Child and Family Welfare: International Comparisons of Child Protection*, Family Service, and Community Caring Systems, University of Toronto Press, Toronto.

Hearn, J., Pöso, T., Smith, C., White, S., Korpinen, J. (2004) (for full details – see bibliography).

Katz, I. and Hetherington, R. (2006) 'Co-operating and communicating: a European perspective on integrating services for children', *Child Abuse Review*, 15(6) pp. 429–439.

Lorenz, W. (2008) (for full details – see bibliography).

The website for SocialPedagogyUK.com provides up-to-date details of practice developments, research and training on social pedagogy.

Chapter 7

Youth justice, policy and practice

Bill Whyte

Summary points

- UK jurisdictions vary a great deal in the way they respond to young people involved in crime.

- After a decade of greater convergence through increased criminalisation, the *United Nations Convention on the Rights of the Child* (UNCRC 1989) and its associated guidance is beginning to impact on the changing face of youth justice practice with its emphasis on child-centred youth justice as an integral part of children services provision.

- European practice standards in the form of Council of Europe (CoE) rules should set the future framework for youth justice practice in the UK aimed at decriminalising young people, diverting them from formal processes and dealing with them separately from adult systems.

- Youth justice policies are expected to be harmonised within the expectations of childcare frameworks focusing on prevention, early and effective intervention, working with families and social networks, managing high risk, victims and community confidence.

- Practitioners require specialist skills and knowledge to address the complex needs of children and young people who display offending behaviour and to work with their families and social networks.

Introduction

Approaches to dealing with children and young people who break the law vary much more widely in the UK than the equivalent justice systems for adults. In addition to cultural and institutional differences, systems vary in their structures and age jurisdiction as well as in the underlying normative and value assumptions underpinning policy and practice. Each jurisdiction shares a commitment to prevention, early intervention and better integrated and coordinated provision for young people involved in crime. All promote multidisciplinary responses, although approaches vary greatly in practice from area to area. The same emphasis is apparent on effectiveness in reducing reoffending, in the use of standardised need–risk assessment alongside a growing emphasis on families, victims and the harm caused by criminal behaviour, but these are pursued in contrasting ways.

One accompaniment of political devolution has been an increased politicisation of youth justice in the last decade. The emphasis on individual responsibility and accountability, due process and just deserts often associated with a retreat from welfare sits in tension alongside principles of best interest, shared responsibility and the use of non-criminal and extra-judicial processes recommended by the UNCRC and its associated guidance.

Even so, practice has to be grounded in a comprehensive theoretical and evaluative framework irrespective of political preferences. Currently, the concepts of inter-disciplinary and multidisciplinary practice are promoted by all UK systems as providing future directions (Whyte 2008). While these concepts provide some consistency to the direction of travel at a policy level, the orientation of practice to a consistent, unified or even identifiable child-centred practice paradigm has proved elusive within the political climate that has dominated UK policy.

These variations in UK systems of youth justice raise many ethical challenges for practitioners. This chapter will identify the policy context and international principles, values, theories and practices which should direct intervention in the twenty-first century.

Policy and practice in UK jurisdictions

The manner in which each country has responded to young people's offending cannot be understood in isolation from that country's historical development, which makes comparative analysis complex, if not problematic. Youth justice systems have tended to be evaluated against the two dominant paradigms: *welfare* (special responses to children and young people) or *justice* (equal rights under the law). These generate tensions in how best to reconcile community well-being and punishment with the need to consider the best interests and the rights of the child or young person. As with all ideal types, models are seldom found in a pure form, and most jurisdictions combine elements of both approaches.

The 'welfare model' is often associated with child development and change through socio-educational intervention rather than prosecution and punishment. In contrast, the 'justice model' assumes that children and young people (above a certain age which varies between jurisdictions) should be held solely accountable before the law for their criminal actions. In the justice model the degree of culpability should be assessed and any punishment made proportional to the seriousness of the behaviour. Between the two models the contrast is strongest where there is a separation between practice systems dealing with the care and protection of children and young people (*child welfare*) and responses to offending by children and young people (*youth justice*). Questionable assumptions about maturity and capacity of criminal intent are factored into systems' responses.

The systems in England, Wales, and Northern Ireland tend to be more 'justice' oriented. They have the age of criminal responsibility set at 10 (12 in Northern

Ireland), but deploy systems of diversion from prosecution and restorative approaches for young people up to age 17. Nonetheless, all children and young people, aged 10–17 years, when dealt with formally or compulsorily for offending, are likely to be dealt with in criminal youth courts. Commentators suggest that, despite an emphasis on welfare within justice in England and Wales in the 1960s and 1970s, current policy and practice reflects a 'new youth justice' philosophy stressing individual criminal responsibility which struggles to secure a 'best interests' approach required by children's legislation and the UNCRC. The separation of family courts dealing with care and protection from youth courts could be argued to have reinforced criminalising principles because of the strong emphasis on individual responsibility of offenders, parental irresponsibility, victim reparation and punishment:

> . . . in England, for children and young persons coming before the courts, there is now a deliberate institutional separation between the 'care jurisdiction' (dealt with by the family proceedings courts) and the 'criminal jurisdictions' (dealt with by . . . the Youth Court.
>
> (Bottoms and Dignan 2004: 25)

In Scotland the age of criminal responsibility is lower at eight, but few young people under 16 will appear in a criminal court, youth or adult. Instead, most are dealt with in Scotland's integrated, welfare-based Children's Hearings system, which also deals with care and protection cases. This integrated approach claims to view young people who offend not as criminals, but as young people whose upbringing has been unsatisfactory and where responsibility for their offending behaviour should be a shared one between the young person, the family, the community and the state. Where possible, resolutions, even formal ones, are sought without recourse to criminal proceedings.

Scottish youth-justice services are delivered by Local Authority Social Work Services, where specialist youth justice social workers are generally located within either children and families or criminal-justice social work teams. The comparable service system in England and Wales was established by the *Crime and Disorder Act* 1998. It places duties on local authorities to provide youth justice services and establish multidisciplinary youth offending teams (YOTs) with an emphasis on prevention and diversion from prosecution. YOTs are made up of representatives from the police, probation, social services, health, education, drugs and alcohol misuse and housing officers, and a YOT manager is responsible for coordinating the work of youth justice services. This multidisciplinary approach is intended to respond holistically to the needs of young people who offend. YOTs work with a range of services, the voluntary and commercial sector and child-protection agencies. The multidisciplinary approach is intended to support shared knowledge and skills, to overcome cultural interagency tensions, to avoid duplication and to improve consistency in provision.

The legislative framework for youth justice in Wales is the same as in England. However, since the establishment of the Welsh Assembly, its policy development has created a distinctive framework for youth justice services that is notably different from England. Local, multidisciplinary YOTS operate but the funding arrangements are different, as is the configuration of community-based services vital to the prevention of youth offending.

The Youth Justice Board (YJB) was originally established by the 1998 Act to oversee local YOTs in England and Wales. However, in 2000 the commissioning of custodial provision for children and young people was transferred to the YJB from the Home Office. It has been argued that this centralist approach undermined local initiative, resulting in a tendency to 'spread the net', i.e. place more young people in custody (Burnett 2005). Currently around two-thirds of the YJB's budget goes on the cost of custody for young people. Despite a recent reversal of this trend, proposals to disband the YJB could kick-start reform to ensure fewer young people end up in institutions and may see a move towards practice better directed by UNCRC principles.

While youth-justice provision in Northern Ireland has been greatly influenced by developments in England and Wales, it has its own distinctive characteristics. Following a recommendation of the Criminal Justice Review 2000, the Youth-Justice Agency (YJA) was launched on 1 April 2003 as an Executive Agency, with the principal aim of reducing youth crime and building confidence in the youth-justice system. YJA works with children aged 10–17 years who have offended or are at serious risk of offending and delivers a range of services, including diversionary interventions through a network of 17 community-based offices and multi-disciplinary teams. Youth courts deal with young people who are prosecuted for criminal behaviour. The most distinctive feature of practice is the Youth Conference Service. Principles of restorative justice (discussed later in the chapter) have been placed at the heart of the system and involve the use of 'youth conferences' at which the young person, victim (or victim representative), professionals and others are brought together to discuss the offence and its repercussions, and to agree on an action plan. Youth conferences are fully integrated within the formal criminal justice process pre-conviction (a diversionary youth conference) and post-conviction (a court-ordered conference). Conferences usually adhere to designated timescales (within 30 days for diversionary conferences and four weeks for court-ordered conferences) and normally result in an agreed conference plan. Most plans, in turn, are endorsed by the Public Prosecution Service or courts and thereafter completed by the young person (Chapman and O'Mahony 2007).

Children or offenders first?

In all UK jurisdictions, children's legislation reaches to the age of 18, yet many, if not most, young people involved in crime are 'criminalised' in some way long before that age, despite research evidence suggesting that early criminalisation is one of the best predictors of sustained criminality. These circumstances present day-to-day challenges for practitioners concerned with effectiveness, with values and with ethical practice. They must contend with variable definitions and statutes on what constitutes 'a child' and 'a youth'. These vary across the UK, as do demarcations between those who are and are not deemed 'fully criminally responsible', or between those considered best dealt with in criminal proceedings and those not.

In a criminal justice paradigm, no one else need accept any share of responsibility for a young person's action despite the intentions of children's legislation and

UNCRC principles. Indeed criminalisation can be seen to absolve adults and service providers from accountability for 'failure'.

Example 7.1

Ally is 12 years old. He has been caught stealing CDs and video games from a local store along with two friends on a Tuesday afternoon. This is the first time he has come to the attention of the authorities. In what ways, if any, would a child-centred welfare or a justice approach to practice differ in response to this behaviour?

International standards

All UK jurisdictions stand accused by the UN Committee on the Rights of the Child (UNCRC) for over 20 years of poor child-centred approaches to youth crime, of high levels of criminalisation and detention of young people many with public-care backgrounds. The near-universal ratification of the UNCRC has placed importance on 'a level playing field' for all children through progressive universal provision and early social intervention measures. Benchmarks for practice have been set by international agreements and regulations. Article 3 of UNCRC requires that:

> in all actions concerning children, whether undertaken by public or private social welfare institutions, courts of law, administrative authorities or legislative bodies, the best interests of the child shall be a primary consideration.

The qualification of 'a' primary rather than 'the' primary consideration can find expression in quite different practices which invoke the public interest as overriding the interests of the child when it comes to criminal matters for relatively minor, even if persistent, offending. The preamble to the UNCRC makes reference to the importance of additional international instruments, such as the Beijing Rules 1985 and Vienna Guidelines 1997, which provide directing principles for youth welfare and justice practice. It stresses the dynamic nature of the framework and that it expects it to be continually fleshed out and developed on the basis of research and practice-related evidence. The international practice model recommended is one of diversion as far as possible from criminal proceedings up to the age of 18, stressing the value of early preventive intervention.

The UNCRC is not incorporated into law in UK jurisdictions. Nonetheless, international law requires that the UK should adhere to the spirit and principles of the Convention. It should represent the standard for measuring any appropriate system of youth justice, particularly as the European Convention of Human Rights (ECHR), which *is* incorporated in UK law, does not comment on whether there are, or should be, positive obligations on states to safeguard or promote the welfare of children and young persons (Jackson 2004). Despite this, it is difficult to argue from evidence on the levels of criminalisation and detention of young people under the age of 18 in UK jurisdictions that the obligations implied by the UNCRC have featured greatly as a childcare or criminal-justice practice priority.

The UN Committee on the Rights of the Child monitors application of the treaty. Representatives of the UK government first met with the Committee in 1995. It published a list of concerns and criticisms regarding the UK's performance, along with a comprehensive set of recommendations on how better to meet practice obligations and protect children's rights. In revisiting these concerns in 2002, the Committee remained highly critical of UK practices and expressed disappointment that the majority of the recommendations from 1995 had not been acted on (Harvey 2002). The third UK report (2008) continued to point out perceived short-comings and is essential reading for practitioners.

One criticism has been of the age of criminal responsibility, which is unusually low in all UK jurisdictions compared with most European countries. In response, the UK delegation has argued that the low threshold allows for early intervention while recognising children's responsibility for their crime. The UK government also defended its treatment of young people in detention by arguing that children's legislation, although providing protection and guarantees of services for children up to the age of 18, did not apply to those detained in custody. However, signal judgements of the High Court in England, following judicial reviews instigated by the Howard League, have confirmed that English, and by extension UK, jurisdictions cannot designate young people under 18 as 'ex children' simply by their entrance to the criminal justice system. On 29 November 2002 the High Court held that the Children Act 1989 did apply to children held in custody. In July 2007 a further Court of Appeal decision in the case of J, who was 15 when she committed the offence leading to detention, confirmed that the local authority should provide her with the care due under Section 20 of the Children Act 1989. This meant in effect that local authorities have the same duties to children who leave custody as to 'children in need'. This judgement highlighted that 'local authorities across the country are failing to provide proper assessments and care plans for vulnerable children' entering and leaving detention, particularly 'where children are in danger of returning to precisely the same situations that led to their crimes and imprisonment in the first place' (Howard League Press release, 26 July 2007).

These decisions confirm that young people involved even in serious crime do fall within the children services policy framework and are entitled to after-care support to ensure their personal and social integration and long-term desistance from crime. However, giving practice expression to these duties is a difficult matter without multi-disciplinary protocols and shared resources between criminal justice/probation, youth justice, children's services, housing, education and employment, leisure and health-related provision. Nonetheless, this is an area that practitioners can influence by ensuring young people involved in serious offending are provided with appropriate assistance.

European standards

If UK politics have ensured that practice standards have remained ambivalent towards UNCRC benchmarks, it could be argued that this should be less so in the context of the ECHR, which has been incorporated into all UK domestic legislation. Nevertheless, the Commission of Human Rights (CoE 2005) noted that the UK tended to consider human rights as excessively restricting the effective administration of justice and public protection. The Commission stated that it was difficult to avoid the impression that

> juvenile trouble-makers are too rapidly drawn into the criminal justice system and . . . too readily placed in detention, when greater attention to alternative forms of supervision and targeted early intervention would be more effective.   (CoE 2005, para. 81)

It commented that extensive programme development appeared to have made little impact on the numbers detained, noting that the UK had among the highest rates of juvenile detention in western Europe, high rates of reconviction following release, a shortage of appropriate psychological care and inadequate educational assistance for young people. It suggested 'young adults should leave prison with something other than advanced degrees in criminality', and drew the conclusion that preventive intervention was '*minimal*' (para. 94).

Council of Europe Guidelines and Rules further strengthen the position of young people involved in offending (see Recommended reading). In particular, they stress the importance of children not being subject to adult criminal proceedings, irrespective of the gravity of their crime, because 'child-friendly' approaches promote social integration and desistance from criminality. These European policies also stipulate that, with some exceptions for serious crimes, records should not be disclosed on reaching the age of majority.

Approaches to effective practice

Good practice needs to be based on evidence about effectiveness as well as UK and international policies. Following extensive reviews of existing research, Andrews et al. (1990) found that the most effective forms of intervention aimed specifically at offending behaviour are likely to conform to a series of broad principles directing practice. These can reasonably be applied to youth justice practice alongside child-development principles, and provide evidence-based yardsticks in designing 'customised' supervision programmes.

Efforts should be made to match the level of service to the assessed level of need and risk (*risk principle*), a principle consistent with the ethics of children's legislation (*no order/minimal intervention principle*). Programmes that provide intensive services for individuals at low risk of future reoffending are likely to use scarce resources unnecessarily and may draw them into formal systems to their detriment (*net widening*).

A priority for intervention should be to alleviate those factors that are judged to sustain and support criminality (*criminogenic-need principle*). There is now little disagreement in the criminological literature about factors affecting the extent and nature of offending, such as age, gender, criminal history, early family factors, schooling and criminal associates. However, there has been much debate about which factors are more readily open to change (dynamic), and when changed in a positive direction are likely to be associated with a reduction in reoffending. While these factors will vary between young people, the most promising changeable targets identified in research include antisocial attitudes, habitual criminal patterns of thoughts and feelings, personal control issues, criminal peer associations, criminality in the family, problematic parental style and familial affection, schooling and leisure activities. These require interventions and opportunities to be provided by a wide range of agencies.

People change and learn in different ways and, not surprisingly, evidence points to the importance of matching programme delivery and practitioner skills to the characteristics of young people and their needs (*responsivity principle*). A crucial element in responsivity is the nature of their working relationship with practitioners and how it is utilised to model authority, positive social relations and to support motivation, participation and cooperation. The most successful structured programmes are, generally but not exclusively, directed by behavioural or social-learning principles. They include a cognitive component focused on challenging attitudes, values and beliefs that support antisocial behaviour, provide pro-social modelling, rehearsal, role playing, resources and detailed guidance and explanation. Theories of change suggest that 'ultimately effectiveness depends on the individual's active participation in the process of change' (Chapman and Hough 1998, para. 4.15).

These three core principles have become known as the RNR (Risk-Need-Responsivity) approach and became the centrepiece of the risk-assessment and risk-management paradigm which dominated thinking in the 1990s and into the 2000s.

This approach reflects evidence which suggests that effectiveness is likely to be greatest where there is:

- a focus on the nature and consequences of the offending behaviour;
- an emphasis on problem solving and behaviour change, cognitive development, personal and social skills;
- a diversity of methods of intervention;
- use of positive authority;
- an emphasis on community integration.

Additional principles distilled from research highlight that programmes in the community seem to fare better than those in institutions (*community-based principle*); that effective interventions tend to be those that employ a skills-oriented approach, using a range of (multi-modal) methods drawing from behavioural, cognitive or cognitive behavioural sources (*modality principle*); that effective interventions are strongly influenced by effective workers, who are warm, optimistic and enthusiastic, creative and imaginative and who use their personal influence through quality interaction with young people (*relational principle*); that there is a strong relationship between clarity of objectives, theoretical base and methods employed within planned supervision and its overall effects (*programme integrity principle*).

Empirical evidence supports inter-disciplinary practice which attempts to incorporate social, educational, health and behavioural sciences and skills into provision, but it has not readily highlighted the operation of innovative multidisciplinary practice solutions. This is likely to require practice which incorporates shared values and perspectives and which links practitioners from different disciplines and clients to meaningful planned activities ('joined-up' approaches'). Often studies highlight different professionals exploring the same issues, largely unaware of practice experience or research generated by other disciplines – 'each doing their own thing' – with client–professional relationships and interdisciplinary approaches retaining their discipline-based ('turf') affiliations.

Evidence suggests that the RNR principles can or will only make an important contribution if they are set within a framework of values that recognises the importance of social and cultural contexts in providing social education and developmental opportunities for young people. In other words, directing practice by RNR principles is likely to be a **necessary** but not a **sufficient** requirement for practice aimed at reducing reoffending.

In reality, most young people involved in offending have a mixture of strengths and weaknesses and a variety of resilient qualities; many are survivors in many senses of the term. It is important that interventions operate in ways that help young people maximise their personal strengths and social resources, where they exist, as well as helping them acquire and/or utilise their cognitive capacities – their ability to connect their thinking, feeling and behaviour. Critiques of RNR are emerging (Ward and Maruna 2007) which stress that too narrow a focus on risk and criminogenic need decontextualises offending and is likely to underplay the young person's developmental needs and neglect them as a whole.

Desistance and social integration

If ending offending or desistance is the intended outcome of intervention, approaches need to be embedded in empirical understanding of how young people desist. For instance, many adolescents engage in crime and other forms of rule-testing, and most 'grow out' of such behaviours. Abnormalising them is not helpful. Asking why young people stop offending, rather than asking why they start in the first place, may assist a positive and strengths-based approach to assessment and intervention (see Chapter 19).

What emerges clearly from desistance research is the importance of being able to shed the self-image of 'offender' and assume the identity of a pro-social citizen. The process of positive identity reinforcement afforded by the establishment of a positive set of social bonds appears to be a crucial element in the desistance process. Policy in all UK jurisdictions recognises the need for integrated child/family/youth provision to ensure that all young people, irrespective of social background or personal circumstances, have access to services that will enable them to realise their potential and achieve a successful transition to independent adult status.

The language of risk factors (Farrington 2007) is now widely used in practice, but the notion of risk(y) processes is underemphasised. Practitioners need to exercise caution as the risk-factor-prevention paradigm individualises offending, suggesting that risk factors are 'modifiable' by the individual alone rather than by society. In reality, the vast majority of risk factors appear to be beyond a young person's control. While practice aimed at prevention and desistance will require changes within individuals, effective practice should incorporate the connections between social structure, personal agency and identity, and aim to meet needs, reduce risks and (especially) develop and exploit strengths and build resilience in the context of family and community. It is important for practitioners to identify potential points of risk where young people may become detached from meaningful provision essential to build their personal and educational resources (human capital) or support resources (social capital). This highlights the importance of access to educational, social and recreational services, in addition to more specialist youth-justice services.

Restorative practice

Many of the aspirations of restorative practice articulate well with the requirements for desistance and better personal and social integration of young people involved in offending. There is no universally accepted or concise definition of restorative practices in justice, and they vary greatly in their apparent intention, Marshall's definition appears to encompass the generally accepted principles:

> a process whereby all the parties with a stake in a particular offence come together to resolve collectively how to deal with the aftermath of the offence and its implications for the future.   (cited in Braithwaite 1999, p. 5)

The emphasis on involving those most affected by crime has resulted in an increased use of restorative practices across UK jurisdictions. Restorative practices operate on the premise that crime and conflict create harm for individuals and communities, and that a restorative approach can heal fractured social relationships and help strengthen social bonds. If conflict is viewed as an opportunity for individuals and communities to take shared responsibility for harm done, it can be argued that it is in the best interests of young people to understand the harm and its consequences on themselves and others as an important element in their social and moral development. It is equally valuable to have a positive opportunity to share in the resolution of harm with the support of family or significant others as a way of promoting their sense of personal control and self-efficacy, at the same time as strengthening the positive aspects of their social support networks. In this sense restorative practices can be holistic and integrative.

The term 'restorative' is used for a plethora of activities within adult and youth justice including mediation and reparation, family group conferencing, restorative and community conferencing, restorative cautions, sentencing and healing circles, community panels and other communitarian associations (Braithwaite 1999). Some people regard developments in restorative practices as a new paradigm, whereas others see them as ways to salvage the existing criminal justice paradigm by providing more meaningful and 'humane' practices alongside punishment and retribution (Daly 2003).

A frequently asked question is do restorative practices work and do they help stop reoffending? Many studies indicate, with varying degrees of caution, that diversion to restorative practices in justice can reduce reoffending, and that all involved in the process generally feel more satisfaction when compared to traditional methods. However, the evidence in regard to young people who offend is equivocal (Sherman and Strang 2007, p. 70). Nonetheless, studies produce consistently promising results as regards victim satisfaction, offender satisfaction, restitution compliance and reoffending.

A recent update of a meta-analytic review (Strang et al. 2010) shows no reduction in the number of people committing offences (prevalence), but an overall reduction of offending of 27 per cent of crimes in the community (frequency). In other words, restorative practices seem to reduce the extent of reoffending, but in themselves are unlikely to lead to desistance. The findings suggest that restorative practices work best for most frequent offenders, better for violence than property offences and better for adults than for youths. The implication is that such practices are wasted on minor offences.

Conclusions and implications

The importance of multidisciplinary and whole-agency responsibility is emphasised by policy (see *Every Child Matters* (2003) and *Getting it Right for Every Child* (2005a)) and is a further step towards practice directed by the UNCRC and research-based effectiveness principles. Effective change management requires good strategic planning, which is not possible without an accountability framework built into action planning through regular and structured reviews. These should 'harvest' evidence of progress, hold providers to account for delivery and be able to blow the whistle on service failure, unmet needs and shortfall as well as holding young people and families accountable.

It is clear that UNCRC principles and practice should apply to young people involved in offending up to age 18, and international requirements raise three important issues for practitioners. The first relates to the transitional nature of childhood and youth. Children and young people are still maturing, not only in biological terms, but also in respect to their intellectual, social, emotional and moral development. No matter the seriousness of their misbehaviour, they do not have the capacity to make fully informed moral judgements in the same way as adults. While not without moral awareness or responsibility, they may not always fully understand the wider practical and ethical implications of their behaviour.

Similarly, young people are less able to implement personal decisions, because they lack personal agency and material resources, and often have very little influence over the identity of those adults who are responsible for supporting them (parents, caregivers, teachers and social workers). Because of this, it is important that practitioners strike the right balance between respecting young people's capacity for personal agency and their ability to resolve their difficulties, while at the same time recognising the harm they may cause themselves and others. The status transition from dependent childhood to independent adulthood is becoming more extended, complex and risk-filled. Despite the diversity of structures, families have a crucial role to play in supporting young people's positive transition, and practitioners, as representatives of the interests of the wider community, have responsibility to provide appropriate support and help.

Second, international committees suggest that human rights issues do not feature strongly in UK youth-justice practice. Criminalisation, levels of secure accommodation and custody, and the lack of models of effective through- and after-care, challenge practitioners about the ethics as well as the relevance of practice. Finally, and directly related to the first two, the challenges of addressing young people's problematic behaviour effectively require greater focus on diverting young people up to the age of 18 from criminal justice systems and providing effective child-centred approaches to those young people who find themselves dealt with by criminal justice.

Desistance literature stresses that multidimensional and multidisciplinary service input is required to support individual, structural and integrative change. A range of agencies can contribute to helping difficult young people not only access material opportunities such as continuing education, employment and constructive leisure, but also the corresponding social bonds of stable family life, pro-social friendship networks and fulfilling personal relationships. Such approaches are crucial if young people are to shed their 'offender' identity, which tends to be reinforced by criminalisation (McAra and McVie 2010). While a risk-factor-prevention paradigm (Farrington 2007) has a contribution to make, the evidence increasingly points to the importance of an integrated or social educational practice paradigm directing the use of core practice skills to engage young people, their family and social networks to access services that will give them a chance to desist from offending, realise their potential and achieve a successful transition to adulthood. This is in the best interest of the young people and in the best interests of the community and their victims.

Exercise

With colleagues or fellow students, consider what adjustments need to be made by a young person aged 15 with a history of offending, who is returning to the community from custody or a residential placement. What resources are likely to be in the young person's social network and home community that might be used to support and maintain positive change? Which tasks and roles might usefully be undertaken by social workers, police, teachers, housing professionals and others, separately or together? How should their work be guided by principles derived from international standards and research?

Recommended reading

Practitioners should be familiar with international guidance.

UNCRC

http://www2.ohchr.org/english/law/crc.htm

Council of Europe Rules on Juveniles subject to Sanctions and Measures (CM/Rec 2008 11E)

https://wcd.coe.int/ViewDoc.jsp?id=1367113&Site=CM&BackColorInternet=9999CC&BackColorIntranet=FFBB55&BackColorLogged=FFAC75

Council of Europe Guidelines on Child Friendly Justice Strasbourg [CJ-S-CH (2010) 3 E]
http://www.coe.int/t/dghl/standardsetting/childjustice/default_en.asp

http://www.coe.int/t/dghl/standardsetting/childjustice/CJ-S-CH%20_2010_%209%20E%20-%205TH%20DRAFT%20COE%20GUIDELINES%20ON%20CHILD-FRIENDLY%20JUSTICE.pdf

Part II

COMMUNITY AND PARTICIPATION

The chapters in this part provide some of the theoretical and practical context in which collaboration among professionals in engaging with children and young people takes place. Children cannot be successfully or fairly treated without due regard to their objective circumstances and subjective understandings and these are crucially connected to networks of relationships – their loyalties, affiliations, self-perceptions and identities – which constitute their 'social being'. It is the fact that children are influenced by and participate in diverse and complex communities, that often requires a multi-faceted and collaborative response. It does so especially where more than immediately presenting problems are to be tackled, and when the young person's capacity for active citizenship is an objective to be pursued.

There is an extensive academic literature on what is meant by 'community'. Plant (1974 quoted in Little 2002) warned that the term 'is so much a part of the stock in trade of social and political argument that it is unlikely that some non-ambiguous and non-contested definition of the notion can be given.' Nonetheless, the ambiguity does not prevent the term from being frequently linked with services to be delivered 'in the community' (we have community medicine, – policing, – education, – social work, – schools, – law-centres) and there is now a UK Department for Communities and Local Government. This suggests we should be careful to determine what sense of community is being taken for granted.

The phrases 'in the community' or 'community-based' tend to denote that a service is located in an ordinary setting outside a large institution such as a hospital. Community-based professionals may still work predominantly with individual self-referred members of the community, but others adopt a broader approach seeking to work 'with the community'. In this wider sense, there are three principle meanings of community distinguished in the social policy literature:

- the (local) neighbourhood;
- an interest association;
- civil society at large.

We should notice that 'the community' is usually held to be distinct from the immediate family or household, even though these are the people with whom children commune most intimately. There is a case for regarding the family or household as the most fundamental form of community, when it comes to engaging with children in their 'communities'. Aristotle taught us to regard the household as the fundamental unit of community (*koinonia*) of 'economics' for meeting the purposes of life – breeding, nurturing, sustaining and educating (Brendan Nagle 2006). Other theorists have insisted that the kinship association beyond the immediate family – clan, tribe, nation – are the most important community of cultural inheritance and identity that state actors should acknowledge and respect. What weight ought to be given to biological or cultural inheritance (and whether they are connected) is a subject wider than we cover, but we should acknowledge in passing that biological inheritance is of some relevance to health, and public policy often expects to take account of cultural inheritance and ethnicity (in adoption placement policy, for example).

Chapter 8 explains that support for families is at the centre of the partnership of professional collaboration focusing on children's early years. The Sure Start programme provides a model of inter-agency collaboration which includes partnerships with the voluntary sector. The assessment of different levels of need and the location of services in Neighbourhood Centres recognises that, although services are 'client focused', some neighbourhoods are better able to call on informal local supports than others. We learn that the 'community development model' requiring centres to 'respond flexibly to locally expressed need' did not survive national evaluation, and the demand of cost-effective, evidence-based working. This illustrates a commonly encountered tension between the requirement for efficiency of universal services and the hard-to-measure demands that arise from the different capacity of neighbourhoods to provide informal support.

All services are territorially organised, but even those with a coverage or catchment area small enough to correspond with a neighbourhood-based community may not fit well with locally perceived neighbourhoods. Similarly, the various understandings of professionals about the community or communities they serve may differ in size, scope and boundaries from those experienced by children or parents. The relevant neighbourhood for young persons will be subjectively delineated according to the places they conduct their lives, which may be the street, tower block, playing fields and local shops. What counts as 'local' depends not just on distance from home, but to a large extent where people feel safe to go.

Chapter 9 analyses the concept of community from the lens of significant relationships and social networks rather than territory. The message for professionals working with children is to view their network of relations as potential resources of support to be tapped into. Research shows that grandparents often play a key role in providing stability. Local neighbourhoods provide promising sites for developing supporting relationships, including schools, leisure centres, childcare facilities, and places of worship. Shared activities produce communities of interest that provide the basis for building positive connections.

Gilligan reminds us that adults do not have a full sight of what is happening in a child's world; peers may know more than parents. Mobile phones and the internet are increasingly important means of communication in young people's social networking, alongside face-to-face relationships. Virtual communities can contribute both to child safety and increasing risk (Wolak et al. 2003).

The police service above all recognises the importance of knowing where distinctive neighbourhood divisions lie, and community policing consists in working with both the public and other agencies to identify threats and to develop strategies for prevention. Chapter 10 points to some of the dilemmas of community policing where a balance has to be struck between investigating crime and bringing individuals to justice and gaining the confidence and cooperation of communities. This is especially sensitive in neighbourhoods and among groups where trust in the police is lacking. Following the findings of the Lawrence Inquiry about 'institutional racism', it is important that the police are perceived to be even-handed in their treatment of minority ethnic and religious communities (Foster et al. 2005).

The need for the composition of police forces to be broadly 'representative' of the communities they serve has been recognised for many years. This was especially an issue in Northern Ireland where the Royal Ulster Constabulary for historic and political reasons lacked credible neutrality among Catholics (Mulcahy 2006). This raises a broader issue applicable to all public services – whether professional communities should aim to be culturally diverse, granted that they cannot be proportionally representative, and qualification for the job must come first.

The chapters on policing and social networks remind us that some 'communities' and 'associations' can be problematic as well as facilitative for active citizenship. There are some neighbourhoods not only where positive support and role models are lacking but where antisocial behaviour is reinforced and criminal behaviour common. The negative influence of antisocial peers is most evident in youth gangs, but Carnochan et al. also acknowledge there are positive elements in gang membership – friendship, loyalty, peer-group approval and a sense of identity – which must be recognised and where possible constructively rechannelled. The model of inter-agency working within communities applies even when these are deemed 'antisocial' from the perspective of the wider community at large. It is unhelpful in policy terms to project errant youth as antisocial outsiders from which 'the community' must be protected (e.g. Scottish Government 2003). Such exclusion is likely to make antisocial behaviour harder to overcome.

Three of the chapters in this part focus in different ways on the role schools play in providing a site for community partnership working, for promoting young people's democratic participation and developing their capacity to exercise the rights and responsibilities of active citizenship. While the school itself must be an educative and facilitating community, it should both be open to actors from outside the school and support students to carry their civil engagement and voluntary service to communities beyond the school.

Chapter 11 discusses the role of what Dyson calls 'full service and extended schools', a generic term for what are sometimes called 'community' or 'community-focused schools' – those offering services and activities to children and families over and above the core role of classroom teaching. What such schools offer is variable, but will include partnerships with other children's services which seek to improve the well-being of families and disadvantaged communities. These schools facilitate communication between agencies and permit speedy holistic interventions which avoid lengthy referral procedures. Dyson points out some limitations. The first is in expecting such schools in themselves to bring about significant improvements in the attainments of all students and provide solutions to neighbourhood deprivation, which in fact require much more commitment of resources beyond the school. The school-centric approach also tends to leave education professionals in charge, when what is needed is an equal partnership with other agencies, with local people also participating in the 'co-production of solutions.' Dyson endorses a different model based on partnership with communities beyond the school and shared decision-making that does not invest control solely in the hands of the school. Arguably, this formulation is applicable to all schools.

The school itself is a complex hierarchical community which may be more or less democratic/autocratic. Its openness and responsiveness to outside agencies and to engage with parents and the 'community' it serves will depend in part on the flexibility of its management. The Chapter 12 analysis of forms of young people's participation is not confined to educational institutions, but nurseries, schools and colleges are key sites for learning about cooperative participation and sharing in decisions. Tisdall's starting point is the obligation which organisations have to comply with Article 12 of the UNCRC to give young people a voice that is listened to. How do people working with children ensure that participation is 'meaningful, sustainable and productive'? Early research on pupil councils showed when they were 'tokenistic' and encouraged 'cynicism' rather than learning about democracy (Alderson 2000). It is vital therefore that children's views are listened to and respected. At the same time, part of what must be learned is that democratic participation should balance different views and interests – it does not necessarily lead to an individual's desired outcome.

What does mark a difference between children and adults is that the former are not considered *necessarily* to be the best judges of their own interests and this makes a difference in how they are to be treated. This is at the heart of the issue of children's representation, discussed in Chapter 13. In everyday circumstances parents are deemed to represent their children's interests, until and unless there are grounds for setting aside this presumption. When courts have to reach contested decisions involving children, there is a major dilemma concerning children's participation. Should their views instruct the position taken by their legal representative or should the representative's judgement of their best interest take precedence? US experience of a highly formal adversarial judicial shows that this can be an arbitrary matter. The dilemma identified is one which applies beyond judicial settings. For example, medical professionals have their own codes of conduct in relation to consent to treatment when there is disagreement among relevant parties. Courts have made decisions about when parental representation may be disregarded, but this does no more than give a legal answer to a complex moral question.

The opportunity for members of the public to engage with children's services is an understated theme in this part, although it is clear that the time constraints on professional engagements with young people makes it always desirable to harness community support, whether through recognised volunteer organisations, or informally by individuals or networks of friends and neighbours.

The discussion of children as citizens in Chapter 14 goes beyond contemporary debates about children's individual rights to link with a body of political theorising which relates what we expect of our children to our aspirations for 'democratic society'. The recent promotion of citizenship education in schools arose in part from an increasing dissatisfaction with pressures for schools to orient themselves towards producing functionaries for the competitive market economy. Education for a healthy democracy requires much more, including the need for young people to engage in voluntary service and participate in community life beyond the school. This places them on equal footing with fellow citizen volunteers.

Lockyer's argument is that education for democratic citizenship is an objective not confined to the remit of schools. He suggests all adult citizens, professionals and public, share an obligation to assist in equipping young people to be fit for active citizenship. It is an open question how far we are able to deliver on the ideal and create a vibrant, interactive citizen community at large, which includes multiple communities of interest across neighbourhoods. What is without doubt is that it will not be achieved if providers of children's services focus only on the individual child removed from their social context and their communities.

Although we do not include a specific chapter on community and public health in this part, there is an unequivocal message from government reports and epidemiological studies (detailed elsewhere in this book) linking poor child health with living in disadvantaged circumstances. Health risks to children vary greatly depending on which type of neighbourhood they live in and what kinds of community association they have. In Chapter 16, Helen Roberts elaborates the factors which increase or diminish the risk to children's health and welfare; poor parenting associates with low income, lack of education and employment, plus poor housing and physical environment. The remedies lie in public policy which makes provision both to address the problems of deprivation and improve civic amenities beyond what can be delivered by any particular service. However, engagement with disadvantaged families in children's early years remains critical, as Chapter 8 stressed.

In this context, the pivotal role of health visitors and community nurses merits iteration. The increasing emphasis on health promotion and preventive advice should not detract from the crucial importance of home visiting to assess parenting, identify risks and providing practical support (Wilson et al. 2007). Health visitors recognise their need be better trained to exercise diagnostic judgement. In the last analysis community and public health is an issue of citizenship education, and as such is for all agencies of government, central and local to promote.

It is a recurring theme of the chapters in this part that the health and well-being of children require an environment in which families are adequately supported. Adults and children tend to thrive in supportive and resourceful communities. These are more likely to exist in a society at large where the inequalities between rich and poor are least great (Wilkinson and Pickett 2009). Regrettably, over the past decade in the UK relative deprivation – the income gap between wealthy and poor – has been increasing. In this context public professionals work to mitigate the impact of inequality on children's lives. This requires a response beyond individual remedies to harness and build resilient communities, which must be a work of partnership between all agents of government and civil society – professionals and citizens, children included.

Reflective exercise

1. What different sense or forms of community are most important from the point of view of enabling children and young people to participate in decisions that affect them?

2. Discuss whether communities of professionals facilitate or inhibit working together with families and fellow citizens in neighbourhood communities.

3. How helpful is the idea of a 'big society' in understanding and promoting community involvement with services and children's participation?

Chapter 8

Centre-based services in the early years

Eva Lloyd

Summary points

- Centre-based early years services have multiple aims, including the provision of childcare and early education, family health promotion, support to reduce family poverty, safeguarding 'at risk' children. The best way to reconcile and balance these disparate elements remains a matter for debate.

- Contemporary Children's Centres and their immediate predecessors, Sure Start Local Programmes, combine features of two post-war models of social-welfare-oriented, early years centres, as well as of integrated early education and care centres.

- Child health services were relatively recently reintroduced within centre-based early years provision, notably in the Sure Start initiative.

- The National Evaluation of Sure Start was one of the first major studies to provide robust evidence for the effectiveness of interprofessional working and partnerships with parents in centre-based early years provision.

- Only in the 30 per cent of the most disadvantaged areas do Children's Centres offer early education and childcare provision as a core service; recent research suggests their sustainability is at risk.

- Despite major policy and practice developments relating to centre-based early years services in recent years, the early year service system as a whole has not been truly reconceptualised.

Introduction

Centre-based early years services have multiple aims, which may include the provision of childcare and early education, family health promotion and family learning activities, support to reduce family poverty and safeguarding children deemed to be 'at risk.' For several decades such services for young children have been at the forefront of efforts to integrate care, education, health and family support functions. Nevertheless, debates continue about how to reconcile and balance these disparate elements, with corresponding implications for the professional backgrounds and orientations of staff. The chapter's main focus is on tracing continuities in policy and practice between different forms of centre-based early years provision and Children's Centres, with particular reference to the positioning of early education and childcare provision within them.

In many countries childcare and early education services embody different historical traditions, which have continued to influence the organisation of early childhood service systems as well as the vision, approach and programme aims reflected in the services themselves (Kaga et al. 2010). In Britain separate strands of centre-based early years services are aimed at different populations of children and families. Children's Centres and some state-funded nursery schools are located within disadvantaged areas or target provision at children in families experiencing disadvantage. Childcare and early education, sometimes combined with some of the parent-support services listed above, are available to a wider population in early years centres run by private businesses or not-for-profit organisations.

Britain's policy and practice in operating a social-welfare-oriented, centre-based early years system in parallel, rather than integrated with, different early education and childcare centres is relatively rare among European countries. It contrasts, for instance, with universal and integrated models of early childhood service systems supported by either education authorities, as in France, or by social welfare authorities, as in Nordic countries (Penn 2009).

This chapter will highlight how two different models of centre-based early years provision have influenced the current shape of Children's Centres. The first model has its roots in early education provision, such as that traditionally provided in nursery schools and nursery classes attached to primary schools, as well as in the combination of childcare and early education offered in contemporary community or private day nurseries.[1] The second, social-welfare-oriented, centre model has traditionally placed a greater emphasis on working with families experiencing disadvantage, particularly where there have been concerns about children's care or development. Social work professionals have often taken a lead role here.

The social work or community development framework within which social-welfare-oriented early years centres have been operating contrasts with the education-led model staffed primarily by education professionals and childcare practitioners. Services within this type of early years centre now often extend to adult education and parenting support, for example, but the provision of early education and childcare remains its primary purpose. Many state nursery schools have over time been transformed into this type of multi-purpose early years centre.

The greater emphasis on integrated working between diverse professionals in centre-based early years provision stems from the provisions of Section 17 of the Children Act 1989. This Act introduced the concept of 'children in need' and a local authority duty to safeguard and promote their development (Aldgate 2002). Schedule 2 of the Act identified a clear role for so-called 'family centres' in enabling health and social welfare professionals to deliver 'family support' to such children and their families, including interventions aimed at preventing serious family problems. Notably, it also introduced a duty on local authorities to provide daycare to such children as part of a programme of preventive measures.

---

[1] This chapter deals mainly with policy and practice in England after devolution in 1998, although many of the developments reviewed here also occurred in the other three UK countries.

The Children Act embodied a response to calls for the philosophy of partnership working to inform national policy, primarily in relation to safeguarding children from abuse and neglect. This encompassed partnership working with parents and reflected a growing recognition of parental rights. The case example below illustrates partnership principles in action in a contemporary Children's Centre.

Example 8.1

Jennie Berwick Nursery School and Children's Centre nestles in the centre of a small inner-city estate in one of England's poorest and most socially divided boroughs. On all sides of the building, doors open into a lovely garden, with open play spaces as well as mysterious nooks and crannies. Jennie Berwick has been around for over half a century. Keeping the description 'nursery school' in its name reflects the centre's proud roots in one of the oldest forms of provision for young children.

Open for 48 weeks of the year, the centre delivers nursery education integrated with childcare for children aged 6 months to 5 years, health services, family support, parenting programmes and advice for parents wanting to take up work, training or further education opportunities. The centre also offers 'marketed' childcare places in its day nursery alongside its local authority-funded 'community' places, creating a socially integrated mix of children and families.

A key principle is that centre staff need to build trusting relationships with the community and the parents and children using its services. The centre's director thinks that good interpersonal relationships are also an essential precondition for successful inter-agency and interprofessional working. That is why she is delighted that the Local Authority Children and Families Team have recently been reorganised on a 'patchwork' basis. For the centre's family-support workers this means more frequent and more meaningful contacts with the senior social worker, helping them deal with children and families with multiple problems. She acts as the interface with the borough's Children's Services Department. As Lead Professional she can access the case record system forming part of the Integrated Children's System (ICS), which supports the assessment, planning, intervention and review process for children in need. Up to a third of all Jennie Berwick places are reserved for children designated as 'in need.'

The benefits of close working relationship between professionals within and across centre boundaries can be illustrated by the story of one particular family. Elaine, a first-time mother, and her 18-month-old daughter Daisy had been referred by her GP to the Children and Adolescent Mental Health Service (CAMHS) because of Elaine's postnatal depression and its effect on her daughter. The CAMHS psychologist then referred the socially isolated pair to the centre, since progress remained slow and Daisy seemed as unhappy as her mum. During the first few 'Stay & Play' sessions they attended, Elaine just sat in the middle of the floor clutching Daisy, both of them sobbing quietly. The family-support practitioners, the other parents and their children all showed ample understanding, patience and flexibility.

Both Elaine and Daisy responded well to the involvement of an experienced art therapist who works at the centre several days a week. Daisy also benefited from an early education place, funded by a pilot programme run nationally at that time. Her social withdrawal and lack of interest in her surroundings had initially raised concern as possible signs of autistic tendencies, but they soon disappeared. Elaine found employment eventually and Daisy proceeded to do well at school, with some continuing support from the art therapist.

Early years centres: the education-led model

At the turn of the twentieth century, nursery centres developed by innovators like the McMillan sisters aimed to promote poor young children's educational and social development alongside their physical development. They were convinced that children's ability to learn was dependent on their physical and emotional well-being. The McMillans and others acted in response to the desperate physical conditions under which many three- and four-year-olds attended Victorian primary schools. Nevertheless, these efforts could not prevent a persistent divide opening up between nursery education and childcare provision, which would persist until late in the same century.

Early education remained a low policy priority for central and local government for a very long time. Unevenly distributed across the country, it was found primarily in disadvantaged areas. Early education, where available, was delivered by qualified teachers in freestanding state nursery schools or nursery classes attached to state primary schools and in a small number of private nursery schools and classes (Penn 2009).

Over half of 4-year-olds were admitted to reception classes of infant and primary schools, although the first term after children reached their fifth birthday has been the compulsory school starting age since the 1870 Education Act. Until recently most 3-year-olds and those 4-year-olds not already in school merely had access to part-time playgroup provision, staffed by leaders without teaching qualifications and by volunteers (Statham et al. 1990).

Early years centres integrating childcare and early education only began making a comeback as 'combined nursery centres' around 1970, well before the introduction of a universal early education entitlement in 1998 (Pugh 2006). In other European countries the integration of care and education had long been seen as indistinguishable. Strong arguments for such integration in British early years provision only gradually reappeared (Penn et al. 2004). Emerging findings of an important longitudinal study which investigated the effectiveness of early education and care in terms of children's cognitive and socio-emotional development, the Effective Provision of Pre-School Education project, helped rekindle this interest (Sylva and Taylor 2006).

Cooperation between education and care professionals working together within such early years centres can evoke tensions. This is the legacy of a divided workforce, including graduate teachers and largely unqualified childcare practitioners, all with different levels of pay. Early childhood workforce developments since 1997 retain this teacher/childcare practitioner split (Cohen et al. 2004). It has even persisted despite the first Labour administration's recognition of the primary role of education, as evidenced by the transfer of central and local government responsibility for early childhood and other children's services to Education Departments, renamed Children's Services Departments in the Children Act 2004.

The introduction of universal part-time early education for 3- and 4-year-olds as part of the Labour Government's 1998 National Childcare Strategy marked a reversal in the fortunes of nursery education. Early education, funded by the Nursery Education Grant, is still offered in state nursery schools and classes, though the number of nursery schools has dwindled. But, additionally, it can also be delivered in different early years centres. These include private-for-profit and not-for-profit childcare businesses. Childminders, too, can deliver early education, provided they are part of a childminding network associated with a Children's Centre. All these providers must meet Ofsted registration requirements, which include the delivery of the Early Years Foundation Stage, a curricular and regulatory programme introduced in the 2006 Childcare Act. The input of qualified teachers is not mandatory.

The implementation of the free early education policy was completed by 2004 and is now being rolled out to targeted 2-year-old children (Smith et al. 2009). This British reliance on a mixed market economy in which private for-profit and not for-profit providers deliver both childcare and early education, alongside state nursery schools and primary school nursery classes is virtually unique in Europe (Lloyd 2008).

At an early stage of implementing its 1998 National Childcare Strategy, the new Labour government also piloted Early Excellence Centres, often developed from state nursery schools. These added a range of parent-support services and adult education to their existing integrated early education and childcare provision, and appeared to have a beneficial effect (Bertram et al. 2002). This raised the hopes of early childhood advocates that Early Excellence Centres might become the model for new types of centre-based early years provision being rolled out. However, as described below, the Children's Centre model places a greater emphasis on health and social care compared to childcare and early education.

The Neighbourhood Nursery initiative (NNI Research team 2007) was developed at around the same time to test out the sustainability of early education and childcare provision in disadvantaged areas. After the withdrawal of their initial funding, though, many closed. Although different in major respects, both initiatives proved to be notable influences on the reconceptualisation of centre-based early years provision under New Labour.

Early years centres: the social welfare model

Social-welfare-oriented, centre-based early years provision was once exemplified by different types of family centre, run either with local authority financial support by national voluntary children's organisations or by local authority social services departments themselves. The latter had often been under health agency management. Such centres continued to be staffed primarily by nursery nurses, though increasingly with teacher input and social-work-trained managers.

Family centres increased in popularity from the late 1970s onwards as a site for 'two-generation' early intervention programmes with vulnerable young children under five and their parents. The Children Act 1989 identified three models of family centre. These broadly represented a taxonomy of family centres grounded in a conceptualisation of a hierarchy of social welfare interventions responding to different levels of family need (Holman 1988; Hardiker 2002).

1. *Client-focused centres* undertook therapeutic work with referred parents and children on the basis of focused assessments of child/parent interactions in cases where children had suffered or were at risk of suffering abuse.

2. *Neighbourhood-focused centres* delivered multiple interventions, including day-care, baby clinics, and group activities such as parenting support and outreach work. Parents might get to attend via referrals from GPs or health visitors.

3. *Community development centres*, provided additional resources to local communities, such as credit unions and adult education, to help them address social disadvantage.

This chapter will only differentiate, following Smith (1996), between 'resource based open-access' neighbourhood centres on one hand and 'client-focused' centres working specifically with families referred by social workers, GPs or health visitors on the other. The first type used to be run by mostly voluntary sector agencies with some financial support from local authorities. The latter were provided by local authorities themselves or by voluntary sector agencies on their behalf. Attendance might be compulsory for parents with children on the child protection register, risking social stigma. The power balance between parents and professionals working together was affected by the type of centre.

Resulting tensions were well illustrated by Ferri and Saunders (1991) in their evaluation of neighbourhood-based family centres operated by Barnardo's. They identified challenges for parents and professionals inherent in jointly determining objectives for the families' attendance. Conflict was mostly associated with differing perceptions of what constituted a family problem. As attendance was voluntary and Barnardo's staff were committed to a consensual approach, parents could exercise 'negative control' over the nature of the work undertaken (Ferri and Saunders 1991: 123).

Health and social care practitioners tended to construct family problems as primarily located in personal and family functioning, so that interventions might fail to address the association with neigbourhood characteristics and wider social and economic factors, including racism. Black and ethnic minority families, despite identified needs for support, were less likely to attend family centres than white families (Butt and Box 1998). For a long time, conceptual issues arising from the gender imbalance in such family centre work, where mainly female practitioners worked principally with mothers and their children, would also remain below the policy and practice radar.

In contrast Save the Children's UK centres reflected an ecological model of children's well-being, taking account of community and wider contextual influences on family welfare. Save the Children's family centre work was based on the premise that social inequality lay at the root of social problems, including many instances of child abuse (Lloyd 1997: 144). Childcare provision and holiday play schemes featured prominently until the agency reassessed its role and methods in the early nineties.

This provision reflected the view that multiply disadvantaged mothers would benefit from some respite from round-the-clock childcare duties, while children might gain from opportunities to socialise with adults outside the family and with peers. Active attempts were being made in some centres to involve fathers as well as mothers. Among the professional staff, youth and community and childcare practitioners outnumbered social and family support workers. Service users participated in deciding on the kind of provision that best met their needs.

This approach to community development was seen as strengthening the centres' community base and fostering community perceptions of these centres as a community resource. This empowering role for parents and communities via a community development approach would subsequently be incorporated in the Sure Start initiative.

Effectiveness studies

Emerging research evidence suggested that the outcomes for highly stressed families of using 'open access' centres, particularly when this included childcare provision, might be at least equivalent if not better than the outcomes for families referred to 'client-focused' centres. In an important study of the short-term outcomes of referral to social services, Gibbons (1991) found that, compared to a range of other practice interventions, only the provision of childcare had a significant positive effect on children and parents.

Subsequently, Smith (1996) came to a similar conclusion in an evaluation of open access and client-focused family centres, provided by the Church of England's Children's Society in disadvantaged areas with high levels of unemployment and/or a low-wage economy. She found considerable similarities between the families using these two types of centre, although families referred to the client-focused centres, particularly those headed by lone mothers, were slightly more socio-economically disadvantaged. Like Gibbons before her, Smith (1996: 178) concluded that open access centres might be at least as effective as client-focused ones, if not more so.

Although tentative, this conclusion would also be reflected in the conceptualisation of the Sure Start initiative. These two types of centres employed different types of professionals. By implication there appeared to be little evidence of a differential impact of interprofessional working related to the type of professionals engaged in it. The manner in which services were provided appeared the more crucial factor, Statham, 2000.

In the mid-nineties an important synthesis of 20 child-protection studies commissioned by the Department of Health also suggested that enhancing a child's wider quality of life formed the best protection against abuse. For the next ten years the need for children's social welfare services to refocus on the appropriate balance between safeguarding and promoting children's well-being was to affect the nature of interprofessional working in family centres. Then the *Every Child Matters* agenda led to even greater change.

Every Child Matters introduced a major structural reform plan for all children's services. Given legal force in the 2004 Children Act, this entailed an emphasis on multi-professional working in integrated teams, both at central and local government level, to improve both early childhood provision and other targeted children's services previously described as 'family-support services'. Its ultimate aim was the reduction of the health and educational attainment gap between poor and better-off children.

By 1993 the evidence-based practice movement in social welfare had begun to make inroads on practice approaches, as evidenced by the establishment of the Evidence for Policy and Practice Information and Coordinating Centre (EPPI-Centre) at London

University's Institute of Education, which undertakes systematic research reviews and promotes new review methods. This was modelled on the same movement in medicine, the international Cochrane Collaboration, which was already operating. The use of evidence-based policy and practice became a hallmark of the first Labour administration after 1997. An evidence-based approach also informed the Sure Start Centre model after 1998 (Glass 1999).

The Sure Start initiative

The 1997 Labour government's early interest in reducing the health and educational inequalities between poor and better-off children resulted in a Treasury-led cross-departmental Review of Services for Young Children involving eleven separate government departments. This was informed by research evidence on the success of the American two-generation, early intervention programmes. The review identified a major gap in good-quality early years provision for children under four, who were increasingly at risk of poverty and social exclusion through multiple disadvantage.

The result was the high-profile Sure Start programme. Although initially conceived as a pilot, by 2000 the programme had doubled in size and been implemented nationally. Soon embedded in the 20 per cent most deprived areas, it was expected to reach up to a third of poor young children. Centres were open to all children aged under four and their families in Sure Start communities, thus offering non-stigmatising provision (Melhuish and Hall 2007).

Sure Start centres, eventually known as Sure Start Local Programmes (SSLPs), were intended to increase community access, promote improved interprofessional and inter-agency cooperation and generate new ways of working. Overseen by local multi-agency partnerships, the centres employed a community-development approach, involving local parents in the design of the centres' programme. The model therefore required a reconfiguration of the relationship between parents and professionals. Even so, official programme guidance recommended adopting evidence-based interventions. The centres' 'core offer' included:

- outreach and home visiting;
- support for families and parents;
- support for good quality play, learning and childcare experiences for children;
- primary and community healthcare and advice about child health and development and family health;
- support for people with special needs, including help getting access to specialised services.

Noteworthy in this package were two things: first the introduction of child health services, and second the absence of packages of integrated early education and childcare provision, as delivered elsewhere. Childcare was embodied by crèche facilities and play and learning opportunities in 'drop-in' play sessions for parents and children. Only a few years later Sure Start centres were reorganised to include childcare facilities.

Its community-development approach did distinguish the Sure Start initiative from the US centre-based demonstration programmes on which it had been modelled. The 524 UK Sure Start centres embodied several characteristics of the two early years-centre models discussed above, alongside a wide variety of alternative approaches. These centres' effectiveness and cost-effectiveness were explored in a major evaluation.

The National Evaluation of Sure Start

The National Evaluation of Sure Start (NESS) became the largest controlled process and impact evaluation of a complex intervention programme undertaken in the UK to date (Belsky et al. 2007). Outcomes were to be assessed against specified targets in children's social, emotional and cognitive development, their health and their families' and communities' functioning. Local programme evaluations also took place alongside the national one. Nevertheless, the evaluation generated a wealth of encouraging and, at times, inconclusive findings on partnership working between professionals, parents and communities.

Here I only summarise key findings relating to partnership working. Given the variations likely to arise from local programme autonomy and the lack of a tightly specified model, the evaluation constructed a rating of programme implementation proficiency. A measure was designed to study to what extent the programmes had been implemented in accordance with the original intentions – in other words, had remained 'faithful' to these. Among programme domains also rated were partnership functioning, multi-agency teamwork, reach strategies and the creation of an environment that empowered users and staff. Better-implemented programmes, which had adhered more strictly to the original implementation guidelines, were found to have a greater beneficial effect on the children and families (Melhuish et al. 2007).

Of particular interest is the evidence for the impact of staffing patterns on centres' effectiveness. Health-agency-led Sure Start Local Programmes were found to be associated with improved outcomes for child and family well-being. This finding was replicated in the cost-effectiveness evaluation (Meadows 2007). These findings on the effectiveness of health agencies and staff in child and parent outcomes were reflected in the additional emphasis on health that was to characterise the subsequent Children's Centre programme. From 2004 onwards this took the Sure Start concept to the next level.

Other Sure Start programme features found to be effective, such as user empowerment through the community-development approach, did reinforce the message of earlier studies of early years centres (this aspect was not linked to health agency leadership). From a parent partnership perspective, it was found that black and minority ethnic communities in Sure Start areas could have been more effectively targeted, particularly since they are more likely to be affected by poverty than the rest of the population (Craig et al. 2007). This issue had previously been noted (Butt and Box 1998), while a review of studies exploring effective ways of engaging BME parents in services (Page et al. 2007) stressed the importance of recognising diversity within and across ethnic communities in formulating responses to local needs. Doubts were also expressed whether or not this integrated service model allowed social work professionals to engage optimally with the most socially excluded families featuring child protection issues (Carpenter et al. 2005).

From a policy perspective, the fact that the Sure Start programme was implemented without reference to simultaneous developments in early years policy and practice attracted serious criticism. Clarke (2006) and Penn (2007) argued that the programme reinforced the divide between universal and social-welfare-oriented early years provision. One of the UK's major experts on prevention and early intervention questioned whether Sure Start's design was suitable for addressing child poverty and could be meaningfully evaluated at all (Rutter 2006).

Before the emerging lessons from NESS could be meaningfully integrated into existing and future models of centre-based early years provision, the policy landscape changed yet again. In 2004 the Ten Year Strategy for Childcare announced the national roll-out of the Sure Start Children's Centre programme, a rather diluted version of the Sure Start initiative.

Sure Start Children's Centres

By 2010, 3500 Sure Start Children's Centres had been established as planned in every English community, managed by local authority Children's Services, health agencies and voluntary sector partnerships. The present coalition government has stated its intention to keep the programme, but to increase its focus on the neediest families. One key difference between Sure Start Children's Centres and SSLPs is their concentration on key services, rather than responding flexibly to locally expressed need, as the Sure Start initiative set out to do.

Though the community development approach has been abandoned, the Sure Start emphasis on child and family health services has been strengthened. Since 2008 all Children's Centres provide the 'Healthy Child Programme' delivered by multi-agency teams, as part of a drive to meet public-health priorities such as reducing childhood obesity and adult smoking rates. The centres' core programme also includes parenting advice and support such as help with job finding through links with *Jobcentre Plus*, the government's employment support agency.

However, this latest early years centre model only partially integrates care, education and health functions. Only in the 30 per cent most disadvantaged areas did early education and childcare remain as a core service until recently. Under the Childcare Act 2006, early education and childcare must be delivered by private-sector childcare businesses, employing a business franchise model of service delivery.

A planned evaluation of Sure Start Children's Centres is going ahead; risks to their viability are identified in some smaller studies. They operate on a much reduced budget, compared to the original Sure Start programme's funding. Persistent financial problems resulted (NAO 2006; NAO 2009). Among centres in the NAO study offering early years provision, 53 per cent reported operating at a loss. The 2008 Childcare Providers Survey (Philips et al. 2009) revealed that 58 per cent of early education and childcare in Children's Centres was provided by local authorities themselves, contradicting the provisions of the Childcare Act

2006. Finding childcare business partners to deliver this type of service is difficult in disadvantaged areas where the childcare market fails to operate efficiently. In late 2010, in response to this situation, the coalition government removed altogether the requirement for Children's Centres in deprived areas to offer full daycare. Instead, centres were given greater freedom to determine and respond to families' particular needs in their locality. However, at the time of writing, the duty on local authorities to meet childcare demands remains.

The most recent Ofsted report (2009) on Sure Start Children's Centres suggests that cooperation across daycare and other services was not particularly effective in 17 out of 20 centres investigated. The most problematic links were those with *Jobcentre Plus*. Although the Ofsted study reported positive short-term impacts on children and parent, more robust studies of longer-term impacts on children and parents are as yet scarce. Research is notably lacking on Children's Centres' work with families where safeguarding children is an issue. It is too early to assess the longer-term outcomes of Children's Centres on the health and well-being of children, families and their communities.

Conclusions and implications

British early years practitioners and academics have long and frequently argued for a comprehensive and universal early years system in which more targeted social welfare services would be fully integrated and which would be distinguished by truly collaborative working between families and professionals (Tizard et al. 1976; Moss and Penn 1996; Chandler 2006). Instead the divide between universal and social-welfare oriented early years provision stubbornly persists.

Despite major developments in policy and practice relating to centre-based early years provision, the early year service system has not been truly reconceptualised. British early years policy continues to favour an early-years-service system distinguished by progressive universality. This term refers to the fact that some services are universal, while additional resources are targeted at those children and families seen as most in need of support. This is mostly accomplished via a segregated system of provision, as in Children's Centres.

Research evidence confirms the challenges of professional partnership working and parent professional partnerships within current forms of integrated, centre-based, early years provision (Melhuish et al. 2007). But evidence is strong for the potential longer-term benefits of partnership working within centre-based provision for children and their families in disadvantaged areas and elsewhere. Such lessons have not yet been translated into the Children's Centre model, however.

What can we learn from this overview about the position of early education and childcare within centre-based early years provision? Although since 1997 there has been considerable reform to the diverse and fragmented early-years-service system (Cohen et al. 2004), not every early-years-service system divide has been bridged to date. Early education and childcare featured in the earliest forms of centre-based integrated early years provision for disadvantaged children, but its viability is at risk in its most recent incarnation. It seems especially paradoxical that quality provision of this kind remains a vulnerable service, despite extensive evidence for its positive impact on disadvantaged children's well-being and life chances.

Exercise

Discuss how well young children's multiple needs are met by the current mix of centre-based early years provision in Children's Centres operating in parallel with private centre-based early years provision and primary school nursery classes.
What changes may be desirable?

Recommended reading

http://eppe.ice.ac.uk

> The national evaluation of Sure Start is a valuable and easily accessible source of all research reports on this major project.

Belsky, J., Barnes, J. and Melhuish, E. (eds) (2007) *The National Evaluation of Sure Start. Does Area-based Early Intervention Work?* Bristol: The Policy Press.

> The contributions from the leaders of the thematic evaluation teams provide retrospective critical insights into the Sure Start programme's planning and functioning.

http://www.education.gov.uk

> The Effective Provision of Pre-School Education (EPPE) project site provides access to all reports on the first major European longitudinal study of a national sample of young children's development (intellectual and social/behavioural) between the ages of three and seven years.

www.dcsf.gov.uk/everychildmatters/research/publications/surestartpublications/1854/

> This government website lists current Children Centre practice guidance and provides useful links to specific guidance and to associated research reports.

http://www.dh.gov.uk/en/Publicationsandstatistics/Publications/
PublicationsPolicyAndGuidance/DH_107563

> This Department of Health site currently lists comprehensive practice guidance on delivering child and family health services in Children's Centres via the *Healthy Child Programme*. This contains references to pertinent research.

Chapter 9

Children, social networks and social support

Robbie Gilligan

Summary points

- Informal social relationships are crucial for individual well-being.
- It is important for professionals to understand how social network ties affect individuals they are working with.
- Strong ties are often supportive, but can also be demanding and exclusive.
- Weak ties can widen opportunities and may be particularly helpful for children and young people with problematic family relationships.
- When a child or parent lacks positive connections, a key professional role should be to facilitate new links and energise existing or lapsed relationships.

Introduction

This chapter is concerned with the importance of informal relationships for children and for their long-term competence and well-being. Particular attention is given to vulnerable young people and those in care.

Close human relationships exert at least as much influence on children's health and social inclusion or exclusions as formal interventions or services (Jahnukainen and Järvinen 2005). Particularly valuable are relationships that incorporate the following qualities:

> individualised responsiveness, mutual action-and-interaction, and an emotional connection to another human being, be it a parent, peer, grandparent, aunt, uncle, neighbour, teacher, coach, or any other person who has an important impact on the child's. . . . development.
> (National Scientific Council on the Developing Child, 2004)

Such relationships are a key channel for the flow of social support. Enduring, meaningful and sustainable relationships arise within social networks. Generally, it is neither feasible nor appropriate for professionals to be party to such in-depth relationships. Professionals should certainly have *good* relationships with the children and families with whom they work but, by their nature, professional relationships generally tend to be short term or fleeting. In their work professionals should strive to be 'friendly' in their approach, rather than to become 'friends' with the service users they meet. The professional plays largely a backstage role, supporting the players on the main stage to find mutual support, to negotiate their parts and their understanding of the shared script in the ongoing drama of the relevant person's life.

Practitioners tend to overestimate the relative significance of their own influence in people's lives. For example, a representative survey in a disadvantaged district in Dublin found relatively high levels of contact with GPs and teachers, but the proportion of families having contact in the previous year with other services was low, under 5 per cent with respect to each type of service (Axford and Whear 2008). Equally, professionals may sometimes overlook the importance of social networks in the lives of the people with whom they work. Particularly where there is poverty or social exclusion, it may be too readily assumed that networks are weak. Fagg et al. (2008) caution against

> stigmatising whole populations by assuming that they all share the social disadvantages of their community in the same degree, or that they generally lack social skills or social capital resources.

Even where a network may appear absent in a person's life, questioning may reveal 'dormant' members who with patience and gentle tact may be drawn back into a more active role. The 'social network' provides an important lens through which to seek to understand the life and circumstances of a child and their family. Broadly, three categories can be identified of network relations affecting children and young people:

1. the presence of network relations and support is readily visible;
2. availability of support is less obvious, but there is at least dormant potential waiting to be tapped;
3. the child or family is truly socially isolated without actual or potential connections to others.

The third group are typically a small minority but their situation calls for serious attention, in terms of building alternative forms of support, which initially at least may be more dependent on formal systems of support. Children leaving care or young lone parents are two categories of young service user where the absence of any informal support would be a particular concern (see Chapter 23).

Who are the people who may be members of social networks?

In the UK and Ireland, family ties tend not to be as extensive as in the past, but close family members remain vitally important in social networks, especially grandparents and siblings. The *Growing Up in Scotland* study has found that grandparents are the most common source of support for the parents of young children, with this being especially so for lone parents and even more so for younger parents under 20 years of age. After grandparents, the next most likely sources of support for these parents were neighbours, friends and siblings (Growing Up in Scotland 2007). Family ties may extend beyond the immediate biological family, with additions arising from remarriage, new partners or fostering, for instance.

The importance of family relationships remains true even in circumstances where strain and conflict have been, or are, present between some or all of the members. Where family difficulties occur, it should not be assumed that such issues pervade the whole set of connections in the extended family. There may be people within any one part of the family network who are unaffected by the strain, or who are functioning well and who wish to make a positive contribution to others in need in the wider network. The quality of relations may prove very fluid, waxing and waning in response to shifting circumstances and perceptions. Family members may get on well most of the time, but even where they fall out this strain may not last forever.

In the case of children and young people themselves, relations with grandparents may be especially important when there are difficulties. Close relations with grandparents have been found to be protective for adolescents in stressful conditions (Flouri et al. 2010). Both Swedish and English research has shown that among children brought up apart from both parents, those cared for by grandparents tend to do best and stay longest (Sallnäs et al. 2004; Farmer 2010). Grandparents may also play a crucial role when children are dispersed (Example 9.1).

Example 9.1

Six children were placed in care, each in separate placements. Their grandparents were meticulous in staying in touch with each child, bringing them together from time to time and in always keeping each child up to date with what was happening for the other five. The children derived great benefit from this contact with their grandparents and siblings while they were in care. In later life all six siblings are still in touch with each other, an achievement that would seem in no small part to be due to the efforts of the grandparents.

Brothers and sisters are usually very significant for children and young people, especially in times of difficulty and when relationships with parents are difficult:

> [Findings] suggest that sibling affection is protective (against stressful life events) regardless of the age gap found between siblings and the gender composition of the dyad . . . and of the quality of the parent–child relationship . . . the provision of security and comfort once ascribed mainly to parental figures *may* [emphasis in original] also be a role that siblings can fulfil when children experience stress caused by life events'.
>
> (Gass, Jenkins and Dunn 2006)

Young care leavers sometimes gain help from older siblings who play a 'quasi-parental role, providing advice, guidance and practical support' (Wade 2006, p. 45). It cannot be taken for granted however that siblings are a key source of support, as shown by an Irish study of young people in need living at home (Pinkerton and Dolan 2007).

In addition to blood relatives, other people may also be important sources of support – friends and their families, in particular. Quasi-siblings may also be important in the case of young people in care. One example is the 25-year-old son of a foster carer who helped a boy placed with his parents to settle in by coaching him in the use of his personal gym equipment.

Small (2006) reminds us of various places in the local neighbourhood that may be promising sites for children or their parents to develop supportive relationships, including schools, community and leisure centres, childcare facilities, places of worship and workplaces. Seemingly chance or short-term encounters may have long-lasting benefits (Example 9.2).

Example 9.2

Chris spent part of his boyhood in residential care in a rural area in Australia. When he was thrown out of his care setting at the age of 14, a local farmer who knew of his plight offered him both a job and somewhere to live. They had strong disagreements, and before long Chris left. However, when he was 19, they bumped into each other again. The farmer was prepared 'to give it another go' and this time it went well. The farmer became a life long mentor to Chris.

This real case shows how a young person in need may obtain help without any prompting or involvement by formal services. The story also illustrates that networks carry latent possible connections, but it is the agency of the social actors that brings alive the helping potential.

Finally, it is important to remember, especially in relation to children, that important network members need not be human. Many studies have shown the importance of pets to many children. The world may divide into those who love and hate cats, like or dislike dogs, but being close to an animal of any kind can promote the social engagement and mental health of the owner (Wood et al. 2005; 2007). The advantage seems to derive not only from straightforward companionship offered by animals, but also they may serve as a conduit to other human contact (Cairns 2004).

Significance of social networks – positive and negative

Informal relationships can deliver social support, be a source of positive role models and provide help in a crisis. Social support may operate in two ways. First, there is perceived *support* where the value lies in people having a conviction that support will be accessible when required from relevant network members. This in itself may be very powerful as an aid to coping. There is also *enacted support* where the person actually receives help when needed.

These positive network functions in turn promote well-being and foster resilience in adversity. A large Irish study demonstrated the value of key relationships in promoting positive health. The researchers found that '(good) parent, sibling and friend relationships were independent predictors of positive health' (Molcho, Nic Gabhainn and Kelleher 2007). Having 'a greater number of supportive relationships was strongly associated with positive health' for the young people. Benefits of supportive relationship may extend, of course, beyond health to material support as in the giving of lifts, paying for holidays or lending money.

Friends may, under certain conditions, play a positive role in all sorts of ways. A young person in care, for example, acknowledged the part friends had played in encouraging him to stay on at school, rather than leave when legally free to do so (Tilbury, Buys and Creed 2009). The lifetime risk of ever being bullied or victimised has been found to be linked to the capacity to have friendships (McMahon et al. 2010).

Informal relationships can deliver support, but they may also be double-edged or worse. Take the example of life in residential care centres for children and young people. There are positive accounts of the role of young peers in residential care (Emond 2002), but there is also evidence of abuse by fellow residents (Gibbs and Sinclair 2000). While often a channel for transmitting support, social networks may also become a source and driver of victimisation. Children may find that peers in school, in children's homes or in the neighbourhood subject them to various forms of abuse (emotional, physical, sexual or racist).

Another possibly negative feature of social networks relates to their potentially confining nature. Close-knit communities may provide mutual aid, but also inhibit access to wider opportunities beyond the physical confines of the community (White and Green 2011). In some instances, this strong sense of boundary between known insiders and stranger outsiders may serve both to confine insiders and exclude or demonise outsiders. Deprived working-class young people might in theory benefit from educational and employment options beyond the local area, but they find it hard to leave behind their close ties to family and friends (MacDonald et al. 2005). One study found that immigrant women enduring domestic violence were discouraged by ethnic leaders from raising their case with 'outside' legal or other public systems (Bui and Morash 2007). A further example of the potentially dark side of social networks and social capital lies in the genesis and sustenance of criminal networks (MacDonald et al. 2005). Whether mainly positive or negative in their overall impact in a given situation, the message for professionals is still clear – social networks matter.

The importance of both strong and weak relationships

A key concept relevant to social support and social networks is social capital (see Chapter 22). This is understood as the reciprocal set of connections, norms and obligations shared between network members, whether at the level of individuals, households or neighbourhoods/communities. Persons with good social support as represented through measures of social capital have better health than people with lower social capital (Borgonovi 2010).

A common distinction in discussions of the concept of social capital is between 'bonding' and 'bridging' social capital. Bonding entails strong connectedness with people similar to yourself in important ways. Bridging social capital, on the other hand, involves fewer close contacts with people who are different from yourself. Bonding capital may provide a lot of support, yet may sometimes prove restrictive. Bridging capital can help in moving on from a predicament, in finding additional resources to break out of a stalemate. Researchers studying the coping experiences of survivors of the devastating Hurricane Katrina in New Orleans found the distinction reflected in the responses of the people they interviewed.

Participants described a process through which close ties (bonding) were important for immediate support, but bridging and linking social capital offered pathways to longer term survival and wider neighbourhood and community revitalization.

(Hawkins and Maurer 2010)

Similar to the distinction between bonding and bridging capital as features of a network as a whole is the contrast between strong and weak ties with individuals in a network. While it is important to have at least some relationships that are close (strong ties), it is worth remembering that less intimate contacts (weak ties) can still prove of great value. Weak ties carry fewer demands and may be less stressful. They open up new connections, information and opportunities. The importance of weak ties was first examined in an American study on job-seeking where people often found jobs through contacts with people not very well known to them (Granovetter 1973). Indirect contacts, like friends of friends, may perform a similar function. A consistent finding from the research on resilience in children facing adversity is the protective power of a positive relationship with even one supportive adult, who was not originally a family member or close friend.

In the past, frequent face-to-face contact was crucial for the maintenance of strong ties. Increased access to an expanding range of communication forms has had a major impact on who has meaningful connections with whom and on the capacity to remain emotionally close while physically at a distance. The internet, the phone, Skype and so on allow people to connect – and, very important, *feel* connected in new ways. The intersection of transnational migration and technology emphasises this point. A study of the intensive interaction between Filipina mothers working abroad and their children at home in the Philippines uses the term 'long distance intimacy' to reflect the character of changes in family relations made possible by technology (Parreñas 2005). One example cited is of mothers working abroad sending daily text messages to their offspring at home. Mobility of family members need not involve foreign travel. For 'internal' as well as international migrants, making connections from scratch in a new location may be a challenge, especially in the absence of a strong base in the community of origin or when lacking even weak ties with people at the destination.

Young people can be active in building, activating or regulating network connections for themselves and their families

Young people are not necessarily passive onlookers in the business of developing social network connections in their lives. Children and young people may help to generate connections and social capital, not only for themselves, but also for their family (Weller 2009). In a British study of families and social capital:

many parents suggested that they had established more networks and friendships in the local area through their children than by any other means – via antenatal classes, nursery and the primary school, or through their children's friends' families. Some parents found firm friends through their children's connections and in one case went on holiday together.

(Weller and Bruegel 2009)

Children may also serve as sources of social support to vulnerable adults, as has been found, for example, in the case of women in substance-abuse treatment programmes (Tracy and Martin 2007).

Yet, it is not the case that all are equal in any given network. Different members may have, or be granted, different levels of knowledge about each other's circumstances. Children and adults in the same family may broadly share the same network, but there may be important differences in their knowledge of the reality of relations within the network. For example, some parents are not aware of bullying in their children's lives (Willams et al. 2009). This is an important reminder that adults do not have full sight of what is happening in their child's world. Children may be selective in whom they confide about certain types of information. On some fronts, and at certain ages, peers may know more than parents, and on others vice versa.

Young people may use their agency to determine who in their network knows what about them – they may choose to remain silent about certain things with certain people, as in the case of 13-year-old Ruth, a lone asylum seeker from Eritrea:

> I cry sometimes but I keep it to myself. I never talk to no one about my mum and my family. My friends at school don't know about me living with a foster carer. They just think I live with my mum. But my friends at church know. (Chase 2010)

Adults may also be selective in their help-seeking, as in this case of a mother participating in a family literacy programme in the US, who found she could confide in the teacher who offered valuable emotional distance:

> Sometimes . . . it's not someone in your family you would want to go to, you know. Sometimes it has to be an outsider to where you can go ask things a little better and they can help you understand it or help you take care of it a little better than a person that's related to you. (Prins et al. 2009)

Building positive connections where they are lacking or insufficient

It must be acknowledged that it is not a simple matter to build new connections for children or family members from scratch. It is not easy for the person involved to generate such connections on their own initiative. Nor is it easy for a professional to take on this task. Often the key may lie in repeatedly scanning the horizon for latent connections that the person may already have – or used to have, since sometimes relationships that have lapsed can be revived positively. It may be easier to reawaken connections, rather than generate completely new ones. Potential or dormant ties may lie in extended family, neighbourhood, faith community, workplace, sports club and so on.

In the case of building new links, Power's (2007) study of inner city families in the UK revealed how important schools were in helping immigrant families to forge connections in their new communities of residence. For these otherwise isolated families, primary schools represented a potential 'entry point' to *local* connections and resources:

> The families' high dependence on schools as a source of support, contact and community reinforcement, over and above education, reminds us of the interdependence of welfare structures and communities, of social support and individual progress, of local institutions and families.
>
> (Power 2007: 187)

School events and routines afford recurring opportunities for casual social interaction with potential peers. Dropping and collecting children at the beginning and end of the school day, or accompanying them to various school gatherings may provide the gentle unobtrusive beginnings of familiarity, acquaintance or even friendship with fellow parents. These contacts may also offer potential for sourcing vital information about relevant developments, facilities or entitlements. Following up such information can lead on to shared encounters and experiences that sometimes prove a seedbed for an emerging supportive connection.

One mother emphasised how much friendships and networks formed through school meant to her:

> When we see one another on the street, it's almost like an old brother or sister we haven't seen for a long while and it's a big excitement.
>
> (Cited in Weller and Bruegel 2009)

The researchers noted that such networks provided a wide range of resource including friendship and support.

However, the picture may not always be so benign. Opportunities to find additional members for the network may be constrained by a range of factors. A sense of threat or danger in the local neighbourhood may, for example, discourage a child from spending time outside, thus limiting opportunities to form new friendships serendipitously, as in this example:

> I don't really go and play out because the last time I played out someone was trying to pick a fight with me. So I don't really like to play out anymore. I like to stay inside and play games inside so I don't really . . . I've witnessed lots of fights but it's not really safe for me to go outside and start playing with other people . . . because usually you see big boys around . . . 14 and 15 carrying these pocket-knives . . .
>
> (Tor, age 11, South London, quoted in Holland et al. 2007)

This quotation is a powerful reminder that the character of a social network may sometimes be influenced by forces beyond the actions of the social actors in the network. Yet even in unpromising circumstances, good may sometimes prevail as in Example 9.3.

Example 9.3

A young boy was growing up in very difficult family circumstances in a very run-down housing estate. At the age of 11, his school enrolled him in a local choir. This simple action by a teacher proved a turning point in his life. He thrived in this faith-based choir which began to serve as a proxy family in many senses. This support allowed him to go on to do well in education and he is now employed as an academic.

As this example shows, opportunities to build connections may lie beyond the family and school life – through acquiring valued social roles in the domains of recreation, work or community life. Social roles serve to integrate the person playing the role into social networks. Crucially, they also play a part in helping the person to accumulate bridging social capital – that is, links beyond the core of their daily routine experience and connections.

The role of professionals in supporting and building positive influences of social networks

In many circumstances, it is helpful to talk with children about who is in their network, what kind of relationships they have with whom, who they turn to for confiding or help. This can aid assessment and may act as a springboard for identifying informal sources of help or discussing how to modify key relationships. Various standard tools are available, such as ecomaps and genograms, which can help structure discussion and provide a comprehensive overview. Sometimes, though, an open-ended approach will be more productive or acceptable to the child (Gilligan 1999; Hill 2002).

Cohen (2004) makes the case for:

> a broader view of how to intervene in social networks to improve health. This includes facilitating both social integration and social support by creating and nurturing both close (strong) and peripheral (weak) ties within natural social networks and reducing opportunities for negative social interaction.
> (p. 676)

Professionals have key roles to play in affirming the value of ties to network members and helping nudge people towards the development or renewal of ties. Professionals working in certain settings, such as schools, may have a head start in terms of organic opportunities to nurture ties unobtrusively. However, in reality, every professional has many opportunities to transmit encouraging messages about the positive potential of informal ties through social networks. Decision-makers can also serve this end by avoiding actions which may erode informal social connections for people involved (e.g. when placing children far from their home community for social or educational reasons).

The characteristics of an individual's social network may change in different ways – positively or negatively – over the course of their lifetime. In addition, the person's perception of members and their significance may vary over time and over various stages of the life course. In making professional decisions about, for example, restricting or ceasing access and contact between parents and separated children, it is important that a longer-term view is taken. Such decisions may impact in the long run on the young person's emerging social network. A point-in-time perspective as a basis for judgement has limitations. Life is more like a permanent video than a single photograph. Even the most unpromising circumstances can change dramatically, sometimes unexpectedly. The passage of time may lead to the reduction (or aggravation) of problem behaviours or the mellowing (or hardening) of attitudes. Daughters opposed to contact with their fathers in their early teens had gradually changed their mind and by late teens had begun to be interested in a stronger connection or understanding with their father. Discerning work with children and families will leave space for relations with key others to be reappraised or revived. It should also be noted that, where contact with either or both parents is suspended or blocked, this may also mean erasing contact with the relevant extended family (e.g. paternal grandparents), unless managed carefully.

Conclusions and implications

Whether as teacher, health visitor, social worker, GP, psychiatrist and so on, it is important for professionals in their overall approach to attend to the importance of social networks – their bright and dark sides. Practitioners should understand the stresses and supports, strengths and weaknesses in social networks – not only within the family or even the neighbourhood, but including significant people beyond. Network assessment can often help identify resources that will complement and aid the professional's role in problem-solving, teaching, stress relief, therapy and so on. Especially when involved with a child or family on a longer-term basis, regular 'checking' of the family's social network is useful. Positive qualities can be strengthened or energised and new opportunities identified to nurture helpful connections.

In many contexts it is valuable to be aware of and support not only individual's networks, but those present in the local area. Many sites such as leisure facilities or faith centres and roles like volunteer and employer can help stimulate social ties. Groups and meetings can bring people together for mutual support. Then it is helpful to bear in mind the value of weak as well as strong ties, bridging as well as bonding capital. In this light, support groups can benefit from diverse memberships – where support is not compromised by the risk of ghettoising, which looms where group members are exclusively composed of people with stigmatised status.

Exercise

Speak with a child or parent you are working with or know well about the key people in that person's network. Identify which relationships are perceived as emotionally supportive, helpful with practical matters, stressful, conflictual or neutral. Consider how the nature and strengths of ties could be altered for the benefit of the person concerned.

Recommended reading

The following illustrate the application of ideas about social networks and capital in social work, health and education contexts:

Gill, O. and Jack, G. (2007) *Child and Family in Context: Developing Ecological Practice in Disadvantaged Communities*, Lyme Regis: Russell House.

Morgan, A. and Haglund, B. J. A. (2009) 'Social Capital does matter for adolescent health', *Health Promotion International*, 24(4) pp. 363–72.

Fenwick, T. and Edwards, R. (2010) *Actor-Network Theory in Education*, London: Routledge.

This text considers use of material objects and technology along with human subjects.

See Hill (2002) for indications about network properties and instruments to capture them participatively.

Chapter 10

The police, the community and multi-agency work for children and young people

John Carnochan, Malcolm Hill and Raymond Taylor

Summary points

- Professionals working with children are often required to work directly or indirectly with the police.
- Community policing involves working in and with communities and is central to the delivery of effective policing in the United Kingdom.
- Besides intervention to address both crime and antisocial behaviour carried out by children and young people, police play a central role in child protection and safeguarding the welfare of children.
- Interventions to reduce levels of violence require the police to work collaboratively with other professions and in some areas utilise preventive strategies similar to public-health measures.

Introduction

Children encounter the police in a variety of ways. They will see them patrolling on foot, bicycles or by car. For many, the first direct contacts will be in school when officers deliver presentations about safety. Not uncommonly children and other family members are victims, perpetrators or witnesses of crimes that require investigation and as a result will have experience of engaging with the police in their own homes. When children are subject to ill-treatment in the home or elsewhere, the police are often called on to provide emergency protection or take them to a safe place. Hence, any professional dealing with children may need to work with the police or provide guidance and support in contacts with them.

This chapter discusses police functions both in general and with respect to children, young people and families, and outlines recent changes in approach. Different forms of collaboration with other agencies are considered. Policing in relation to child protection and violent crime gang activity are also reviewed.

The police role in general

Policing is a devolved responsibility, and separate legislation governs the police in different UK jurisdictions, though the main principles and elements are very similar. In addition to this, all statutes and police actions need to comply with the UK Human Rights Act 1998.

Since the police service was formed in the early nineteenth century, its main tasks have been to guard, watch and patrol. Their main duties[1] are to:

- prevent crime;
- protect lives and property;
- preserve peace and order;
- take lawful measures when an offence is committed and help bring offenders to justice;
- serve court warrants;
- give evidence in court.

It is important to note that the police do not prosecute – this is the responsibility of the Crown Prosecution Service (England and Wales), Procurator Fiscal (Scotland) or Public Prosecution Service (Northern Ireland). First offenders in England and Wales are normally referred to Youth Offender Panels, while children and young people in Scotland who commit offences are dealt with by the children's hearings system (see Chapter 7).

Community policing

The policy discourse across the United Kingdom is explicitly community-focused in relation to large areas of public service, such as social services, education and health. Likewise, the dominant model of policing in the UK is Community Policing. This approach is core to effective problem-solving through enforcement, public reassurance and focused response policing. As noted by MacKenzie and Hendry (2009) Community Policing has a number of distinctive characteristics which include:

- visible foot patrol;
- public/neighbourhood meetings and liaison;
- partnership working;
- public satisfaction surveys;
- neighbourhood watch coordination;
- youth work.

---

[1] see e.g. The Police (Scotland) Act 1967 Section 17.

Community Policing involves engaging in dialogue with the public and other agencies, proactively and regularly, rather than in response to incidents, in order to reduce the likelihood of crime taking place. The police are there not only to apprehend people who have committed offences but also to help and advise others and to problem-solve. The Community Policing approach recognises that protecting members of the public and preventing crime are responsibilities that need to be shared with other agencies and citizens as a whole. For example, the police work with local authorities to develop community safety strategies and give guidance to individuals and neighbourhood watch groups about 'target hardening', i.e. measures that make it harder to burgle or steal cars, for instance (Gilling 2000).

In the United Kingdom, Community Policing developed initially in the 1980s. Officers were allocated to small areas (beats) with the purpose of getting to know key people in the locality and attend community meetings. In relation to children and young people the police exercise their Community Policing responsibilities by carrying out educational and advisory functions, usually in collaboration with teachers or youth workers. This typically includes meeting youth groups and talking to children in school classes (Donnelly 2008). More recently, the Metropolitan Police in London have set up youth panels who are consulted about priorities to establish safer neighbourhoods. Also, attempts have been made to engage with young people and take account of their views at national levels. For instance, in Scotland consultation has taken place with the Youth Parliament, and a statement issued recognising young people as citizens entitled to fair and equitable treatment (Strang 2005).

In Coatbridge, Lanarkshire, Strathclyde Community Police have fostered strong links with the voluntary sector, the public sector and businesses. One Community Sergeant has been the catalyst for bringing disparate groups and interests together, thereby enriching existing community networks, developing capacity and strengthening social capital within the town (see Chapter 22). A successful venture has been the Coatbridge Festival, which replaced the traditional police open day, thereby opening out an existing, long-standing police initiative into a much broader community event. The planning that goes into the festival, and spin-off developments such as the family sports day, help build relationships across the community, benefit the local economy and contribute to a sense of civic pride. This police officer's knowledge of local young people, including those whose behaviour brings them into conflict with the law, has reinforced his determination to make a difference to the community he serves.

Child protection and safeguarding children

In England *Working Together to Safeguard Children* (2010) sets out how organisations, agencies and individuals working with children should work together to safeguard and promote their welfare in accordance with the Children Act 1989 and Children Act 2004. Similar arrangements are in place in other legal jurisdictions within the United Kingdom.

The police have a vital role to play in safeguarding children as part of their general duty to protect lives. In extreme and emergency situations, the police are often the first agency to be called as they have the powers to remove a child to a safe place if that child is in immediate danger. If a child is ill-treated by a stranger, familiar person or family member, the perpetrator will often have committed an offence such as assault or an indecent act with a minor. The police are required to investigate the alleged crime and take necessary lawful actions to deal with it. Dilemmas may arise when the police duty to pursue the offender may conflict with a child's own wishes – for example, wanting the abuse to stop but not wanting the abuser to go to jail (Beckett 2007).

It is now standard practice for allegations of harm to children to be jointly 'investigated' by police and social-work personnel. In the past, the police gathered evidence in relation to a suspected crime towards the children, while social-work services assessed and acted to protect the children. Now contacts with children and their families for both purposes are combined and coordinated, in particular to avoid duplication and reduce the stress on children. Similarly, medical assessments are carried out jointly by NHS and police doctors. If a child needs immediate medical treatment, this takes precedence over any investigative requirement.

When there are grounds for suspecting that abuse has taken place, police will be involved in information sharing and case conferences to assess the risks and needs of children who have been abused and to plan appropriate action. Chief Constables have a duty to ensure there is effective cooperation and collaboration between the police service and its child-protection partners. At times this responsibility includes identifying if organised crime is taking place, in the form of child pornography or prostitution.

When allegations of abuse are made, these are frequently responded to by specialist units that have been established within individual Police Authorities (see Example 10.1). Specialist child protection teams select officers who are able to work sensitively with distressed children and young people. Officers within these units will generally agree with their social services counterparts how individual investigations will be carried out. A number of forces have also developed child-friendly facilities where children can be interviewed in an environment that is non-threatening.

Example 10.1

In 1989 Central Scotland Police created the Family Unit as part of the first joint police and social work collaboration in the United Kingdom with a remit to deal with child protection. The Family Unit is made up of a detective sergeant, six detective constables and two acting detective constables, who operate in plain clothes and use unmarked vehicles. They work closely with colleagues in social work, health, education and a range of voluntary organisations. The unit deals with all aspects of safeguarding children, including physical, sexual and emotional abuse as well as neglect. It also acts in situations where children are living with parental drug or alcohol misuse or in environments where domestic abuse is taking place.

Young people who 'run away' from their parental home or a placement in care are at serious risk of exploitation, and not uncommonly the police are the first public agency to identify them, whether on the street or in some other location. Lancashire police constabulary have developed an initiative in partnership with care providers and local authorities to reduce the numbers of children running away from care and to minimise the negative consequences (Fitzpatrick 2009). Likewise, as part of their duty to assist where individuals in a public place may be putting themselves at risk, the police can encounter young people who self-harm or attempt suicide. Some forces (e.g. Lothian and Borders) have developed guidance and training for this, as well as protocols for cooperation with mental-health agencies.

The police role in relation to children and young people involved in crime and antisocial behaviour

Children are deemed to have criminal responsibility once they reach a certain age (10 in England and Wales, 12 in Scotland, 12 in Northern Ireland). Younger children may be dealt with under care and protection procedures when they commit 'crimes'. The police have duties to investigate alleged crimes and the power to charge offenders when there is legal ground to do so. They will normally give evidence in subsequent hearings. If a court issues a warrant to secure the attendance of a young person, then the police will seek out the individual and accompany him/her to court. Besides dealing with offences and offenders, the police also have a responsibility to prevent crime, which requires different forms of intervention discussed in a later section of this chapter.

Since the Police and Criminal Evidence Act 1984,[2] children and young people being interviewed by the police have been entitled to legal advice and to support from an appropriate adult (often a parent, but sometimes a trusted professional). In England and Wales measures were put in place to strengthen the training and accreditation of lawyers who took on the legal representative role (see Chapter 13). Observations of such interviews have shown that legal advisers and parents are often passive, leading to concern that young people may need better or different kinds of assistance to state their position and avoid incriminating statements. The role to be adopted by an appropriate adult is uncertain. Research in Northern Ireland revealed different perspectives on this and sometimes serious tensions among legal advisers, social workers, parents, young people and police (Quinn and Jackson 2007).

In lieu of charging, the police are able to give official reprimands or warnings,[3] normally to young people who have committed minor offences, are remorseful and/or are relatively new to offending. Warnings are usually issued by a senior police officer at a police station in the presence of a parent. Their aim is to stress the importance of the wrong-doing, even though no formal charge is being made, and to deter from future offending.

[2] In Northern Ireland the Police and Criminal Evidence (NI) Order 1989.
[3] Warnings only in Scotland.

A prominent innovation over the past 20 years in response to both adult and youth crime has been the approach known as 'restorative justice' (see Chapter 7). The key idea is that, instead of or in addition to formal action, the offender is encouraged to make some kind of reparation or expression of regret either to the victim of the crime or to the wider community. One option is that a meeting or restorative conference is arranged and facilitated by specially trained police or a mediation agency. Here a young offender and their victim meet, each with a supporter they have chosen (Hoyle 2008; Liebmann 2008). Victims who have participated in restorative justice conferences have mostly reported high satisfaction. Restorative justice has been particularly widely used in Northern Ireland, where the Justice (NI) Act 2002 introduced youth conferences for all types of offence (Hoyle 2008). In England and Wales, Youth Offender Panels may agree a contract including an act of reparation. Some schools also use a restorative conference approach to deal with bullying and violent behaviour.

In relation to antisocial behaviour, police and community support officers in England, Wales and Northern Ireland may enter into a contract with parents. They can order groups to disperse or individuals to desist, failure to do so being a criminal offence. Also on-the-spot fines can be issued to anyone over 16 (over 10 in some areas).

Cooperation with other agencies and the community

In 1996 the Association of Chief Police Officers (ACPO) in England and Wales adopted a policy committed to partnership with other agencies and a focus on crime prevention. The subsequent Crime and Disorder Act 1998 promoted partnership working and this has been a feature of legislation and policy ever since. ACPO policy on children and young people (2010) recognises that a significant minority of young people lack confidence in the police, and that enforcement has limitations and early intervention is desirable. The ACPO strategy commits the police to working in partnership with other agencies in line with *Every Child Matters* (see Chapter 1). ACPO adopted a tiered approach similar to that used by health services. This begins with core activities appropriate for all children and young people and progresses from targeted services to specialist and priority intervention. In certain places police have worked with community organisations to reduce abuse, assaults and property damage, as in the Southwark Mediation Centre Hate Crimes Project (Liebmann 2008).

In Scotland the Local Government Scotland Act 2003 places a statutory obligation for the police to work in partnership with local communities. Additionally, *Getting it Right for Every Child* requires the police to work closely with other agencies through early intervention so that children obtain help when they need it to reduce the likelihood of future problems, including offending.

In relation to some matters (such as safeguarding children) the police have an important role in inter-agency collaboration but others take the lead, whereas the police usually dominate crime prevention partnerships (Gilling 2000). The police play a major part in Youth Offending Teams, while legislation introduced by the last Labour government required the police to work with local authorities to produce strategies for dealing with antisocial behaviour. The police work with local authorities, prison service and health boards with respect to violent and sexual offenders through a strategic body known as Multi-Agency Public Protection Arrangements (MAPPA). This reflects the community, preventive and partnership themes noted above. The Scottish Police Service has developed a protocol with the Crown Office and Procurator Fiscal Service in relation to domestic abuse. This promotes best practice and consistency of approach in the investigation, reporting and prosecution of cases, with a view to improving the service particularly to victims.

Campus policing and relationships with young people

School liaison is a long-established practice. Police officers regularly visit schools with an explicit remit to promote awareness of road safety, drugs or stranger danger. These visits also serve to promote a positive image of the police not linked to arresting criminals. Research by Hoare et al. (2010) noted that the vast majority of children (83 per cent) had seen a police officer or community support officer in or around their school – and provides evidence of the effectiveness of these interventions. Further to this, many extended and community schools have a police officer present on a full- or part-time basis (see Chapter 11). In parts of Scotland an intensive form of campus policing occurs, with part of the cost paid for by local authority educational services. A school cluster (secondary and associated primary and nursery schools) has a dedicated police officer, who is based there and takes part in the School Management team. Campus officers spend a lot of time interacting with children – formally in class and informally at break times. The campus police officers may help with Duke of Edinburgh and other awards and activities. They also attend parents' evenings to be available to give information and advice. Not only do the friendly relations enable the police to engage better with families, but they also gain early intelligence about potential crimes or gang activities from children, teachers or local shopkeepers. Another key role that has been identified is the transition from primary to secondary school, where a police officer can assure Primary 7 pupils that he/she will be a familiar face when they move up to secondary school.

An independent evaluation of campus officers revealed that many teachers, parents and children were initially concerned that officers would become involved in school discipline, focus on gathering intelligence or give the school a bad reputation, but such worries soon disappeared to be replaced by positive feedback (Black et al. 2010). The presence of police increased feelings of safety among both pupils and staff. As Brown notes, police were able to spend time with groups of children in a range of activities. Campus officers also gave helpful information to staff and advice to parents. As other research has shown (Norman 2009), however, children's favourable attitudes to the individual officers on campus did not necessarily generalise to the police more widely.

Getting to know children and young people informally helps build positive relationships. Research has shown that young people tend to view the police favourably when they have contacts unrelated to suspected crime or antisocial behaviour, but a significant minority hold negative views either because they resent the police intervening in actual criminal behaviour or because they feel unfairly picked on as suspects (McAra and McVie 2005; Norman 2009). This has been prominent among black and minority ethnic populations in areas where they feel they are singled out for attention and body searches (Sharp and Atherton 2007).

Antipathy also tends to be greater in parts of Northern Ireland on account of the political history. One study found that over 40 per cent of young people living in North Belfast said they had been stopped and questioned for what they felt was no reason, or experienced verbal harassment by the police (Byrne et al. 2005). Another study in Northern Ireland found that a majority regarded the police as honest and helpful, but many saw them as disrespectful and one-fifth said they had themselves been treated in an unacceptable way (Radford et al. 2005). The perceived power of the police and the pressure on officers to seek evidence and confessions make it inherently difficult to establish open and honest communication in encounters where young people are suspected of a crime or believe this to be the case (Drury and Dennison 1999). The police across the UK have attempted to overcome such tensions by seeking to establish friendly relationships in non-adversarial situations. When young people feel that officers listen to their concerns, then confidence in the police improves (Norman 2009).

In the remainder of this chapter we deal with two subjects that have evoked widespread public and media concern – violent crime and gang activity.

Violent crime and children and young people

Across the UK, levels of reported crime have come down steadily since the mid-1990s. This is based not on convictions, which cover only a small proportion of crime, but on population-wide reports. Homicides have decreased. Violent crime has also decreased, but less rapidly. These trends apply to both adult and youth crime (Pople and Smith 2010).

Children can commit violent offences and can also be victims of crimes committed by adults or other children. Commonly the same individual child will be both offender and victim, whether on a single occasion (by taking part in a fight) or on different occasions. Violent crime is a particular problem in Scotland, where, for instance, young men aged 10–29 are five times more likely to be victims of homicide than in England and Wales.

Violent crime can have a serious impact on victims, many of whom are children. The crucial element of violent acts to qualify as crimes is an intention to harm. The law specifies a spectrum of violent crimes from assault to murder. In this regard bullying can be a crime.

Only 30 to 50 per cent of violent assaults known to accident and emergency services are reported to the police (Sheridan and Moller 2005). Many children are seen at hospital as a result of attacks, almost half of which took place in school (Carnochan and McCluskey 2010). The Home Office and ACPO have sought to improve notifications by hospitals of knife-induced injuries, to facilitate understanding of the problems and helping responses. In Cardiff and parts of Scotland questionnaires are completed about injuries resulting from violence.

Towards a new coordinated approach to violence

It has been recognised that simply responding to alleged crimes or assaults is not an effective policy, and it is this insight that has driven the Community Policing model discussed earlier. For example, it is known that many crimes do not come to the attention of the police and some perpetrators are not caught. Some of the people who evade formal charges may pose a bigger risk than those who are caught. For these reasons it is important to understand the circumstances that lead to criminality and tackle the underlying causes. In short, it is better to think and act preventively and work with teachers, health professionals, social workers and others so that children are less likely to be violent.

Following research about the high level of violent crime in the west of Scotland, Strathclyde Police set up a Violence Reduction Unit (VRU) in 2005 and it became a national unit in 2006, with the remit to target all forms of violence, from bullying to suicide. Violence to and by children and young people is a prominent part of its work.

The VRU has adopted a public-health model with a focus on communities and populations as a whole to promote community health to prevent the 'disease' of violence from occurring or recurring (World Health Organisation 2002; Carnochan and McCluskey 2010). A public-health model involves the utilisation of research evidence about causes of violence and factors that increase or decrease the risk of violence, in order to devise ways of preventing it. As far as possible interventions should also be based on evidence of effectiveness. This approach requires working with other agencies to tackle the root causes of violence, particularly in localities that police intelligence shows to have high rates of associated difficulties such as drug or alcohol misuse and trafficking (Carnochan and McCluskey 2010). Another aspect of violence-reduction work is advancing public awareness about the nature and causes of violence.

The VRU places emphasis on early intervention, since research shows that the tendency to violence is often acquired at a young age (Tremblay 2010) and is more difficult to tackle once it has become entrenched behaviour in an individual or group (see Example 10.2 at end of chapter). Initiatives that promote parental sensitivity and empathy can be critical in households where poverty and aggressive relationships are rife (see Chapter 18). Similarly, violence intervention strategies, including anger and stress-management programmes, are required in locations where violence comes to the attention of agencies other than the police, notably hospitals and surgeries.

As in health promotion work, several levels of prevention are recognised:

- **Primary prevention** – preventing violence or other antisocial behaviour from occurring in the first place. Focused on children from pre-birth through to high school age and their parents, services include parent support and education programmes, intensive pre- and postnatal support, early years' enrichment.

■ **Secondary prevention** – preventing the escalation of violence and antisocial behaviour toward serious criminality. Focused on children of secondary school age (11–18). Activities range from offering positive educational/recreational opportunities for young people to more formal youth justice measures.

■ **Tertiary prevention** – preventing violent offenders reoffending, e.g. through offender programmes within prison or coordinated by Criminal Justice Authorities in the community.

Many of these preventive initiatives rely on vital input from education, health or social work professionals. For instance, a key feature of young people living in deprived estates is the poverty of employment prospects, with children often failing to acquire at school the 'soft skills' and cultural capital necessary to be accepted for the jobs that are available (Warhurst and Nickson 2007).

Gangs

It is important to recognise that the media and others may exaggerate the significance of gangs, and label phenomena as gang activities when they are not (Alexander 2008). Mostly when young people 'hang out' in groups, they are chatting or enjoying themselves with no intention to threaten others, even though some adults will feel concerned. The great majority of young people do not belong to gangs and most of those who engage in offending as part of groups are not in a gang.

Nevertheless, gangs of young people in the sense of coherent and persistent groups with a propensity to commit crime and threaten perceived outsiders have been a prominent feature of large cities in the UK and elsewhere for many decades. Over 150 gangs are thought to exist in London (Alexander 2008), while around 55 gangs were recently identified in the East End of Glasgow alone, with 600+ members altogether (VRU 2010). Use of crime pattern analysis indicates that the nature of gang activity in Glasgow has changed considerably in the past 5–10 years. There are fewer inter-gang fights and less defending of territories.

Gangs may be based on area of residence, religion, football club allegiance or ethnicity. Some have names, structures and history that have persisted over several generations of members (Alexander 2008; Broadhurst et al. 2009; Deuchar 2009). Most young people in gangs are boys, but some girls belong too, having learned aggression from parents and others as a means of survival in 'rough' areas (Batchelor 2009).

Gangs provide members with friendships, a sense of belonging and protection. These membership benefits act as a considerable barrier to giving up, unless an alternative support network and lifestyle are available. Many gangs engage mainly in low-level troublesome behaviour, but some are aggressive to non-members and especially to those seen as part of hostile or rival gangs. In certain areas knives and guns are carried and sometimes used. This has resulted in high-profile murders, usually of other children, in places like London, Liverpool and Glasgow (Alexander 2008). Attacks and injuries lead some to give up weapons, but result in others thinking these are vital for defence (Bannister et al. 2010). Parents and children living in areas with territorial gangs cite them as one of the main threats to their children's well-being and as seriously restricting the times and places where younger children may safely play or traverse (Turner et al. 2006). Gangs rarely originate in schools, but in a minority of schools they contribute to incidents of absence and violence, as well as impacting on journeys to and from school (Broadhurst et al. 2009).

Police responses to gang activity

Until recently police reacted to gangs by dealing with individuals involved as offenders (arrest) or victims (support). Now the approach is more group-based and preventive by 'getting in among them'. The aim has shifted from attempting to break up gangs or remove members to altering their behaviour in a pro-social direction. This involves challenging gang members to stop violence, and making available alternative activities like football and basketball, especially at the times of day and week when gang members would otherwise be at a loose end. One such initiative in Dumfries and Galloway received favourable reports from young people and was followed by a reduction in complaints about the police (Donnelly 2008). Some individuals will be referred to specialist agencies for intensive support and others to violence-reduction programmes. A police presence in schools can help to defuse incidents, disperse groups and aid information-sharing with teachers (Broadhurst et al. 2009).

Several police forces in cities like London and Manchester have set up special units to tackle gangs or violence more widely. Glasgow's Community Initiative to Reduce Violence (CIRV) has deployed a range of ways to reduce violence by adults and children (Carnochan and McCluskey 2010; VRU 2010):

- intelligence gathering and analysis;
- intensive engagement with gang members seeking pledges to give up violence;
- dispersing groups who cause alarm or distress and directing young people to youth clubs and groups;
- mentoring;
- help accessing educational and employment opportunities;
- diversionary football league on Friday evenings (managed by a private company);
- enforcement operations against persistent offenders (targeting and arrest).

Violence by members of these gangs who engaged with CIRV decreased by one-half in a year, compared with an 18 per cent reduction for those who did not engage.

The CIRV was modelled on 'problem-oriented policing' developed in Boston and Cincinnati which combines a stick and carrot approach. This includes strong enforcement of the law (zero tolerance of violence) with multi-agency work and diversionary activities. Such work may be conceptualised in terms of social capital (see Chapter 22), which recognises that gangs provide young people in deprived areas with compensatory support, inclusion and identity, so that intervention should aim to provide different means of obtaining such resources through social and educational initiatives (Deuchar 2009).

Through CIRV in Glasgow, police are working closely with partners in health, education, social work, community safety, housing and the local community to help young gang members find a way out of their violent lifestyle. This change will not happen quickly – breaking out of a pattern of behaviour is hard and will not happen overnight. While it will be some time before it is known how successful the work of CIRV has been, evidence so far suggests that considerably less violent behaviour is occurring among those young people from the East End of Glasgow who, despite their often very violent past, have pledged to change their behaviour and engage with the CIRV programme.

Conclusions and implications

To protect children from abuse, reduce crime and violence, the police, other agencies and voluntary groups must work more closely, establishing partnership arrangements that are founded on delivering positive outcomes rather than being designed to make the jobs of professionals easier or the cost of services cheaper. Information-sharing is a fundamental component of effective partnerships and this requires good relationships among the individuals involved, with working arrangements that respect each agency's role and remit while at the same time acknowledging the importance of shared values.

The police often have vital information that can assist others in a better awareness of situations, in order to understand the risks involved. They can also provide advice and where necessary take law-enforcement action. However, in the long run problematic behaviour will only be reduced through the actions of individuals, families, schools and other agencies in the community. Real change will require action at individual, community and societal levels.

In this example based on intelligence compiled by the police on an anonymised real case, we see show how individual, family and neighbourhood factors and life events combine to predispose an individual towards violence.

Example 10.2 David's story

David was born to a mother who was dependant on alcohol. During early childhood, David and his family moved several times, mainly as a result of domestic abuse, always living in socially deprived wards. Nursery staff were concerned about poor care at home. For a time David lived with grandparents. Also living in that house were three adults who between them had over 120 previous convictions mostly for drugs, violence and dishonesty. At secondary school David started to get involved in local gangs, was a frequent truant and was disruptive when present. He was described as being 'outwith parental control'. During his teens he abused solvents, broke into houses and stole cars. He was eventually charged with multiple violent offences and sent to prison.

Exercise

Consider Example 10.2. Which kinds of agencies and professionals would have had contact with David and his family at different points in time? Remember adult and family services (like housing) as well as those with a focus on children. When might the police have been involved and for what reasons? How might coordinated action have modified David's journey into crime and violence?

Recommended reading

Mackenzie and Hendry (2009) provides an overview of Community Policing.

ACPO (2010) sets out principles for police work with children and young people.

Wallis and Tudor (2008) offer a useful guide to the principles and methods of restorative meetings and referral orders.

Violence Reduction Unit (2010) discusses strategies to tackle violence.

Chapter 11

Teachers working with the community and other professionals: full service and extended schools

Alan Dyson

Summary points

- Schools in many countries offer services and activities to children, families and communities over and above their core role of teaching students in classrooms.
- Such 'full service and extended schools' have the potential to make significant contributions to the lives of children and families experiencing disadvantage.
- They have less to offer as a way to raise attainment in the short term.
- Their potential can be maximised through thoughtful design and planning, targeting and evaluation.
- More might be achieved if their work were aligned with an overarching area approach to disadvantage.
- Schools also need to escape from the deficit perspectives they tend to use.
- The emergence of these schools raises important issues about the relationship between schools and other community agencies, and about the respective roles of teachers and other professionals.

Introduction

In countries across the world, schools are being developed that look beyond their classrooms and try to engage with the whole of their students' lives. While their main concern remains with teaching and learning, they see the way their students learn as inseparable from how they develop as people, and therefore from the lives they lead outside the classroom, among their friendship groups, in their families and in their communities. For these schools, therefore, it is not enough to teach well. They must also do what they can to ensure that children are healthy, confident and socially adept, that their families are stable and supportive, and that the places where children live are safe, well-resourced and rich with opportunities. It is, of course, impossible for schools to achieve all of this on their own. They therefore develop partnerships with other children's services, with community agencies and organisations and with local businesses. For some of them, this means that they change from being institutions whose sole task is to educate children to being agents in the development of whole communities.

Such schools have appeared in a wide range of countries including the USA, Canada and the Netherlands. They go by many names – full service schools, community schools, broad schools, all-day schools. In the absence of an agreed name, I use the term 'full service and extended schools' in this chapter. They have also emerged in the different administrations of the UK – as extended schools in England, full service and extended schools in Northern Ireland, integrated community schools in Scotland and community-focused schools in Wales. The range of names signals different emphases, and variations occur even within the same administration. In some places, the schools focus particularly on children's learning. In others, they focus on health, or leisure and cultural activities or on opening up their facilities to community use.

While this responsiveness to local conditions makes sense for schools that are trying to engage with families and communities in particular areas, it raises important questions for those who are going to lead such schools, and for the teachers and other professionals who are going to work in them. In particular, in the absence of a single, proven model, how can schools know what they should be offering, or how effective their work is likely to be, or even what it is they should be trying to achieve? It is with these questions that this chapter is concerned.

Full service and extended schools in action: some examples

Despite the variations between schools and across administrations, there is a recognisable pattern in the forms of provision that most full service and extended schools offer. The definition of 'community-focused' schools provided by the National Assembly for Wales (2003: 3) captures the essence of this as well as any:

> A community-focused school is one that provides a range of services and activities, often beyond the school day, to help meet the needs of its pupils, their families and the wider community.

We can see what this means in practice in the example of 'Clark' school, one of the participants in the 'full service extended' schools initiative which ran in England between 2003 and 2006 (Cummings et al. 2011).

Example 11.1 Clark School

Clark is a non-selective school for secondary age (11+) students serving a large, highly disadvantaged, inner-city catchment area. The community it serves had, school leaders reported, experienced decline, neglect, low levels of aspiration and adults who had a poor experience of education. These conditions were echoed in the school where, according to teachers, many students displayed signs of low self-esteem and low aspirations, while levels of attainment were poor. In response, the school focused heavily on providing students with support to deal with their personal and social problems. During the initiative it developed a much wider range of provision. This included:

▶

- An on-site multi-professional team focusing on students' behaviour and well-being, that is able to work with students in the school and in its feeder primaries, and with families. The team comprised a nurse, an 'emotional well-being' worker (social-work trained), an 'inclusion' officer, learning mentors, family support worker and the school's full service coordinator.
- A community police officer based in the school and partnerships with a wide range of local agencies.
- An 'alternative curriculum' off-site for older students who were not doing well in the mainstream curriculum.
- A student support centre on site offering personalised curriculum opportunities and learning mentor support.
- A breakfast club where students could eat before the start of the school day.
- A school radio station, with broadcasts planned and presented by students.
- 'Learning for life days' focused on a range of broader issues affecting children, such as sexual health.
- A luncheon club for elderly residents, run at a local community centre by students following the alternative curriculum, a senior citizens club on the school premises and plans to provide adult learning opportunities.

Although different full-service and extended schools might not offer precisely the same pattern of services and activities as Clark, they tend to select from a common menu of provision. Many offer extra-curricular activities to extended the range of children's learning opportunities and engage them in ways the standard curriculum might not. They stay open for longer hours and more weeks in the year. Most – particularly in highly disadvantaged areas – provide non-educational services to promote children's all-round development and address problems that might interfere with their learning. They develop partnerships with non-educational agencies to provide these services. Many seek to engage families with their children's learning and to support them through any difficulties they might experience. In addition, some work with community members and organisations to mobilise resources to support children and to make the school's resources available to the community.

What can full service and extended schools achieve?

Because full service and extended schools are very diverse in aims and methods, evaluating outcomes from such schools is challenging. Nonetheless, there is convincing evidence that they can, under favourable conditions, have some important impacts (Cummings et al. 2007, Cummings et al. 2011). In particular, they can help children facing significant disadvantages to stay 'on track'. They can support them with their personal and family problems, re-engage them with education where that engagement has been lost, help them to achieve useful skills and qualifications and ensure that they move on from school towards further education, training or employment. For some children, the intervention of the school maybe literally life-changing. Schools can have similar impacts on parents and families. They help stabilise families, build the confidence of parents, help them see themselves as learners and place them on a trajectory towards gaining qualifications and, ultimately, gaining employment. In turn, parents are likely to be more confident and effective in supporting their children's learning.

There is evidence of less dramatic, but nonetheless important 'cultural' effects on wider school populations. Students can begin to feel more positively about themselves, take on leadership roles and experience an enriched range of learning opportunities. The ethos of the school and the nature of students' engagement with the school can, accordingly, begin to change. Similarly, there is evidence of actual and potential impacts at community level. Adults facing significant disadvantages can, like parents, be set on upward trajectories of growing confidence, qualifications and employability. More generally, it seems likely that the consistent availability of full service and extended provision will, over time, have wider effects across whole communities and will contribute towards making the areas served by schools safer, more cohesive, more attractive to employers and so richer in opportunities.

Finally, there is clear evidence that full service and extended provision brings benefits to schools as institutions. Partly, this is because schools acquire more positive local reputations, find it easier to persuade families to send their children there and are able to marshal a wider range of resources in dealing with children's difficulties. Partly, it is because becoming a full service or extended school is often part of an overall package of school development which produces rises in overall levels of performance as measured by student attainments, behaviour and attendance. It is not unusual for schools to embark on the development of full service provision because they have reached a crisis point in their existence, and to complete that process as thriving and popular institutions.

It seems clear that full service and extended schools achieve the most significant of these impacts through a combination of access to children and their families and multiple streams of intervention that other agencies find hard to replicate. We can see what this means in practice in case Example 11.2, which is an account by a Connexions (careers advice service) worker of what it was possible to do for a troubled and troublesome girl in a full service extended school in England.

Example 11.2 'Clara's' story

Clara was referred in Year 9. Her behaviour in school was aggressive towards teachers and staff. She wasn't staying in lessons. She was a substance misuser, was disaffected with school and at risk of exclusion. So the work I did involved home visits so that parents were involved, and I did self-esteem and anger-management sessions [with the pupil] and linked in with the inclusion team so she could do four GCSEs in the unit [the inclusion unit in school where students get 1:1 support to complete GCSEs] and I supported her to and from her work placement. I also referred her to the substance misuse worker who comes into school . . . The inclusion team and I got her a taster course at an FE college in hairdressing and beauty so her timetable was a flexible package, so she did this and had sessions to do her GCSEs . . . When she left Year 11 she came here [the school] to apply to do an NVQ in early years. Her attendance has been brilliant and now she is looking to work in social care and I've linked her with the social worker [in the FSES] to get a grounding in the job . . . It's really boosted her self-esteem and she is now thinking of helping other young people who she says 'were like me'. It's so great when it goes like this. It's the multi-agency staff that's given this input.

(adapted from Cummings et al. 2007: 52–53) Crown copyright material is reproduced with permission under the terms of the Click-Use License

What we see here is that, like all schools, full service and extended schools have regular, direct access to children as part of their core educational business, and can fairly readily extend this so that they have access to families. Problems in children's lives often show themselves in classrooms, perhaps in the form of misbehaviour. While most schools have limited resources with which to respond to those problems, full service and extended schools typically employ a range of staff who can work with children and their families outside classrooms and off the school site. They also tend to have access to professionals from other agencies who are based at the school or who work closely with the school. This means that they can tackle underlying child and family problems by deploying a range of professionals working from a variety of perspectives. In this case, for instance, the counselling offered by the Connexions worker is supplemented by specialist input from a substance abuse worker, a modified curriculum, work experience and social work support.

There is often little in terms of the individual interventions that full service and extended schools typically deploy that is different in kind from the standard practices of child and family services. The key seems to be that interventions are not deployed singly, but in clusters. Provided these clusters are well-targeted, they can be mutually supportive, so that gains in one domain – say, anger management in this case – can be supported by benefits elsewhere – in family dynamics, say, or in engagement with learning. Moreover, because of the partnerships they build up with other agencies, full service and extended schools are able to marshal such holistic interventions speedily, and without the need for lengthy referral procedures. This means that early intervention (doing something before problems reach crisis point) becomes a realistic option rather than simply an unattainable ideal. So in this case we see interventions being deployed before the girl is excluded rather than afterwards, when it might have been too late. It also means that interventions are possible for a much larger population than those who would receive services through the traditional referral routes, which tend to filter out all but the most acute cases.

Limitations of full service and extended schools

Despite the great potential of full service and extended schools, it is important to recognise what they are unable or unlikely to achieve. Research has identified two major limitations in these schools' achievements. First, although attainments often rise rapidly as schools develop their approaches, there is little evidence that it is the full service and extended provision itself which brings about these rises. Evaluations of full service and extended schools in the UK, for instance, have found rises in overall levels of school performance but only limited (if any) gains in student attainment relative to schools elsewhere (Cummings et al. 2007, Sammons et al. 2003). Likewise, in the USA a combination of school reform and out-of-school services in the much-trumpeted Harlem Children's Zone (Tough 2008) has produced significant gains in attainment for children attending the Zone's schools – yet siblings who receive the same services but attend unreformed schools outside the Zone show no such gains (Dobbie and Fryer 2009, Whitehurst and Croft 2010).

The explanation seems to be that schools develop their full service and extended approaches as part of an overall package of reform. The package as a whole can bring about dramatic rises in overall school performance, but it seems likely to be the within-school changes that make the short-term difference, rather than the additional services. In systems where schools are under pressure to drive up their performance, many schools will be engaging in such changes. Full service provision is probably best seen as a complement to these efforts, rather than as an alternative. Its role is not to bring about short-term hikes in attainment, but to promote a longer-term engagement with learning, and to secure the all-round well-being of students, families and communities.

The second set of limitations is to do with the capacity of full service and extended schools to make a substantial difference to social and educational inequality. As critics of other efforts to tackle this issue have pointed out (Power et al. 2005, Rees et al. 2007), there is little prospect that interventions at neighbourhood or area level will make much difference to widespread inequalities that have their origins in underlying social and economic structures. Giving schools some limited extra funding so that they can employ adults other than teachers or reconfiguring existing services around schools is unlikely on its own to have much impact on the gross inequalities between social groups or between areas. This is not to say that full service and extended schools cannot have important ameliorative effects, particularly at the level of targeted individuals and families. However, they cannot substitute for strenuous efforts at national – even international – level to create a fairer society.

How full service and extended schools can become more effective

There is now enough experience internationally with full service and extended schools for it to be clear what makes such schools more and less successful (see, for instance, Coalition for Community Schools (no date), Cummings et al. 2007, Dryfoos et al. 2005). One key feature would seem to be clarity of purpose. Obvious as it might sound, schools need to know what they are doing – or, more accurately, *why* they are doing what they are doing (Cummings et al. 2011). When schools begin to develop full service provision, particularly in the context of funded initiatives, they are typically presented with multiple opportunities to set up activities and services. The temptation is to develop these opportunities in an *ad hoc* manner, seizing on those that are closest to hand, or seem most likely to solve a short-term problem. The consequence is that a random array of provision is developed that has no core purpose and, very often, is unsustainable in the longer term. It is important, therefore, that schools develop their provision in a careful and coherent manner. This implies widening the focus of decision-making from planning how to get things done – something at which school leaders tend already to be adept – to thinking more deeply about how any actions relate to aims and outcomes.

There are a number of planning frameworks that can help with such a process, but the use of approaches such as logic modelling and theory of change seems particular appropriate (Kellogg Foundation 2004, Connell and Klem 2000). These approaches are often described as 'theory-based' because they focus not just on practicalities, but also on the assumptions and hypotheses, which form the theory underpinning action. They call for a searching analysis of the situation that the school faces, an identification of the outcomes that are aimed at in the long term, and a clear articulation of how, precisely, the action that is planned will change the situation over time to produce these outcomes.

A second key factor in success is a schools' ability to target disadvantage effectively. Most (though not all) full service and extended schools serve populations facing significant economic deprivation and the social and educational disadvantages which arise from that deprivation. Typically, therefore, they try to target many of their services and activities on those children and families facing greatest difficulties, but often in a somewhat *ad hoc* way (Cummings et al. 2010). A more robust targeting process is needed, which draws on 'objective' data as well as personal knowledge and which is clear about why particular children and families are targeted for particular interventions. This is, of course, much more straightforward where the school has already developed a robust 'theory' to underpin its provision. Moreover, simply making provision available is not enough. Schools and their partners typically have to work hard over sustained periods of time to ensure that the children and families access the services and activities from which they are likely to benefit. A lengthy process of trust building is often necessary, and involves the school in going more than half way to engage people who might initially be suspicious or lacking in confidence.

It is important for schools to be able to manage resources in creative and efficient ways. Frequently, full service provision depends on a multiplicity of short-term and unsustainable funding arrangements. Schools need, therefore, to develop a more coherent, long-term resourcing strategy. This might involve designating a staff member other than the head or principal as the coordinator of full service provision, with the explicit task of pursuing sources of funding. Even more important, it might involve identifying resources other than financial ones, particularly in the form of expertise and personnel from other agencies. It follows that building partnerships with other agencies is a major strategy that schools can use to ensure the sustainability of their provision (Cummings et al. 2011). Such partnerships, however, take time – sometimes many years – to develop, and they depend on the partners becoming convinced that it is in their mutual interest to work collaboratively.

Schools also need to know how to use their resources to maximum effect, and to demonstrate to governments and other resource providers that their investments are worthwhile. This is particularly challenging given that the multi-stranded nature of full service provision and the lack of good measures for many of its intended outcomes make it difficult to know 'what works'. Schools can deal with this challenge at the planning stage by ensuring that individual components of provision are, so far as possible, evidence-based and that the 'theory' underpinning the school's work is coherent. They can also do this as provision unfolds by ensuring that it is supported by evaluation. The theory-based approach to planning can play a dual role by forming the basis of a 'theory of change' evaluation (Dyson and Todd 2010). Once the intended outcomes of provision are identified, it becomes possible to think about the kinds of outcome measures that are appropriate to what the school is actually trying to achieve, rather than assuming that attainment outcomes are all that matter. Likewise, once there is a clear articulation of how particular actions are expected to produce those outcomes, it becomes possible to assess whether or not those changes are taking place long before the outcomes themselves become apparent. External evaluation is lengthy and is often not affordable. Schools themselves can monitor changes using data they have, like participation rates in services and activities, feedback on participant satisfaction, case histories of children and families, reports from class teachers on children's achievements and behaviour.

Finally, the success of full service provision is likely to depend heavily on the nature and quality of leadership in the school. While all school leaders need to be focused on improving teaching and learning, those in full service and extended schools must additionally act on the basis of a principled commitment to tackling disadvantage, promoting equity and seeing their schools as engines for social justice, rather than simply as mechanisms for enabling students to pass academic tests (Cummings et al. 2007, Muijs et al. 2008). In particular, this implies a willingness to develop real partnerships with other agencies and schools serving the local area, rather than seeing their school as an autonomous institution pursuing its own interests in isolation.

Beyond full service and extended schools

Where schools display this combination of principled leadership, clarity of purpose, skill in targeting and resource management, and evaluative capacity much can be achieved. Despite this, however, there is a fundamental reservation about whether such a school-centric approach is the best route to take in tackling social and educational disadvantage. Although school leaders are often enthusiastic about what they can achieve, there are, as we have seen, real doubts about whether schools have the capacity to make much difference to deep-rooted social and educational inequalities. Even at the local level, there is not much that they can do to increase people's income, create employment opportunities, build better houses, reduce crime levels or establish better transport links for disconnected estates and neighbourhoods. Moreover, the approaches adopted by schools are typically shaped not by the children, families and communities on whose behalf they supposedly work, but by education professionals who sometimes appear to hold somewhat negative, deficit-oriented views of local people (Cummings et al. 2011).

It may be, therefore, that the next stage in the development of full service provision will be to move away from a school-centric approach towards more strategic approaches located at area (neighbourhood, say, or local authority) level. Such approaches should involve schools closely, but need not be driven by school leaders' priorities, nor restricted to what can be provided in and by the school. 'Area-based' initiatives have a long history in the UK and are far from unproblematic (Lupton 2010). Nonetheless, they make it possible for a wider range of resources to be deployed than those that can be marshalled by the school, and for an area's needs to be considered from many more perspectives than that of education professionals. The Harlem Children's Zone, referred to above, is an example of what an area approach might look like. However, the recent emphasis in the UK on integrated services and 'joined up' policy has given rise to many less well-publicised examples in the UK, often – though by no means always – led by local authorities (e.g. Barnsley Metropolitan Borough Council 2005, Knowsley Council 2008, Rowley and Dyson 2011).

Moving away from school-centric approaches means, of course, that non-education professionals help to shape strategy, bringing to bear different sorts of knowledge of the local area informed by different kinds of interactions with local people. This is likely to moderate the negative views that are sometimes found in schools. There are other ways in which education professionals can avoid falling into the trap of focusing exclusively on the supposed deficits of the disadvantaged populations they seek to serve. So-called 'assets-based' approaches to community development are well-established outside the world of education (Foot and Hopkins 2010), but their principles apply equally to school–family–community relations. In other words, the focus of schools' work might be on how to build on the capacity of local people to tackle their own problems, on tackling the environmental barriers to their using their strengths, and on maximising the opportunities for them to lead productive and fulfilled lives. Again, there are many examples in the UK and beyond of such approaches beginning to emerge, and of new sets of relationships developing between schools and the people they serve. In these examples, local people become co-producers of solutions with professionals rather than simply the beneficiaries of their benevolence (Cummings et al. 2011, Mediratta et al. 2009). As a result, schools come to be seen less as hubs from which professionals deliver the services they deem to be necessary and more as resources that families and communities can use to improve the quality of their own lives. This can apply in any area, not just disadvantaged neighbourhoods. The ultimate implication, therefore, is that full service and extended schools become a universal resource rather than one targeted only at those who are most disadvantaged.

Conclusions and implications

In this chapter we have seen how schools in many countries are offering additional services and activities to children, families and communities. Such 'full service and extended schools' may not offer a 'quick fix' for raising attainment in the short term. However, they have the potential to make significant contributions to the lives of children and families experiencing disadvantage. This potential can be maximised when:

■ they are based on a robust and explicit 'theory' of how they will generate their outcomes;

■ they target carefully those children and families who might benefit most;

■ they are able to monitor and demonstrate the effectiveness of their provision.

More might be achieved, however, if the focus shifted from what such schools can provide towards how their work can be aligned with an overarching area approach to disadvantage. More again might be achieved if schools could escape from the deficit perspectives they often apply to the people they are trying to support, and instead engage in a more balanced process of partnership and co-production with those people.

This has significant implications for the teachers and para-professionals who work in schools, and for professionals in community agencies working alongside schools. Over the past ten to twenty years, many countries have tried to focus the attention of teachers and school leaders on teaching and learning – or, more specifically, on ensuring that students perform well in national and international assessments. However, it is far from clear that schools should *only*, or even *primarily*, be about helping students to pass tests. It is arguable that their role should be to help children learn and develop more holistically than a focus on attainment suggests and, indeed, that they should have a role as a resource for the communities they serve and, more generally, as agents of social change.

This, of course, has implications for how other agencies relate to schools – and vice versa. If schools are simply concerned with attainment then they can either operate in isolation from other services or they can see those agencies as instruments for tackling whatever non-educational barriers students face. On the other hand, if schools have a broader social role then some sort of close partnership with other agencies is essential, together with shared decision-making that does not vest control solely in the hands of the school. Potentially this goes well beyond the limited forms of collaboration that have characterised most attempts at inter-agency partnership in the past.

Finally, all of this has implications for the role of teachers and other professionals who work in and around schools. In a situation where schools are narrowly focused on attainment, there is some evidence that importing other professionals and para-professionals to deliver additional services and activities simply encourages teachers themselves to retreat further into what they see as their core business (Edwards et al. 2010). However, any more fundamental rethinking of the role of schools demands an equally fundamental rethinking of the role of teachers and their partner professionals. In particular, if children's learning is understood as being intertwined with all other aspects of their lives, it is inevitable that teachers must, to some extent at least, become involved in those other aspects, just as workers in social care and health must become involved in learning.

All of this may sound improbable in a context where a narrow focus on improving attainment drowns out all other concerns in many countries. Yet, in England this tendency has been accompanied over the last decade by an equal and opposite move towards integrated children's services, area-based approaches and more or less radical reconceptualisations of schooling (DCSF 2007; DCSF 2008a; DfES 2003) and there have been similar developments in other parts of the UK). In some ways these attempts have been problematic, but they indicate that governments may recognise the importance of acting on wider agendas. Moreover, most developments in this field do not need to wait on legislation and government guidance. They stem from local initiatives, where those who organise and deliver services at community level come to the conclusion that their traditional practices are not appropriate to the sometimes challenging situations they face. Even where governments are indifferent, such local initiative may offer the most promising way forward.

Exercise

Think of a school and/or community you know well. What are the needs and potentials in the situation they face? What kind of outcomes would be needed to address these needs and maximise these potentials? What services, activities and interventions might be offered by the school (or as part of a local strategy involving the school) to produce these outcomes? How exactly would these actions bring about changes in the situation over, say, a five- to ten-year time period in order to produce the outcomes?

Recommended reading

Cummings, C., Dyson, A. & Todd, L. et al. (2011).

Provides an overview of international developments in the field, and reports in detail on the evaluation of full service extended schools in England.

Dryfoos, J. (1994) *Full-service Schools*, San Francisco: Jossey-Bass.

This is a pioneering work from the USA, which sets out the case for full services schools and has formed the basis for many developments since.

http://www.continyou.org.uk/

The website of ContinYou, a charitable UK organisation concerned with community learning. It has supported the development of full service and extended schools for many years, and its website contains many useful resources and links.

http://www.teachernet.gov.uk/wholeschool/extendedschools/

The UK government's website offering advice on extended schools and services. Although the guidance relates specifically to England, it contains case studies and other resources with wider relevance.

Chapter 12

Taking forward children and young people's participation in decision-making

E. Kay M. Tisdall

Summary points

- Children and young people's participation in decision-making has become a popular policy and practice demand in the UK. This has been encouraged by international legal obligations, under the UN Convention on the Rights of the Child (Article 12).
- Challenges have arisen in ensuring that such participation is meaningful, sustainable and purposeful.
- Participation is a wide 'umbrella' term, which can camouflage different power relations and include tokenistic activities.
- Particular 'discourses' frame the thinking and practice of participation in decision-making, each with advantages and disadvantages. For participation in 'public', collective decision-making, the predominant types of discourses are: legal; consumer/service user involvement; democratic education; and children's well-being and development.
- Alternative discourses, like transformative performance or political emancipation, are rarely used in the UK.
- In the UK 'voice and choice' are privileged. This undervalues other forms of communication than 'voice'. 'Choice' can be misleading because it associates children's rights solely with self-determination. In 'public', collective decision-making, children and young people's participation may involve children and young people 'being at the table' with other stakeholders, and their views truly influencing the decisions.

Example 12.1

Imagine you are working in a day nursery. The early years inspectors are coming to examine your nursery. One of the inspection standards is:

Standard 5.4: Children and young people will have opportunities to express their views, exercise choice and, where possible, influence the programme (Scottish Government 2005 © Crown Copyright 2012).

You and your co-workers ask: How can we meet this standard? How can we know if we are meeting this standard well?

Introduction

Malcolm (2009), using her own experience as a nursery manager, undertook exploratory research on the questions in Example 12.1. She found that while the rhetoric of participation is becoming more integrated into policy and practice demands, practitioners struggled to operationalise this standard – and evidence it. Yet the standard clearly exercised staff, with it establishing an expectation that they would address participation.

The example demonstrates the 'good news story' for children and young people's[1] participation. In the 1990s the United Nations Convention on the Rights of the Child (UNCRC) was relatively new and the UK's ratification of it only recent (1991). Now, children and young people's rights to be heard and consulted are peppered throughout numerous pieces of legislation. This is evident in the children's legislation of 1989 (England and Wales) and 1995 (Northern Ireland and Scotland) (see Chapter 1). It has been extended, in various parts of the UK, into education, housing and communities legislation. When decisions are being made by public services on individual children's lives – like a court considering what will happen to a child when her parents' divorce or a local authority making decisions about a looked-after child – the child's views must be duly considered. The collective views of children and young people must be considered when planning services, such as the obligations for antisocial behaviour strategies in Scotland (S.1 (3) Antisocial Behaviour etc. (Scotland) Act 2004). Children and Young People's Commissioners, across the UK, promote children and young people's participatory rights (see Chapter 3). As shown in the example introducing this chapter, children and young people's participation is becoming incorporated into inspection standards. Senior courts have now made influential decisions that emphasise that it is not a question of *whether* children and young people should be heard but rather *how* they should be heard (*Shields* v *Shields* (2002) GWD 5-143). Children and young people's participation has become a policy and practice requirement.

Activities have proliferated that involve children and young people in collective decision-making. Pupil councils have become compulsory in Wales, and extremely common elsewhere in the UK (around 90 per cent of schools in England (Whitty and Wisby, 2007) and Scotland (Children in Scotland and University of Edinburgh 2010 a–e). Youth forums and parliaments have developed at local and devolved government levels. A plethora of more informal activities occur, from one-off, large-scale conferences involving children and young people to intensive ongoing work with children and young people by non-governmental organisations and other service providers. Children and young people's participation has indeed become a popular policy and practice activity.

However, this immense growth of activities, policy and legislation is accompanied by tensions and challenges as the rhetoric has moved to implementation. Sinclair (2004) presented a list of tough questions:

[1] The phrase 'children and young people' is generally used in this chapter, following young people's typical preference to be referred to as the latter. Broadly, 'children and young people' is used to refer to children up to the age of 18, following the definition within the United Nations Convention on the Rights of the Child.

1. Is it clear what the purpose of the participation is? Is it purposeful or just a 'tick box'?

2. Which children and young people are included?

3. How do we [adults] interpret what children and young people are saying?

4. How do children and young people's views fit among other stakeholders?

5. Is the participation ethical?

6. Is the participation meaningful to those involved?

7. Is the participation having any impact on decisions?

Asking and addressing these questions may be even more pertinent today. When public services are facing financial constraints, children and young people's participation risks being a 'fad' of the past twenty years. Seed and innovation funding was available when children and young people's participation was novel – now that it has a longer history, activities can struggle to become embedded financially. With the growth of activities has come great concern from children and young people about tokenism, where consultation is a 'tick box' on a grant application or a local authority plan, but where the children and young people see no impact on the actual decisions. Making children and young people's participation meaningful to all those involved, and to demonstrate that it does have some impact on decisions along with other stakeholders, is necessary to avoid children and young people 'turning off' civic engagement. In short, children and young people's participation faces particular challenges in being meaningful, sustainable and productive.

The rest of this chapter interrogates how participation, particularly in terms of involvement in collective decision-making, has developed in the UK. It begins by considering definitions of participation and the limitations thereof. It then considers particular discourses of participation, with underlying values, goals and modes of participation. The chapter concludes by considering what is not included within our particular discourses in the UK and dilemmas that need to be addressed to move on and consolidate children and young people's participation.

Definitions of participation

Perhaps because it is such a popular term, 'participation' has many and varied definitions. A dictionary definition of participation is very broad – e.g. 'The act of taking part or sharing in something'. Within children and young people's participation literature, Hart is a seminal author and, in 1992, defined participation as: 'the process of sharing decisions which affect one's life and the life of the community in which one lives' (p. 5). This definition has the advantage of emphasising the everyday lives of children and young people and their embeddedness in social and local relations. What Hart's definition lacks is an emphasis on impact. The participation right of Article 12 (UNCRC) is more than participation as a process – the views of the child are to be given 'due weight'. Some impact of children and young people's views is thus required. Writing in the context of the UNCRC, Gerison Lansdown incorporates this into her definition:

> Participation can be defined as children taking part in and influencing processes, decisions, and activities that affect them, in order to achieve greater respect for their rights.
>
> (2002: 273)

In the UK a distinction has been made between participation in individual decision-making and in public decision-making. This distinction can be useful but it is also problematic. For example, it might underestimate the many connections between them. Experience suggests that younger children think personally and locally, and that participation at these closer levels provides the platform for thinking more broadly. Norwegian research on citizenship similarly shows that children and young people do not make this distinction between the private and public, but rather rights' understandings flow between the micro-situations of families and peers into the meso-spheres of school and local communities (Kjørholt and Bjerke 2008). The distinction between private and public may be further broken down by the breadth and intensity of involvement of children and young people with digital media (Ipsos Mori 2009). As social network sites take off and people experience 'second lives' on the internet, distinctions between the private and the public become less and less relevant.

But it may be useful to consider a greater and more precise elaboration of the types of activities that come under the children and young people's participation umbrella – and to consider whether all should be covered by it. For example, the phrase 'pupil voice' has become highly popularised in education, to promote children and young people's participation in school settings. But Lundy (2007) demonstrates powerfully the phrase's limitations and how it allows for tokenistic listening and very little hearing and subsequent action. Consultation, which is honest about its limited agenda but highlights where real influence is, might be allowed to carry the label of participation, but it can be distinguished from the intense engagement, dialogue and mutual commitment of a child/young person-dominated, non-governmental organisation like Investing in Children (Cairns 2009). Greater specificity of terms may encourage more honest offers to children and young people to participate.

Framing children and young people's participation in decision-making

In the UK, arguments for children and young people's participation can be divided into four types (Tisdall et al. 2008):

1. **Upholding children's rights and fulfilling legal responsibilities.** These reasons appeal to international children's and human rights obligations, which at least have a moral claim for recognition if not incorporation into domestic law.

2. **Improving services and decision-making.** These arguments relate to the consumer and service-user involvement agenda. The agenda grew out of Conservative governments in the 1980s and 1990s but was further developed under the Labour governments subsequently (see Cabinet Office 1999). The agenda was primarily about adults' involvement – and often parents were the proxy for children (especially in schooling) – but the arguments were made that children and young people were equally consumers of public services and should as such be consulted too.

Table 12.1 Participation discourses in the UK

	Underlying values	Goal	Mode of participation	Characteristic remedy
1 Legal	Moral claim to rights Rule of law	Upholding children's rights Legality	Adults and institutions ensuring rights acknowledged and met	Appeal to court
2 Consumerism/service user involvement	Responsive services Voice/choosing to exit (stop using the service)	Improved consumption/ services	Service providers' consultation, engagement potentially in evaluation, monitoring, inspection	Complaints Inspection Other kind of regulation
3 Democratic education	Commitment to liberal democracy	Increased civic/ political participation	Adults providing training, role modelling, volunteering	None
4 Children's well-being and development	Children's needs and protection	Improved outcomes for children	Being listened to by adults/ adults providing training and opportunities	None

3. **Democratic education.** Addressing the considerable panic about the perceived lack of engagement of young people in formal political processes, children and young people's participation was offered as a way to familiarise and inculcate children and young people into the ways of democracy.

4. **Children and young people's well-being and development.** Children and young people themselves would benefit from participation. For example, participation would increase their self-esteem and teach them useful and transferable skills.

Each of these arguments appeal to particular agendas of policy-makers, professionals and other influential adults, to provide room and support for children and young people's participation.

This chapter seeks to take the above groupings further in their implications for children and young people's participation in decision-making. They each represent a discourse of participation and, as discourse theory suggests (Fulcher 1989), are not neutral vehicles to promote participation, but in fact frame such activities in particular ways with certain possibilities included or excluded. They have underlying values, a primary or legitimating goal and subsequent implications for the 'mode' of participation. If the participation is unsatisfactory, there may be a remedy. Table 12.1 seeks to map these out succinctly. Some sit easily together while others conflict. All have advantages and disadvantages, but some may have particular virtues that would favour one over another.

For example, these types could be considered in the light of research findings on pupil councils[2] in Scotland (Children in Scotland and University of Edinburgh

---

[2] 'Pupil councils' was the predominant phrase used in Scotland during the time period of the research. 'School council' is not used as it invites confusion with adult-led 'school boards' and 'parent councils' in the Scottish context. A working definition of a council is provided by the official Welsh website on such councils: '. . . a representative group of pupils elected by their peers to discuss matters about their education and raise concerns with the senior managers and governors of their school'. (http://www.schoolcouncilswales.org.uk/en/fe/page_at.asp?n1=30&n2=31&n3=69)

2010 a–d).[3] This research involved surveys of all 32 Scottish local education authorities, a postal School Survey of all secondary schools and a representative sample of primary schools, and case studies in six schools. What became evident was that those involved in pupil councils – local authority advisers, schools' headteachers and adult advisers to pupil councils, and pupil council members – had different ideas about what pupil councils were for. The discourses above highlight and organise certain of these differences.

Legal

Scottish law requires pupils' views to be considered in 'significant' decisions about their schooling but pupil councils are not mandatory. In the research, local authority policies and advisers might (or might not) mention the legal requirements and Article 12 of the UNCRC more generally, but within schools these were not mentioned. Some reference was made by a few adult advisers to local authority policy requiring pupil councils but no further elaboration was given.

These findings encapsulate certain of the advantages and disadvantages of the legal discourse. Legal changes, combined with training and information, can give increased attention to children and young people's views in service settings. Legal rights can enable those who are committed to participation to argue their case within their particular setting, to create a 'space' for participation that otherwise might not be there. Some clarity is provided by at least some legal rights – who is the rights claimant? and who has the duty to ensure these rights are met? Rights can be moral claims, and participation can be fundamental to ideas of recognition and social justice (Thomas 2007).

However, the legal discourse has disadvantages. Law can feel unfamiliar and off-putting to professionals far from their day-to-day activities. The requirement to consult can become tokenistic, something that must be done rather than deeply considered. Most children remain unaware of their rights (Willow et al. 2007) and seldom access legal assistance on their own behalf. Certainly, no reported case has yet been taken on the relevant section of the Scottish education law. The court remedy is arguably strong, in a country so wedded to the rule of law, but its effectiveness is seriously diminished as few children would even think to access it. Judicial review research suggests that, even if cases were successfully taken, the impact on front-line services tends to be limited beyond exceptional cases (Richardson 2004). Rights in law do not always translate into practice.

Consumerism

A discourse of **consumer and service-user involvement** was found in the pupil council research, through the interest of pupil council members to make their schools 'a better place'. Further, some local authorities utilised pupil councils as a consultation

---

[3] The research team were: Children in Scotland – Sher, J., Gwanzura-Ottemoller, F.; University of Edinburgh – Milne, S., Tisdall, E. K. M., with Thompson, A., Iliasov, A. and Masaba, S.

network, and case study schools showed how pupil councils were regularly used as consultation forums for school staff's ideas.

Consumerism has a long history of critique, within social policy literature, as being manipulative, controlling and limiting dissent. Individualised consumerism can lead to consultation by service providers on a narrow agenda, but not to radical change (e.g. Prior et al. 1995; Barnes et al. 2007; Cockburn 2009). A consumer's ultimate power is that of exit (i.e. leaving), which hardly applies for many children and young people in *compulsory* education – although they could resign from the pupil council. Another option is complaint, increasingly used within administrative justice, as a means for voice and potential redress. Consumerism has a tendency for 'blaming' the service provider (e.g. teachers) rather than promoting shared responsibilities by all in the school community, including children and young people, teachers and other staff (Whitehead and Clough 2004).

This is evident in interviews with adult advisers, who were worried about pupil councils being 'whinging' forums, and research observations of pupil councils that were dominated by pupil councillors passing on complaints from those they represented. As a complaints mechanism, pupil councils were able to provide a space to raise, but not always to resolve complaints, or for action to be taken elsewhere. The School Survey, for example, showed a wide range of issues discussed in pupil councils, but far fewer resulted in any decisions being made or implemented. In the case studies one pupil council particularly felt consultation fatigue, as policies were repeatedly presented to them that did not seem relevant and took away from what they perceived as their central task – reflecting on their school environment.

More positively, certain pupil councils took particular pride in their achievements – for example, improvements in play grounds and school gardens. At its most positive, the consumer discourse lead to personal problems being recognised as public ones, resulting in collective responses and responsibility.

Democratic education and children's will-being development

The two last types of discourses – **democratic education and children's well-being/ development** – were considerably entwined within the pupil council research findings and they were the dominant ones. Pupil councils were predominantly seen as 'laboratories of democracy'[4] by headteachers/adult advisers, vehicles by which pupils could practice formal democratic practices in terms of representation and meetings. Pupil councillors themselves would gain skills and confidence.

The pupil council research confirms findings elsewhere that children and young people value participation processes, when they are undertaken well, and the skills and positive feelings that result (Davies et al. 2006). These positive personal outcomes may be more widespread than commonly believed. Despite the accusation that pupil councils are about the 'articulate elite' and a minority consideration, a representative survey of secondary school pupils found that at least one-third of pupils have had experience of being a councillor (often at primary school) (Tisdall, 2007). As pupil councils become more prevalent, this proportion is only likely to increase

[4] A phrase coined by J. Sher, one of the research team on Having a Say at Schools.

further. The studies discussed in this section found no significant socio-economic biases in pupil-councillor selection, compared to their school populations.

There can be an emphasis on process and not *actual* influence on decisions. This is neatly captured by the headteacher in School A:

> . . . I think the process in itself is worthwhile. Whereas for them [the pupil council] it's probably the outcomes; it's in their mind. But if we can get them some of their outcomes and allow them to take part in the process at the same time, I think that's a reasonable trade-off.

Pupil councils in the research were more concerned about outcomes (i.e. what actions they would take and goals they would accomplish), while adults involved tend to be more focused on processes within, and the symbolic value of, pupil councils. This did lead to frustration for some pupil council members.

The research suggests certain practical actions could be taken to improve pupil councils in Scotland – from ensuring pupil council elections are fair and perceived as such, to recognising the critical role of the pupil council's adult adviser through training and career rewards. There are obvious dangers of the dominant discourse of democratic education – as Alderson (2000) wrote a decade earlier, having a tokenistic pupil council can have a more negative effect on young people's belief in democracy than having no pupil council at all. But this chapter's analysis suggests that *whatever* discourse chosen for pupil councils, there will be trade-offs between advantages and disadvantages. Given the different views on what a pupil council is for, within even the same school, continued dialogue between staff and pupils on what *their* pupil council is for would be productive – and assist in avoiding staff and/or pupils being frustrated by how their particular council functions.

Alternative discourses?

The four discourses have become so established in UK participation activities that it can be productive to consider what is *not* included.

Commentators working in Asia have criticised the use of children and young people's participation in their countries as **performance**, with participation being equated to an artistic display of children dancing or playing music (Theis 2007; West et al. 2007). Similarly, there have been highly critical comments on children and young people taking the international stage – literally – at UN and other events. While highly emotive, the effectiveness of this on subsequent decision-making has been questioned, along with how well those few children and young people have been selected to 'represent' broader groups (see Ennew and Hastadewi 2002).

We might worry in the UK that at times children and young people's participation is indeed used as performance. The participation rhetoric has led to the need for local or national governments, or other public, private or voluntary organisations to be *seen* to have consulted with children and young people. Not doing so can lead to negative media attention or criticisms from the conference floor – more positively, involving children and young people can garner particularly media and political attention. However, this kind of performance can easily fall into the tokenism that children and young people have come to criticise and fail to impact on decisions (see Tisdall and Davis 2004).

Nevertheless, can we see performance differently? Learning from Brazil and South Africa shows the potential of *transformative* performance, where cultural expressions are harnessed and children and young people engaged by artistic opportunities to develop and express their views. At the most politically obvious are the South African protest songs sung by young activists throughout the 1960s, and more intensively in the mounting struggle against the apartheid state during the 1980s, celebrating political leaders and trade unionists and expressing the wish for their release from prison (Henderson 2010). Today, the transformative potential of performance continues with the community theatre groups of children and young people in South Africa, or the reclaiming of community space through the medium of play in a *favela* in Rio di Janeiro, Brazil (see http://rocinhaludica.blogspot.com/).

Such experiences are suggestive for the UK. For example, participation activities here – when adult-led and adult initiated – are strikingly bureaucratic in comparison. Artistic methodologies are harnessed and there is now excellent practice about engaging children and young people in fun and meaningful ways (e.g. see case studies in Tisdall et al. 2009). Graffiti walls are regularly shown following consultations and role play filmed on DVD etc. However, these are then typically taken into formalised, bureaucratic settings of decision-making with artistic expressions making a sharp contrast to the 'usual ways of doing business'. Do we capitalise enough on children and young people's frequent interest in art, drama, music and the digital media, for its potential to be more child-led than adult-dominated, and particularly its *transformative* potential? Do we know what elements of such activities are transformative (and transformative to what?), for children and young people and their audiences?

Another notable absence in UK discourses is the hard edge of **political mobilisation and emancipation.** Enhancing democratic processes is mentioned but not campaigns for voting rights, political campaigns for particular candidates nor manifesto commitments. Children and young people's participation is frequently bracketed off from political campaigning – for fear of manipulation? – and typically from adult participation in their communities (Morrow 2005). When children and young people do seek to engage – e.g. to attend protests on UK participation in the Iraq war – their engagement is treated as disruptive (see Cunningham and Lavalette 2004). Yet children and young people are integral to the landless movement in Brazil, creating a community where age is not the most relevant criterion. If we truly want to encourage wide public involvement in civic society and politics, do we need to accept that some children and young people can be political, and being so alongside adults?

Conclusions and implications: back to the example

The example on p. 151 encapsulates both the 'good news story' of children and young people's participation – and current dilemmas.

On the one hand, there is an established official commitment for children and young people's participation in matters that affect them. This commitment has been translated into legal rights within domestic legislation. It has permeated numerous policies affecting children and young people, complemented by monitoring and inspection to regulate implementation. Children and young people's participation in decision-making has become a policy and practice expectation.

On the other hand, the enthusiasm for children and young people's participation, and the ensuing proliferation of activities, have raised particular dilemmas in practice. Increasingly the 'how to' engage children and young people creatively is being developed, but the actual impact on decisions remains elusive in many circumstances. The 'how to' at times has been isolated in particular individuals – from the adult adviser to the pupil councils to the growth of participation workers as an employment option – rather than spread throughout the professions and adult decision-makers. Indeed, participation activities need to work as much with the adult decision-makers as they do with the children and young people, for children and young people's views actually to influence change.

Does children's and young people's participation need to lead to change? Democratic theory would show the *symbolic* value of exercises like voting, when individual voters can recognise that their single votes are unlikely to sway a result. Voting instead can be seen as endorsing the process of the democratic system and making a 'quasi-contract' to respect the result, because the individual expects others to do so too (see Singer 1973). Symbolism may well be important to children and young people – certainly school staff in the pupil council research thought having a pupil council did show the school's valuing of participation. But voting has the *potential* to influence change. The problem with children and young people's participation, at its most tokenistic, is that such potential is lacking. If participation is solely symbolic, children and young people report their frustration.

The chapter reviewed the various discourses of children and young people's participation based on legal rights, consumerism, democratic education and children's well-being/development and concluded that there are advantages and disadvantages to each. But any of these can be mechanically 'ticked off', leaving children and young people frustrated and the potential for transformative participation for all those involved missed.

Certain professional groups may be more – or less – inspired by certain of these discourses. Children's well-being and development, for example, may particularly match teachers' aspirations for their pupils while the legal rights and their associated moral claims have attracted non-governmental organisations and youth groups. Referring back to the example at the start of the chapter, it suggests that nursery inspections are no guarantee that children are regularly and effectively involved in their nurseries – although the inspection standard clearly invites nurseries to consider their practices and may inspire them to do so. Participation is relational (Kina 2010) as well as procedural, and all – adults, children and young people – need to share an ethos that values participation if it is ultimately to be meaningful and sustainable. Inter-agency cooperation for children and young people's services provides an opportunity to reconsider children and young people's participation, and to build just such an ethos across professionals, services and spaces.

The standard mentioned in Example 12.1 exemplifies the multiplicity of what comes under the participation umbrella – expressing views, exercising choice and influencing the programme. It risks privileging 'voice and choice' (perhaps because of the consumer discourse's influence?) at the expense of 'listening' to other forms of communication, from movement to behaviour – which in fact early years practitioners are very good at documenting and can be harnessed as 'participation' (Malcolm 2009). It sets up a potential misunderstanding that children's rights generally, and children and young people's participation in particular, are solely about self-determination and autonomy. A close reading of UNCRC Article 12 definitely demonstrates that children's views are supposed to be taken into account in all matters that affect them. Children's views are thus not necessarily determinative, but important views among others' views. The problem to date is that all too frequently children and young people's views have not been included at all, too easily dismissed or only supported when they 'chime' with other evidence and professionals' assessments (May and Smart 2004). Children and young people's participation sometimes is appropriately about choice, but at other times it may be about being one of multiple stakeholders, for example, in policy decisions.

The exploratory research by Malcolm (2009) suggests practitioners' discomfort with involving the very youngest children under the participation umbrella. It is provocative that the Scottish Court of Session (not necessarily known for its child-friendly expertise) in *Shields* v *Shields* underlined the point that it should not be *whether* a child should be heard but *how*. Adult service providers and participation workers perhaps too easily set up age barriers to who is involved, discriminating against the youngest children and their involvement. Why do we feel comfortable, as is frequently seen in consultation reports and research findings, with saying we will only involve those under the age of 12, or the age of 8?

The pupil council findings do suggest relatively simple ways service providers can involve children and young people more effectively. The early years staff can call on a host of methodologies and 'how to' toolkits to involve children productively in their nursery and be evaluated positively by the inspectorate.

However, there are also more fundamental questions about children and young people's participation in the UK. Questions like how such participation can actually become embedded and meaningful to all those involved – from decision-makers, to service providers, to adults, to children – like whether we need to develop a more sophisticated typology of how participation is framed, to exclude some of our current practices as manipulative and tokenistic and to allow for a continuum of involvement that suits the decisions that need to be made. We need to consider whether we are limiting the transformative potential of participation within the UK, by privileging bureaucracy and excluding other participation discourses. Children and young people's participation is fundamentally about respecting them as community members – we need to address our current challenges of ensuring their participation has an impact on decision-making.

Exercise

- What discourses of participation predominate in your service? What are their advantages and disadvantages? What could diminish the disadvantages and enhance the advantages?

■ Discuss with a child or young person experiences of participation in decision-making. What positive or negative experiences were there? What made the experiences positive or negative? What top tips would be useful in your work?

Recommended reading

Miller, J. (2009) *Never Too Young: how young children can take responsibility and make decisions*, London: Save the Children.

One of a range of available 'how to' toolkits, this one is aimed at early years workers. It contains tools and techniques of how to do so, in very practical ways. This is a reprinting of the popular book.

Participation Works http://www.participationworks.org.uk/

An extensive online gateway for children and young people's participation. It is a hub for information, resources, news and networking for the involvement of young people 'in dialogue, decision-making and influence across a wide range of setting'. It is particularly focused on England but has widespread application to those elsewhere, particularly in regards to its resources. It provides information about 'how to' toolkits and training on participation.

Percy-Smith, B. and Thomas, N. (eds) (2010) *A Handbook of Children and Young People's Participation: Perspectives from theory and practice*, Abingdon: Routledge.

This edited collection contains chapters from across the world, discussing contemporary theory and practice on children and young people's participation. It presents examples from a range of different settings from schools to non-governmental organisations.

Tisdall, E. K. M., Davis, J. D. and Gallagher, M. (2009) *Researching with children and young people*, London: Sage.

An advanced text aimed at those doing direct research and consultation with children, who wish to move beyond the (sometimes very good) beginner texts that are now widely available. This book contains five core chapters covering areas like ethics, date collection and dissemination, and 11 different case studies of research and consultation activities. It contains activities, discussions questions, top tips, research tools and practical advice.

Chapter 13

Children's representation

Andrea Mooney and Andrew Lockyer

Summary points

- It is quite common for other people to act on behalf of children, with parents being the main 'representatives' of their children's interests.
- In judicial contexts children, like adults, often need legal and other forms of representation.
- Tensions occur in all forms of children's representation, e.g. how can or should adults' judgements about what is best for children be made independent of their personal or organisational interests; at what age and how should children's own viewpoints figure or take precedence?
- Drawing on American experience, two models of legal representation are discussed.
- Both US and UK experience indicate the need for representatives in legal decision-making settings to have a good understanding of both the law and children's development, needs and communication.

Introduction

The subject of this chapter is child representation – namely speaking or acting on behalf of children. Parents frequently take on this role, especially in relation to young children – for example when deciding that their child will benefit from attending nursery school or explaining to a doctor the symptoms of their sick infant. Occasionally professionals or judges and their equivalents may override the parental representative role in order to safeguard children's interests. This chapter introduces different forms of representation and then focuses on issues that arise with representation in judicial contexts in light of American and British experience.

The general case for a representative to act on behalf of another is that the representing agent is better able to present, promote or protect the interests of represented parties than they are able to do for themselves unassisted. The circumstances in which *adults* most commonly require representation is where matters affecting their rights and interests are to be determined in settings where they may not themselves be fully competent or authorised. In a judicial or quasi-judicial forum, the entitlement for parties to be represented is a requirement of a fair decision procedure. All parties should have equal means to make their case and influence the decision (lawyers call this 'equality of arms').

Children have the same rights as adults to have their interests represented in such settings, but the circumstances in which they are deemed not fully competent actors are broader. This correspondingly requires the scope of representation to be more extensive beyond judicial settings.

One of the implications of children being vulnerable and requiring extra representation is that those who have contact with them, professionals and members of the public, must frequently determine when it is appropriate to deal directly with particular children, and when appropriate to do so through, or with the involvement of, a representative. Although the principle of fairness seems clearly to demand that being less able to present evidence or arguments in their own best interests should not disadvantage a child, it is far from straightforward as to how fair treatment is to be ensured. Both those who are obliged to act for children and those with a duty to provide services for them have difficult judgements to make about how children's interests are to be interpreted and determined.

Parentalism

Adults are normally regarded as capable of making choices: about when to be represented; who might represent them; on what terms and with what instructions. By contrast, children are not presumed in practice or in law to be necessarily the best judges of their own interests. There are no uniform procedures for authorising and prescribing when and how the representation of children is appropriate. Yet there is a culturally universal presumption that their parents or those in the parenting role will usually represent children. Persons recognised to have the primary responsibility for children's care are also generally presumed to act in their interests and, if necessary, on their behalf, unless and until there is a state-authorised decision to locate this responsibility elsewhere, whether permanently, temporarily or for specific proceedings.

The long-standing ideology of patriarchalism meant that male heads of households acted on behalf of all its members. Before women acquired the right to vote, it was assumed that the household had a single interest represented by the male in elections, while fathers also held legal sway over children. Following the extension of the franchise to women in representative liberal democracies like the UK, the patriarchal principle was modified to 'parentalism' – the presumption that the interests of children are included in the votes of their parents (Dahl 1956). However, in practice parents do not necessarily act or vote with their children's interests in mind, which results in the 'problem' of the 'missing child' in political accountability (O'Neill 1994). Furthermore, two parents of the same child may have divergent preferences. These issues in politics are replicated in civil society and domestic life. The same discrepancy of judgement embedded in paternalism or parentalism might equally arise in respect of other decisions taken on behalf of children when more than one person or agency has an obligation to include consideration of their interests. It is not unusual for there to be disagreement about what is in a child's interests – for instance, among family members, social workers, health professionals and others in child-protection cases. Similarly, differences can occur about what weight to give to the views of children themselves and when they are old enough to express them.

The Children Act 1989 and the Children (Scotland) Act 1995 make it clear that parental responsibilities and rights to represent their children normally apply to both married parents with whomever the child resides, unless a court has determined otherwise. On top of this it is commonplace for public bodies to regard parents to be representing their children in all manner of decisions that affect the family as a whole or an individual child. For instance, seeking parental permission for medical treatments or school outings is standard procedure even when the child is capable of giving or withholding consent. The child's right to education in the UK has been secondary to the parent's right to determine who shall deliver it and perhaps what it should include.

The position in the UK is affected by treaty obligations to follow certain international standards. For instance, the European Convention on Human Rights was adopted as part of UK law by the Human Rights Act 1998. This affirms parents' rights to ensure their child's education is 'in conformity with their own religious and philosophical convictions.'

The UN Convention on the Rights of the Child (UNCRC) has been ratified by the UK but not the USA, where strong opposition exists towards the idea of international law influencing domestic policy. The UNCRC recognises that children must have some rights that they share with adults, including the right to independent representation in judicial proceedings where they are accused of an offence or there is a threat to their liberty. Significantly, Article 5 underscores both the right of the child to receive 'appropriate direction and guidance' in the exercise of their rights, and the right and responsibility of parents, in the first instance, to give it. There is an appropriate balance to be struck between 'direction' and 'guidance' (no doubt differently interpreted in different cultures and habitually contested between generations); but the balance must recognise the child's right to express their own views and have them given due weight (Article 12).

It is open to question what becomes of the parental role when the state sees it to be necessary for children to be represented independent of their parents, as in certain divorce or care proceedings. Here courts and/or public officials may take on the role of *parens patriae*, which literally refers to the parental responsibilities of the 'fatherland' in situations where parents may not be able to fulfil their role adequately. When a child is being separately represented does this mean that the child's right to parental direction and guidance is being denied or suspended, or even temporarily transferred? Should an appointed agent for a child continue to recognise the parental presumption to provide direction and guidance by consulting with the parents or take on the presumptive parental role themselves? How can the independence of non-parental representatives be guaranteed?

The rest of the chapter considers situations where the state is intervening in family life or seeking to do so, such that issues arise about who is best able to represent children's interests and how.

The United States: Gault, delinquency and other types of cases

The issues and dilemmas of child representation are similar in different jurisdictions, but can express themselves differently. A comparison of the UK and US shows that, despite their shared juridical heritage, their juvenile justice systems followed diverging paths during the twentieth century. Until the 1960s the American system involved informal processes for dealing with children's offending or care issues, with decisions made ostensibly in the child's best interests. Children lacked any right to independent representation. This changed dramatically following the US Supreme Court judgement in the Gault case.

15-year-old Gerry Gault was taken into custody in Arizona in 1964 on the basis of a complaint that he had made an obscene phone call to Mrs Cook. The boy was held in detention for three days after an informal hearing in Judge McGee's chambers. Several features of what lawyers call 'due process' were absent. Gerry had not received notice of the charge and he did not have a legal representative. Mrs Cook's complaint was reported by a deputy probation officer (i.e. as hearsay). At a similarly constituted and informally conducted hearing a week later Gerry was committed to the State Industrial School with the possibility he might remain there for 'reform' at the state's discretion until age 21.

The case went on appeal to the US Supreme Court, whose groundbreaking judgement changed the direction of juvenile justice in America. The Court's majority opinion was that the lack of due process had produced 'unbridled discretion' for the decision-makers and resulted in a lengthy loss of freedom wholly disproportionate to the original complaint (Watkins 1998; Duquette 2007). The Court determined that henceforward the same protections of due process, which the constitution guaranteed to adult citizens, should apply to children who were subject to a finding of delinquency. They should have a right to counsel (at the cost of the state if necessary), the right to remain silent, the right to bring witnesses, to confront and cross-examine witnesses and so forth. These measures protect citizens against abuse of the *parens patriae* role of the state.

On the other hand, the actual parent or legal guardian continues to have very little part to play in delinquency cases in the US, which leaves the child without parental oversight. With small exceptions, a juvenile delinquent trial is conducted like an adult criminal trial. The child's representative must be an attorney, who handles the case as a criminal defence lawyer would and seeks to avoid harsh sentences, which may include incarceration. The parent may hire an attorney for the child. Even if the parent is paying, the attorney advocates for the child not the parent, and is directed by the child as with any other attorney–client relationship. When the parent cannot or will not make such arrangements, the child is assigned an attorney.

In the United States, as in the UK, children may appear at legal proceedings not because of an alleged crime, but on account of a status offence. By this is meant forms of behaviour such as truancy or 'ungovernability' indicating the child may be in need of public supervision. Sometimes a parent – far from representing their child – is asking the court for assistance with handling a difficult child, and in effect becomes a 'prosecutor' of that child. In such circumstances, the child's views and interests may be very different from those of the parent, so the child requires an independent advocate. In most cases, the court appoints a lawyer to represent the child, while a social worker will attempt to work with the whole family problems. There are marked similarities with UK jurisdictions here.

In yet other cases, a child is brought before the court because the state is directly alleging that the parent is in some way incompetent in the care of their child. In these cases, the parent cannot be trusted to speak for the child. Instead an attorney, a social worker or a volunteer provides representation.

The significant difference between delinquency cases and cases where the child is a victim is that the role of the child's representative in the latter is much less clearly defined. For instance, it may not be at all self-evident whether children will be helped or harmed if the parents are proved to have neglected them. Similarly when it comes to consideration of the disposition or sentence, the child's representative may need to take a view about what is best for the child, separate from that child's own opinion. The US experience exemplifies a dilemma that also emerges in UK jurisdictions, such that comparison is instructive (Duquette 1992). Two distinct models of representation inform how child advocates approach their role in these circumstances in the US.

Two models of representation

The first model of representation can be thought of as 'traditional zealous advocacy'. In both the US and the UK the legal system which includes the juvenile justice system is predominantly an adversarial one. Zealous advocates for each side articulate that side's position, then a neutral fact-finder (either a judge or a jury) determines the just result. An adversarial system such as this requires that each side is well represented by a competent solicitor (or attorney), who takes the client's wishes as their directive and seeks to accomplish the client's wishes, regardless of their own opinions or biases.

Zealous advocacy representation normally works well with juvenile delinquency cases and status offences, where the child's attorney mounts a defence for the child to counter the case made by the state's attorney. In child abuse and custody cases, however, the child is the subject of the case, rather than a party. Most states allow for children to have active representation, but have not modified evidentiary or procedural rules, so it can be unclear how the children's attorneys may question witnesses or in what circumstances are able to present their own witnesses.

Even when an attorney decides to act strictly as a zealous advocate, there are inherent problems. The attorney for the child is often seen as an arm of the court rather than an independent advocate for a client. This has sometimes resulted in a court asking for a report from the attorney, which conflicts with the attorney's advocacy role and ethical rules.

Further, it is often difficult for the attorney to determine what the child's wishes actually are. It is not unusual for children, particularly those who have been abused or neglected to mistrust adults. The writer Mary McCarthy (1957) illustrated this process vividly in her autobiographical account of being treated very harshly as a child by her grandparents, yet colluding with them to present a favourable image of the family to outsiders. Many attorneys acting for children are uncertain about how to speak with a child. Few are trained in child psychology. Gaining the trust of a child is likely to require several meetings, preferably including in the child's own environment, but attorneys can rarely take the time to get to know a child well and gain their confidence. The difficulties presented to a US attorney are not of course peculiar to their jurisdiction, but the less time and opportunity to engage with the client outside the court setting, and the more formal the court process, the harder it is for the attorney/solicitor to be clear about acting on the child's instruction.

The second model of child representation is for the advocate to represent the child's best interest, rather than the child's views about what happened or about which legal disposal they prefer. In this form of representation, the attorney takes as their task to persuade the judge or jury to make a decision that best serves the child's emotional, psychological or physical well-being, regardless of what the child may articulate to their representative. The attorney/solicitor acting in a child's best interest will investigate the case, talk with those who have information about the child and then make up their own mind as to what would be in the child's best interest. The attorney may make this decision without ever speaking with or even meeting the child. Equally they may listen to the child's wishes, if they are old enough and able to express them, but what weight to attach to the child's wishes is a matter for the attorney/solicitor.

When an attorney/solicitor undertakes best-interest representation, they are essentially substituting their judgement for that of the child. The determination of when to act on this model of representation is generally a matter for the attorney alone – very few jurisdictions provide guidelines on how this decision is to be reached. It is normal for attorneys to decide that they must substitute judgement in cases involving young children, especially infants. Even pre-verbal children, though, can indicate their wishes through behaviour, but it is the rare solicitor who is able to interpret the behaviour of a young child. The age and level of maturity at which attorneys judge they do not have to substitute for the child's views again depends largely on the particular views or personal experience of the individual undertaking the child's representation.

Example 13.1

Seana is an eleven-year-old subject of a custody dispute between her parents. Seana loves both parents and wants to spend time with each; both love her and are good caretakers. Seana's mother plans to move with Seana from the family home to the home of the mother's boyfriend. Below we see the implications of the allocation of two different kinds of attorney. These are hypothetical but based on real examples.

Instance 1

The court rota assigns the case to Ms White, a recently appointed attorney. She has attended the basic training that her jurisdiction requires for children's attorneys. Seana attends an appointment in

▶

Ms White's office and says little. Ms. White takes Seana's reticence to indicate limited understanding. She decides she must act in the girl's best interests by substituting her judgement for Seana's. Ms White thinks pre-adolescent girls are best brought up by their mothers and so advocates for Seana to live with her mother. Seana remains unaware of any rights she has to challenge her representation

Instance 2

The court rota assigns the case to Mr Shaw, an experienced attorney working in an office that has specialised in family cases. He has attended in-service training workshops on ethics of child representation, child development, impact of custody disputes on children and communication skills with children. Mr Shaw arranges to meet Seana at the office, in the family home and again after school. At the third meeting, Seana is more relaxed. She explains she would prefer to stay with her father, in her present house and attending her current school where she has good friends. Her father will help her continue seeing her mother. Mr Shaw thinks Seana knows her own mind and has sound reasons for her preference. He advises Seana on how to speak to the court and advocates for her wishes.

More complex and subjective decisions to switch from a zealous advocacy presumption to a best-interests model occur when attorneys come to think during the course of a case that children's wishes involve an outcome that is not best for them (e.g. to return to a parent who will re-abuse them). Usually attorneys act as zealous advocates in opposing a proof of delinquency, then advocate for the child's best interests in the disposition, but on occasion they may conclude that it is not right to try to disprove a charge when it is valid and will lead to the child being given help.

An area of representation that generates much controversy is with regard to custody disputes. Unlike juvenile delinquency or child abuse and neglect cases, no legislative or judicial decisions have indicated how an attorney should act in cases which pit parent against parent, each arguing that their proposed solution is in the child's best interest. Guggenheim (2005) criticises what he believes is an arbitrary but not uncommon practice where advocates make recommendations based on their own subjective perceptions of parents' behaviour, regardless of the parents' abilities to provide good care or the child's own wishes.

Solicitors and attorneys who work with children spend most of their time between the black and white of the two models discussed above, determining whether they should be conducting a 'client-directed' or 'best-interest' representation, or some hybrid of the two. Unfortunately, far too often the decision as to the type of representation is determined not by general principles and the circumstances of the case but by a particular representative's preconceptions or preference – the luck of the draw. This raises questions about the kinds of preparation that attorneys receive for child representation in the US. They quite often consult with teachers, social workers and others about particular cases, but this is not a requirement of the task and only compensates in part for the lack of training in non-legal aspects of the role. A number of states now require specialisation in child-welfare law and have mechanisms for certification of such knowledge (Duquette 2007), but it remains rare for attorneys to have expertise in child and family dynamics. The

University of Michigan Law School has been given federal funding to support ways of improving the quality of child representation.

Scottish experience of child representation

It is helpful to compare representation in the US with that in Scotland because among the UK jurisdictions, the Scottish system embodies the greatest contrast with the US. It remains based on a decision-making forum (children's hearings) that is relatively informal and non-adversarial. It embodies lay community engagement in decision-making and encourages direct participation by children and parents (Lockyer and Stone 1998; also Chapter 7). By contrast, England has like the US witnessed over the last 40 or so years a greater separation of child welfare from youth justice and an emphasis on due process (Bottoms and Kemp 2007; Creekmore 2007).

A distinctive feature of Scotland's children's hearings system is the institutional separation of the adjudication of facts, which constitute its 'grounds of referral', from the forum of decision about the 'disposal' (which in other jurisdictions might be called a sentence). Grounds of referral encompass both offences and care or protection. If 'grounds for referral' require proof, because either parents or children deny them, or if children lack understanding then, these must be established or dismissed by a sheriff (Scottish judge). The hearing of proof, though technically before a sheriff in chambers, is both formal and adversarial (Kearney 2000). All parties are entitled to publicly funded independent legal representation to challenge the grounds and are similarly entitled if they make an appeal. In essence, the child's rights to individual legal representation are the same before the Scottish courts as the US and other UK jurisdictions.

Once grounds for referral are accepted or proved, discussions and decisions about the disposal take place in an informal children's hearing. Hearings were set up with the intention that decision-makers, family members and professionals explore options together and ideally reach a consensus about measures that will meet the child's needs, including the need to address their problematic behaviour. In practice, conflicts of opinion are expressed at hearings and compulsory measures can be imposed, but this follows active participation of all concerned. A key issue, then, is what kind of representation is compatible with the ethos of children's hearings?

The rules that govern the conduct of children's hearings from the outset to date have permitted the child and parents or relevant persons 'to be accompanied by a person . . . for the purpose of assisting . . . in the discussion of the case' (SSI Rules 2002: 11). Representatives are expected to 'assist' in discussion, not speak for the person they represent or instead of them. The child and parents may have the same or different representatives. These elements are consistent with children's hearings being dialogistic discussions in which family members are expected to participate directly. In practice, it has been quite common for there to be a single representative, often a neighbour or family friend, who may simply give 'moral support' or freely share in discussing the case. They are more likely to support parents than children, but have no formal obligation to agree with either. Where there is conflict between children and parents, it is important that someone is available to support or if necessary represent the child, a role that may be undertaken by a social worker or teacher or a specially appointed safeguarder (discussed below).

From the outset of the hearings system, the rules have allowed anyone to be a representative, including solicitors but there was no public funding for them in hearings, and, significantly, there was no concept of privileging their participation as 'legal representatives'. Moreover, many people have opposed legal representation at hearings, either at all or as a routine practice, because it was thought this would bring an adversarial stance at odds with hearings' informal participatory style (Stone 1995 xv). In 2002 the legal position was changed in response to concerns over compliance with the ECHR (Kearney 2000). Legal representation must now be considered by hearings if a child is likely to 'lose their liberty' (e.g. by placement in secure accommodation). In addition, hearings may appoint a legal representative to allow the child to 'effectively participate in the hearing' (SSI Rules 2002 3(1)). Legal representation at hearings is still not the norm, however.

Lawyers do not necessarily introduce an adversarial element into hearings, as most are able to adjust to its consensual ethos (Reid 1998). Nevertheless, their task is to advocate for the child, even if less zealously than is appropriate in the US. The presence of a party under instruction and not free to give their personal views in a debate on the best disposal may well detract from the conception underpinning children's hearings of a 'free, frank and unhurried discussion' in which all give their honest views (Stone 1995 Report para. 109). There may be little added value from a legal representative enabling the child's view to be heard, with parents, non-legal representatives and social workers regarding themselves as having that remit.

Guardians and safeguarders

We conclude with brief attention to individuals who are given the sole role of representing children's interests in legal decision-making forums. Unlike zealous advocates for the child, such persons act independently of the child as well as of parents and public services, albeit with an overriding responsibility for the child's welfare. Traditionally, in England, Wales and Scotland courts could appoint a guardian-ad-litem (curator in Scotland) to undertake this activity, but in recent years these jurisdictions have moved in different directions. In the late 1990s in England and Wales a non-governmental national body was set up (Children and Family Court Advisory and Support Service), which took over the functions of local authorities to provide a guardian service and also court welfare functions. The hope was that CAFCASS would not only provide greater consistency and quality of service, but also be more clearly independent of local authorities, which arguably have a vested interest in care and protection cases. Scotland however has developed a decentralised safeguarder service (Hill et al. 2003). Although the service is organised by local authorities, these have made sure that it is located in a department separate from social work and education, while safeguarders themselves are independent practitioners paid a fee per case. They do not have line managers, unlike CAFCASS staff. A third model is illustrated by Finland, where an independent guardian service is provided by a national voluntary organisation.

Unfortunately, organisational matters have overshadowed professional issues in the work of CAFCASS, with strong criticisms having been made about its failure to cope with the heavy demands for its services (NAO 2010). The imposition of centralised standards and procedures has been unpopular. Children's guardians (Family Court Advisers) working for CAFCASS have independence from other interested parties, but many feel they lack professional autonomy (Timms 2009).

CAFCASS guardians are qualified and experienced social workers. There is no agreed requirement for Scottish safeguarders to have a particular professional qualification, but in practice most are either lawyers or social workers, with a few having teaching or other backgrounds (Hill et al. 2003). In Germany it has been suggested that guardians should have a combined legal and social work background.

Guardians in England and Wales *must* appoint a legal representative (unless the court has already done so), while safeguarders *may* do so. This 'tandem system' deploying both child welfare and legal expertise has been well regarded by legal commentators (Lowe and Douglas 2007). However, Bilson and White (2005) have argued that the guardian role tends to subsume children's wishes within their primary duty of assessing their best interests and that children's participatory rights as citizens might be better served by an advocate alone.

This is confirmed by research which indicates that, despite the CAFCASS Service adopting the UNCRC and seeking 'to put children first', the ethos of the family court is still adult orientated, adjudicating on disputes about children's best interests without giving the 'views and feeling' of children much weight (James 2008).

Contrary to the comments by Bilson and White, safeguarders usually do not see it as problematic that their role involves reporting on what is best for the child and at the same time expressing the child's views (Hill et al. 2002). These aims are not incompatible because, even when a safeguarder's view on what the hearing should decide does not follow the child's wishes, it still serves the child's interests to have their views known and given due weight. Many, though not all, safeguarders explain to the child where their recommendation differs from that of the child.

Both guardians and safeguarders are involved with children only for a limited time and with a focus on the legal decision. Duquette (1994) has suggested that something like the American example of Court Appointed Special Advocates would be useful as they have a sustained commitment to a case. They seek to ensure that care or supervision arrangements are carried out in the child's interests. Such Advocates are not legally qualified and are often volunteers.

Example 13.2

The grounds of referral to a children's hearing in Scotland were based on an alleged assault of a child by foster carers. They denied the allegation and the hearing appointed a safeguarder, whose services were retained by the Sheriff considering whether the grounds were proven or not. The safeguarder took the view that the child's interests were best served by resisting the allegations, so that the child could stay with the carers. The safeguarder instructed a solicitor, who effectively challenged the leading evidence (Kearney 2000, para. 34.06).

Conclusions and implications

Adults represent children in many contexts – in everyday life, politically, when making professional judgements and in judicial and quasi-judicial settings. Children's need for representation varies not only with their age/maturity and the forum in which they appear, but also how far they are assisted to speak for themselves. This requires making adult-orientated institutions more child responsive, as well as promoting the young person's belief that they equally share in the purposes for which public institutions in a democratic society are designed. Professionals must be able to judge when to speak directly to children and when to do so through or with the engagement of representatives. The parental duty to 'appropriately guide and direct' must be recognised, and at times other carers might properly exercise this function, but it must not be presumed to represent, or substitute for, children's expressed views. Representing children involves assessing and making judgements about what is best for them together with skills in communication with children and ensuring the child's viewpoint is effectively heard and taken into account. Dilemmas arise for legal representatives and for those appointed in a guardian role as to how and when best-interests considerations should override the views of the child.

Comparisons between the US, Scotland and England have highlighted questions about what is the appropriate expertise for children's representatives within the legal sphere. A qualification in child law is a prerequisite for advocate roles, but lawyers normally lack formal knowledge about children's needs, parenting and communication with children. Contacts with other professionals and expert witnesses may help in particular cases, but time constraints and the requirement of independence may limit the scope of this. It is therefore desirable that advocates and legally trained guardians should have additional training about children's development and needs. Conversely, those in a safeguarding role whose expertise lies more in child and family dynamics must have appropriate legal advice and training, and know how to share knowledge with courts (in training court personnel or as expert witnesses).

Exercise

Emma aged 8 has been living in foster care for about a year and has been doing much better at her new school near the foster home. However, she has confided in a teacher that she wants to go back to live with her mother so she can see more of her younger brother. Social workers consider that the mother's partner might abuse Emma if she returns home. A legal hearing has been arranged because Emma has been caught stealing from local shops.

Consider what kinds of information and from whom it might be gathered by a legal representative acting for Emma and by a guardian or safeguarder appointed in this case. How might representation of the child's interests and wishes vary in different jurisdictions?

Recommended reading

A British journal entitled *Representing Children* dealt with representation in legal contexts, though it ceased publication in 2007.

Hill et al. (2003).

Duquette (2007).

Timms (2009).

Chapter 14

Taking children's citizenship seriously

Andrew Lockyer

Summary points

- Citizenship concerns the relationship between individuals and the state, particularly their rights and responsibilities with respect to each other.
- Active citizenship denotes taking steps to contribute to democratic processes and social well-being.
- Opinion is divided about how far it is appropriate to regard children as future citizens, citizens now or citizens-in-the-making.
- A major policy emphasis in recent years has been for schools to prepare children for active citizenship, which includes political literacy.
- Children themselves recognise they have responsibilities as citizens.
- The notion of active citizenship also helps in understanding roles undertaken by adults as volunteers.
- All have a responsibility to assist children to be become active citizens.

Introduction

This chapter discusses the recent invigoration of the concept of citizenship education, and explores the implications for those who deal with children and young people of taking their citizenship seriously. Since the origins of democratic government in ancient Greece, who shall be citizens and what citizenship entails have been continually debated. Among the key aspects of being a citizen are the rights and responsibilities an individual has with respect to the state, and vice versa. Where children and young people stand in relation to this subject has a related history that has become increasingly contested and complicated in recent years.

Whether or not children count as citizens is partly related to different senses of citizenship. In a narrow sense, citizenship is roughly coterminous with legal nationality, although the United Kingdom is a multi-national state where 'British citizenship' covers four home nations (Kearney 2006). Increasingly citizenship is used in a broader sense to refer to political and social entitlements. The impetus for the expanding discourse on citizenship is the view that democratic citizenship requires active engagement; citizens should seek to make positive contributions to their communities beyond the private sphere (Oldfield 1990). In the past, these broad forms of citizenship were seen as initially confined to male heads of households and then gradually extended to all adults, but children were seen as lacking the capacity for such involvement. From this perspective, children are not yet citizens.

Changing views of childhood have stressed their rights and have revised thinking about what children are able to do, at least above a certain age (Lansdown 2005). Therefore, increasingly advocates for children regard them as 'citizens now', rather than potential citizens whose active citizenship is to be delayed until they exercise the same rights as adults. An intermediate position regards children as 'citizens in the making' (Lister 2008; Lockyer 2010).

Within the context of professional work with children, ideas about citizenship in recent years have largely focused on the roles of teachers and schools, where preparation for future citizenship became part of the required curriculum in England and Wales and also more prominent in Scotland and Northern Ireland. The driving impetus behind the increasing focus on citizenship was the worry that responsibilities associated with democratic state membership were being over-looked. Besides concern about an apparent drop in interest in voting was a wider acknowledgement that the way we socialise and educate young people is crucial to the creation of a healthy democratic culture (Lockyer 2003). It is increasingly accepted that education for active citizenship requires recognition that children are bearers of both rights and responsibilities. Arguably these matters are not the preserve of parents or formal educators alone, but should be addressed by everyone involved with a child's upbringing.

Citizens now

The idea that children are citizens from birth is generally an acknowledgement that they are born with a *legal identity* as members of a particular state that has responsibilities towards them. The right to have a legal identity is something easily taken for granted, but Doek (2008) pointed out that it is denied to nine million stateless persons, including children. The great majority of children in the UK are British citizens, but asylum seekers, for instance, are not and so their entitlements are weaker and less clear-cut, governed by international treaties rather than citizen rights (Kohli 2007). Conversely, formal British national identity does not necessarily reflect how young people see themselves (Lister et al. 2003). Dual identities like British-Indian or British-Chinese are common, and some prefer to link their cultural identity with a sub-state nationality such as Welsh or Scottish Pakistani, which may focus their political engagement on devolved institutions (Miller and Hussain 2006; Scourfield et al. 2006; Ross et al. 2008). The key is that young people must be confident in their cultural identities – ethnic, religious and national – for them to participate as active citizens (Kiwan 2010).

As the chair of the UN Committee on the Rights of the Child, Doek (2008) made the case for children as citizens now, largely on the basis of legal identity: 'The

Citizen Child is a citizen of today and the full recognition of this fact is one of the fundamental requirements of the UNCRC'. The human right to be 'registered' at birth, which is embodied in Article 7 of the UNCRC, is the entitlement to be a citizen. The right is to a recorded name of at least one birth parent and thereby 'the right to acquire a nationality'. This makes it clear a child's inherited citizenship is tied to their family identity, which is a prerequisite of their state membership.

Doek suggested that the security of the child's national identity is not simply a matter of acquiring passive rights (for example, to protection by one's state) but also a prerequisite for the 'full and harmonious development of the child's personality' which makes it possible for her or him to 'participate fully as active members of their community' (Doek 2008, xv). Thus, the child's right to a specific identity from birth carries much more than a formal legal status. Many commentators share Doek's view that seeing children as citizens from birth is the key to investing them with all the rights that are embedded in the UNCRC. In particular, this perspective expects children and young people's views, just like those of adults, to influence decision-making in schools and other public contexts affecting them (see Chapter 12).

Nevertheless, the UNCRC acknowledges a number of qualifications with regard to children's active rights, which differentiate them from adult citizens in the following ways:

(a) a child's right to have their views taken into account is qualified by the obligation on others to decide on their 'maturity' and thereby what weight to attach to their views (Article 12);

(b) consideration of a child's interests is a primary consideration, which must trump acting on their views, when their views and interests are deemed to conflict (Article 3);

(c) parents have the right and responsibility to provide appropriate direction and guidance in the exercise of children's rights (Article 5);

(d) some exclusively children's rights, like the right to receive primary education, are 'non-elective' (i.e. compulsory) (Article 28);

(e) Children's rights do not include the key democratic political rights: to vote and stand for office.

In short, children's current citizenship has at least to overcome the hurdle of being compatible with their lack of adult autonomy. According to the UNCRC, for those with responsibilities toward children to treat them as if they were adults is to mistreat them. This begs many questions about what is appropriate, but it illustrates that there is a case for viewing children as not yet fully social and political citizens – whether future, partial or citizens-in-the-making is the preferred ascription.

Future citizens or citizens-in-the-making

Thinking about children as future citizens acknowledges both an acceptance that the young are not yet to be vested with all adult rights and responsibilities and recognises the obligation to prepare children to acquire these. However, a widely expressed concern is that focusing on the future status and well-being of the young too often leads to their current entitlements, needs and qualities being overlooked. (Roche 1999; Wyness et al. 2004) For this reason, it may be preferable to think of children as citizens-in-the-making, who progressively acquire the rights and responsibilities of citizens.

However, to fully appreciate the case for deferring citizen status from young people (even if ultimately to reject the case) some of its historical antecedence must be understood. Within the liberal democratic tradition, state membership was deemed to be based on a real or imagined contract between the individual and the state, so a person could only be a member of a democratic community by choice. From this principle, John Locke (writing in the 1680s) concluded that children remain in the domestic household, under the authority of their parents, until they have reached the 'age of reason' when they can decide for themselves whether or not to place themselves under the authority of a particular state (Locke 1689).

This is consistent with the long-standing, pre-modern view that the state is essentially an association of households, and the head of the household exercises an authority in the private sphere that is equivalent to that which the state exercises over its subjects or citizens. Although this domestic paternalism is modified by modern ideas of gender equality such that the state is an association of individuals, there is still an assumption that children remain under the authority of parents within the household until they are liberated.

The separation of the private sphere of the family from the public-sphere state and the resistance of the former to 'interference' from the latter is a much-cherished principle. Parents are deemed to have the liberty to raise their children according to their own values and beliefs (Mawyer 1995). This is often portrayed as an issue of 'privacy' or 'the defence of family life', or even 'religious and cultural freedom'. However, a countervailing principle is that the state has particular duties towards more vulnerable citizens, including children. The upbringing of citizens is properly a shared responsibility of parents and public agencies. When the state provides education, it necessarily places school-aged children partly outside family life and in the public sphere. While parents' rights to choose their child's school and type of educational regime has (with limitations) been embodied in law and by courts, the court's authority has also been used to override parental choice where a child's health and well-being is judged by those with a professional duty of care to be seriously at risk.

The standard argument for compulsory state education in the liberal democratic tradition is that children must receive basic education to maximise their life chances. As Feinberg (1980) expresses it, children have a 'right to an open future' which they should not be permitted to jeopardise prematurely. But this liberal case is only half of the story. It is misleading to present education simply as the young person's right, it is also their duty. Our education system seeks to equip students to be of service to 'society' – their 'communities' – as well as themselves. The aspiration that children should realise their potential and develop their talents for their own advantage is consistent with the obligation of citizenship to contribute to the common good.

It was T. H. Marshall (1950) who first characterised children as citizens-in-the-making. His reluctance to consider children to be fully citizens was because he saw citizenship entailing an equality 'with respect to the rights and duties which the status endowed.' Citizenship had three elements – social, civil and political; it was their unequal political rights and responsibilities that suggests children are not yet fully citizens. It is important to recognise, as Marshall did, that the equality which citizenship entails is more than a formal equality of status – it requires the equalisation of opportunities and burdens, which in turn requires greater social and material equality. A citizen-in-the-making requires material circumstances and education to facilitate the equal fulfilment of their potential.

The description of children as citizens-in-the-making is compatible with them being citizens now, provided that we accept that citizens may have relevant differences alongside what they have in common. Children have some protective rights and educative responsibilities not afforded to adults, just as adult citizens have certain political rights beyond those of children.

Education for citizenship

It could be argued that the introduction of citizenship education as a formal part of the schools curriculum in the United Kingdom during the last decade of the twentieth century was a major admission on the part of government that British citizens were ill-prepared for life in a modern democracy. The requirement to make citizenship an examinable subject in the National Curriculum in England[1] and in the other parts of the UK a cross-curricula subject followed the recommendations of the Advisory Group on Citizenship chaired by Sir Bernard Crick (QCA 1998). This invoked the concept of active citizenship and sought to make a radical impact, with an emphasis on making contributions to the wider community:

> We aim at no less than a change in the political culture of this country both nationally and locally: for people to think of themselves as active citizens, willing, able and equipped to have an influence in public life and with the critical capacities to weigh evidence before speaking and acting; to build on and to extend radically to young people the best in existing traditions of community involvement and public service, and to make them individually confident in finding new forms of involvement and action among themselves.
>
> (Paragraph 1.5)

The impetus behind the report was concern among politicians and some influential academic commentators about a malaise in the functioning not only of our democracy, but also of civic society in general. The report spoke of 'the worrying levels of apathy, ignorance and cynicism about public life', and a decline in 'traditional forms of civic cohesion' (paragraphs 3.5, 3.6). This was thought to apply especially to the young.

Here the Crick Report links to a wider a body of discourse claims about the loss of social capital (Putnam 2000). This is characterised by the weakening of community ties and increased individual isolation, consequent on both the disappearance of some organised groups in civil society and the narrowing of informal social networks.

[1] A National Curriculum Review raises doubts about whether citizenship will be a core subject after August 2014 (see Department of Education website).

Crick himself linked the weakness of British democracy with 'unsocial individualism and the values of consumer society' (Crick 2010: 22). The solution proposed in the Crick Report was to adopt the civic republican idea of citizenship endorsing the ethic of political engagement and civic activism. This requires schools to equip all students for active citizenship.

The purpose of citizenship education as set out in the report is to provide young people with the 'knowledge skills and values' to perform effectively in a participatory democracy' (QCA 1998: paragraph 6.6). It specifies three elements of citizenship to be learned:

1. social and moral responsibility;
2. community involvement;
3. political literacy.

Active citizenship is construed as 'a habitual interaction of all three' strands, while participation may be characterised as the 'glue' (Kiwan 2010)

The notion of learning 'social and moral responsibility' is compatible with a variety of core values and beliefs, and with either discursive or didactic teaching methods (see Chapter 23). Some may interpret education about moral responsibility as inculcating a particular ethical or religious code, but the Crick Report made it clear that moral education should prepare pupils and students to live within a multi-cultural and multi-faith society, and comprise discussion that allows them to make up their own minds on moral issues. Crick (2000) states that young people have a sense of fairness (recognised by primary-school-aged children), which provides a basis for recognising the reciprocity between rights and responsibilities and leads to a more sophisticated understanding of legal and social justice. The two remaining elements, political literacy and community engagement, are now examined more closely.

Political literacy

The concept of political literacy was introduced by Crick and Porter (1978) to move beyond the approach then current to teaching politics in schools. Hitherto, politics teaching had concentrated on the institutions of British government, partly as a way of avoiding political bias in teaching, which successive Education Acts in 1986 and 1996 had prohibited. By contrast, the Crick Report argued that discussion of controversial issues was 'the essence of worthwhile education' (QCA 1998: paragraph 10.4). Learning political literacy encompasses far more than knowledge of government and includes the skills and attributes required to function in equal democratic society.

Although active citizenship had been promulgated by the Conservative Major government, it was the Labour government that implemented the Crick Report and introduced its approach to citizenship education into schools by means of the Citizenship Order of 1999 (Crick 2003). Indeed a former student of Crick, David Blunkett, was the presiding Minister for Education. In England, citizenship education became a compulsory part of the National Curriculum. Elsewhere in the UK it was blended with existing subjects and taught in a more cross-curricular manner, following the 'light touch' prescription to allow schools to be responsive to local circumstances (Munn 2010). In Northern Ireland, citizenship education met with a mixed response. Some saw the concept as an opportunity to improve social cohesion. For others, it was hard to reconcile with a rejection of British identity or with school provision segregated by religion (Wylie 2004).

The Qualifications and Curriculum Authority provided guidance to schools in England, which closely followed the Crick recommendations:

> Citizenship addresses issues relating to social justice, human rights, community cohesion and global interdependence, and encourages students to challenge injustice, inequalities and discrimination. It helps young people to develop their critical skills, consider a wide range of political, social, ethical and moral problems, and explore opinions and ideas other than their own. They evaluate information, make informed judgements and reflect on the consequences of their actions now and in the future. They learn to argue a case on behalf of others as well as themselves and speak out on issues of concern.
>
> (QCA.org.uk quoted by Munn 2010: 91)

Crick saw that this approach required trust in teachers not to 'indoctrinate' their classes, as well as having the confidence and skills to manage discussions in which students learn about the rules and conventions of 'public discourse'. These include what he called 'procedural values – tolerance, fairness, respect for the truth and reasoned argument' (Crick 2000: 68) The 'procedural values' chimed well with the growth of participatory methods like school councils (see Chapter 12) and are also relevant to a range of group and youth work undertaken by professionals others than teachers. These are in fact more than procedural, as they introduce concepts central to the principles and practice of a liberal democracy. Crick (1962) had argued that the activity of politics in a broad sense is a vital safeguard not only against authoritarian government, but also against forms of oppression which come with the exercise of power in civil society – social deference, bigotry and fanaticism. Thus, teaching political literacy was from this perspective very much about the benefits to society as a whole, rather than about children's rights in the here and now. However, Crick saw politics as not being confined to voting and government actions, but as the art of reaching agreement by necessary compromise in all spheres, private and everyday as well as public and momentous. It is present for ordinary citizens 'in the family, the locality, educational institutions, clubs, and societies and informal groups of all kinds' (Crick 2000: 65).

Citizenship education reinforced the use of discursive methods in education, while 'political literacy' added explicit connections to the obligations of citizenship. The Crick Report drew on recent developments in education such as a 'whole school approach' (stressing the interconnectedness of subjects and learning) which includes attention to the 'informal curriculum', opportunities for participating in clubs and societies and school ethos. This means that citizenship education should not be confined to the classroom and to talking about external issues, but should affect all relationships among staff, students and parents. Moreover, Crick suggested that children should be involved in decision-making within the school and wherever possible be given 'responsibility and experience in helping to run parts of the school.' (QCA 1998: paragraph 6.3.1).

The concept of sharing in the goals and purposes of the school on equal footing with teachers is the key to students thinking of themselves as citizen members in a shared learning enterprise. The school, for most young people, is their first, and frequently most influential, experience of a public association. How they are treated and regarded has a major impact on how they function beyond the school. While schools should become more responsive to democratic practice and less unnecessarily authoritarian, it is not necessary for them to be wholly democratic institutions in order to foster political engagement (Lockyer 2010).

Children's and young people's perceptions of citizenship

Not a lot of evidence exists about what children and young people think of citizenship and studies in England showed their understandings to be vague. Nevertheless, voluntary community service is a key element in what they take it to be. A significant proportion of young people see themselves as partial- or non-citizens, because they see citizenship as contingent on such things as having your own home, voting or paying taxes (Lister et al. 2003). A large-scale survey of children and young people found that the majority were interested in current affairs and four-fifths thought they should have a voice in political affairs (CYPS 2003), but a significant proportion adopted a negative stereotype of politicians. Although many young people are indifferent or hostile to conventional party politics, many express a desire for more political education at school and some would like to see a lowering of the voting age to 15 or 16 (Fahmy 2006).

An international project examined children's views on citizenship in six countries in different parts of the world, though not including the UK (Smith et al. 2009; Taylor and Smith 2009). For the most part, children associated the term 'citizenship' (or its equivalent in languages other than English) with nationality or with local residence. Interestingly, they described what it means to be a citizen more in terms of responsibilities than rights. This included such things as the duty to vote and obey the law. Also important was being an active member of the community – caring about your local neighbourhood and being involved with efforts to make or keep it in good shape. Taking responsibility for the rights and well-being of others figured strongly in children's discussions of citizenship in some countries like Norway and New Zealand. Many children also implicitly recognised a model of being citizens-in-the-making as they described acquiring rights and exercising responsibilities in graduated steps as they got older.

A survey of 1000 girl guides revealed that they associated active citizenship most strongly with service to others, which has been a key principle of children's uniformed organisations for many years. The guides were deeply committed to voluntary work and aware of the importance of social issues, especially those that affect men and women differentially, but they tended not to see that these were relevant to politics (Fitzgerald 2010).

One of the main inhibitors of children perceiving themselves as capable citizens is their adopting adult stereotypes concerning themselves as implicitly irresponsible, threatening, or at risk and not to be trusted without supervision, especially in public space outside the home (see Example 14.1).

Example 14.1

In a survey of children's experiences of hospital, all 120 children interviewed as out-patients at three sites reported they would have to be accompanied by an adult in this environment (James et al. 2008). Among the reasons given were that they might:

■ hurt themselves;

■ get lost;

■ find medicines on the floor and eat them or drink them;

■ run off.

Community involvement and voluntary work

As we have seen, both the Crick Report and many children in their statements about citizenship highlight the importance of contributing to the local community. The concept of 'community involvement' was much heralded by the House of Commons Commission on Citizenship (1990), who enthused about involving young people in serving their communities. 'Young people should be offered the experience of working with others to tackle real problems in their local environment.' It was to the mutual benefit of the community and it would give the young person invaluable experience as a responsible member of a team developing essential skills.

This is part of extending the learning experience beyond the classroom and bringing schools into closer contact with local community organisations, including those with experience of working closely with young people. These ideas build to an extent on the concept of 'work experience' which already had a place within the notion of secondary education as preparation for employment; it added the concept that unpaid, freely given service to others was central to the idea of citizenship. The Crick Report suggested there was a strong connection between 'community-centred learning' and political engagement '. . . it could help make local government more democratic, open and responsive' (Paragraph 1.11). However, the connection here only arises when community volunteering has an educative strategic or political dimension. Active citizenship can also, of course, originate in the neighbourhood rather than in schools, as exemplified by the Investing in Children project in Durham, where young people have been supported to develop the skills and competence to engage in consultative decision-making (Cairns 2006).

If service in the community is to be politically educative, it needs to be more than providing help to needy neighbours, or sharing in collective local efforts to make good the lack of public funding. There is a growing recognition that it must be congruent with forms of participatory politics. Similar ideas apply to voluntary work by adults, including parents.

A well-developed component of citizenship education in the US is 'service learning' – namely, acquisition of knowledge and skills through work in and for the community. Similarly, Annette (2010) identified the potential for learning about democratic practice in the programmes for neighbourhood and civic renewal introduced by the last Labour government. This included a partnership strategy for making use of the human resources and resourcefulness of communities in return for some power devolved from government to the people – a principle echoed in the present government's Big Society ideas. Annette insists that community engagement as part of citizenship education must be structured to assist political literacy by involving some aspects of power-sharing.

It may be that voluntary service to the community provides substantive pre-employment opportunities for young people to encounter older citizens and 'civil serving professionals' in a context where they can recognise the value and relevance of active democratic political participation. It is not surprising that citizens-in-the-making readily find common ground with other disadvantaged groups.

Notions of citizenship are applicable to volunteering by adults, which has always played an important part in mutual help and continued to have a significant role after the establishment of the welfare state. The role of volunteer recognises that citizens have obligations to their fellows and that it can be appropriate for help to be offered without financial rewards. There are dangers that volunteers may be exploited or seen as cheap substitutes for professional service, but experience has shown that they can satisfactorily supplement and complement the work of paid professionals. There is, for instance, a long tradition of lay involvement in legal decision-making, in addition to qualified judges, by means of lay magistrates and justices of the peace (JPs) in England and by JPs and more recently children's panel members in Scotland (Reid and Gillan 2007). Volunteers also provide a direct service to children (e.g. as mentors and befrienders) or to parents, as in HomeStart. Although initially one-sided, the relationships can become reciprocal and cumulatively contribute to the building of civil society and social capital.

Bringing various kinds of professionals and local politicians into school, and arranging reciprocal visits, has been an expanding part of the citizenship curriculum (see Example 14.2).

Example 14.2

The Citizenship Foundation in partnership with the Law Society has a successful programme of 'Local Lawyers in Schools' to develop their awareness and understanding of the law. (www.locallawyersinschools. org.uk). This both enables lawyers to 'connect' with their local communities and gives young people a better idea of the law and how it can be used to defend people's rights. Lawyers have found themselves participating in debates about international human rights as well as local issues of law enforcement.

Conclusions and implications

This chapter has discussed how ideas from political philosophy about citizenship have had a direct and extensive impact on schooling. Thinking about when and how rights and responsibilities, in relation to both local community and national politics, are acquired is relevant to anyone who works with children.

It has been argued above that viewing children within the setting of the school as citizens-in-the-making is potentially transformative both to the ethos of the institution and to relations between staff and students. A key element of learning to be a citizen in a democracy is provided by opportunities to be an equal partner in decisions at home, in school and in the community at large. This is a precondition for the reform and improvement of local and national political institutions. These opportunities arise in non-autocratic settings. The more we can reduce the arbitrary and unnecessary exercise of power over children, the more they will be able to contribute to democratic life.

It is also important to consider how treating children as active citizens-in-the-making could affect their relations with other service providers or agencies who engage with young people. What difference might it make to view children as active citizens rather than consumers, or patients, as objects of care, or in need of special measures of supervision or support?

Welfare provision is generally focused on the concept of the individual, whether adult or child, whose vital needs should be met. Although different agencies make somewhat different assumptions, there is tendency, and even a policy imperative for some purposes, to regard them as consumers. The power of consumers lies largely in their entitlement to choose or refuse what is on offer. The notion that recipients of welfare might also be providers, or parties to the corporate decisions which influence priorities of resources allocation is an atypical, if not wholly alien, concept (Donnison 2010).

If children in particular are conceived as citizens-in-the-making, my suggestion is that it is not solely an obligation of educators to assist them to become better, in the sense of more literate and empowered, citizens. For all those able to have views, consulting them on matters that affect them (alone or among others) acknowledges their identity and agency. Giving their views fair consideration and due weight follows. So too does the general duty to assist them to participate in decisions. This is no more than their due as citizens with rights. However, what is often overlooked is to respect them as bearers of responsibilities.

Oddly we are happy to attribute the capacity for moral and criminal responsibility from an early age. We are less willing to recognise children's active-responsibility for assisting family members, siblings and parents, or friends and neighbours. Although there is now greater recognition of young people as a distinctive interest group who have a legitimate voice to be heard via consultation or youth parliaments, this does not generally extend to recognising them as advocates for the interests of others, as young carers, for instance, are able to do.

Viewing children as citizens now requires us also to recognise their democratic political responsibilities. No professional or lay person, any more than the state, ought to be indifferent to the development of the next generation of citizens. In assisting them to be more active and able, we enhance not only their prospects of life in a civilised democracy but ours too, whether we work with children or not.

Exercise

Consider or discuss what difference there might be in your treatment of young people if you were to consider them as fellow citizens, now and in-the-making, rather than as patients, clients, students or consumers. What difficulties might there be for your cooperation with (other) professionals if you insisted on relating to young people as citizen to citizen?

Recommended reading

The Crick Report contains both an excellent review of key issues about citizenship and associated education principle, as well as a blueprint for action.

The Citizenship Foundation http://www.citizenshipfoundation.org.uk is an invaluable source.

Association for Citizenship Teaching (ACT) http://www.teachingcitizenship.org.uk/ provides materials, projects and information supporting citizenship education.

Invernizzi and Williams (2008) covers many issues associated with children, citizenship and the UNCRC.

Crick and Lockyer (2010) is an accessible collection of essays on the implications of active citizenship.

Part III

EVIDENCE AND THEORY FOR PRACTICE WITH CHILDREN AND FAMILIES

This section of the book takes a step back from policy and organisational issues affecting services for children to consider research and theoretical concepts that underpin professional practice. Our choice is inevitably selective, concentrating on ideas and findings of particular relevance to most people working with children.

The accumulation and analysis of research evidence is closely intertwined with theorisation. Sometimes hypotheses are developed from theories and then tested – for example, about the impact of the nature, immediacy and frequency of reward and punishment on children's learning. Alternatively, concepts may be developed to help interpret research findings (see Chapter 1). Often a body of knowledge may develop through constant interaction between evidence and concepts, as in relation to attachment and resilience (see Chapters 18 and 19). Theorisation is important because it provides practitioners with guiding principles and ideas that can inform assessment and action. For instance, Corby (2006) urged practitioners to be open to a range of explanatory theories about child abuse, which he grouped into psychological, social psychological and sociological. The theories have differing implications for the level, stage and nature of professional activities – e.g. separating and/or changing an abuser, treating the family as a whole or tackling social structures and norms. These need not be mutually exclusive.

A distinct form of research that is especially relevant to the work of professionals is evaluation of services or specific forms of intervention. Evaluative studies vary in purpose and design, but most seek to establish whether or not a particular way of working is effective (see Chapters 16 and 17). For this, experimental methods and standardised measures are usually seen as most conclusive, but other approaches are available. It can also be important to find out how well the principles of a programme or agency goals are put into practice and assess the views of service providers and recipients. Increasingly, practitioners are involved in evaluations of their own agency, often engaging young people in the process (Coghlan and Brannick 2005; Tisdall et al. 2009).

Experimental research is well suited to unitary treatments, but when an intervention has multiple components it is harder for studies to disentangle the contribution of different elements (Craig et al. 2010). It must also be remembered that systematic research evidence usually involves findings that the intervention in question produces good results more probably or for more people than an alternative course of action, but there may be individuals for which it is less well suited (Hill 2009b). It appears, for example, that young women often do not respond well to the kinds of cognitive-behavioural programmes for young offenders that experimental evidence has show generally work well for many young men (though not all). Moreover, reliance on standard programmes ignores others kinds of evidence about how young people desist from offending, which indicates individualised influences and pathways (McNeill 2009a).

This Part covers research and theory in relation to children and families, while Part IV examines evidence and concepts relevant to interprofessional cooperation. It is possible to connect the two – for instance, through understanding of systems (in the family, child's environment and service organisations) or through application of ideas about learning (Daniels 2001; Chapter 23). For example, Vygotsky's (1978; 1986) theories on child development and learning, which currently have a strong influence on learning and teaching in schools, have also been influential in theorising how adults work together (Engeström 1999; Wenger 1998) in order to generate understanding, insight and effectiveness in their inter-disciplinary activities.

The first two chapters deal with general features of the population of great relevance to children. First, Jamieson provides an account of changing family relationships and forms which shape children's experiences and identities. The chapter considers the implications of family diversity and disruption for care networks and the time that parents and other adults have available for children. Jamieson notes how differences in family life and resources interact with social divisions of social class and ethnicity. Cohort studies, which follow up large representative samples of children over a number of years, confirm that material disadvantage adversely affects children's educational attainments and parental health, while ethnic differences are complex (Hansen et al. 2010a). Understanding family practices and relationships is critical for many people working with children. Assessment of resources, communication, roles, rules and the setting of internal and external boundaries can provide important pointers to changes that may be needed to improve the care of children, reduce internal conflict or manage external pressures. A range of theories have been developed and applied in more specialist work including family therapy and relationship counselling – for instance, based on psychodynamic, systems or structural approaches to the family (Rivett and Street 2003; Geldard and Geldard 2009). Narrative approaches link perceptions of family history and possibly distortions and secrets to individual biographical identities.

Next, Chapter 16 considers protective and risk factors in child health. Beck (1992) has argued that society has become increasingly marked by risk, with young people facing many uncertainties and a growth in collective and environmental hazards. Moreover, Roberts argues, this has been combined with a tendency to attribute setbacks as personal shortcomings rather than due to external events or circumstances. Children are often described as 'at risk' of harm, abuse or behaving badly. There are two other main senses of the word 'risk'. First, it is often used to denote a hazard or threat. Second, it refers to the chance or probability that something will happen, usually a negative outcome like an illness or accident, though the same principles apply to positive events such as passing exams or winning the lottery. Roberts addresses both environmental threats to children, like traffic accidents, and long-term risks to well-being. She cites evidence about the close link between inequalities in child health and social inequalities and the extent of poverty. Hence, action is necessary on a wide front (not only by health services) if the gap in health outcomes and life expectancy is to be reduced and the negative lifelong implications of issues like obesity and smoking are to be tackled. Roberts concludes that a secure family income, good education, living in a safe environment and good affordable childcare are essential for promoting child health and eradicating inequalities in health. While supporting the use of sound research findings, Roberts highlights evidence about the valuable role that lay expertise can play, so that health and other professionals should understand and tap into the knowledge of parents, children and others, for example about local environmental hazards. This echoes points raised in Part 2 of the book.

Besides 'risk', other key terms that inform both policy and theoretical frameworks in relation to children are 'rights' (considered in Parts I and II) and 'needs', which are crucial to the chapters that follow. They consider what children require from their environment and support services to meet a wide range of their needs – emotional, health, educational, and so on. The topics covered broadly follow an age-related trajectory, starting with infancy and ending at the threshold of adulthood. However, rather than provide a developmental account for which many text books are available, they seek to illustrate important themes involving children, such as mental health, well-being, offending and disability.

Within the family, the relationship between a child and the parents or other caregivers is fundamental. Chapter 17 describes how the close attunement of carers to the needs and moods of infants – and the opposite of insensitivity – have a major impact on social, emotional, cultural and developmental well-being. The chapter illustrates how evidence-based programmes focusing on detailed carer–infant interaction can be very helpful to improve the quality of parenting, especially for young children with additional needs. Quinton (2004) and Hallam (2008) have reviewed research evidence about what kinds of approach to parenting support are helpful, including those aimed at families with older children.

Chapter 18 develops this theme in an account of attachment theory, which is concerned with the nature and impact of children's intimate relationships, particularly with their parents or other carers. Early formulations of attachment theory provided many useful insights about the importance of consistent, responsive care, as Puckering also emphasises, but were also criticised, for example, as overgeneralising about dangers of early short separations and multiple attachments (Hill and Tisdall 1997: pp. 44–45; Davies 2011: p. 111). However, recent research has built an important body of knowledge with implications for all aspects of children's needs, as well as for parenting and later life (Howe 2011). Minnis and Bryce show how understanding of attachment processes can provide a shared language among different kinds of professional. They emphasise the importance for children to have a 'secure base' in order to gain confidence, learn and relate well to others. Insecure attachment patterns are related to problematic care, significant losses or traumas in early life. Children with such experiences often challenge professionals and new carers emotionally and behaviourally, so that understanding of the underlying dynamics helps practitioners not only with assessment, but with learning how to ensure their own responses are constructive. Insights have been widely applied to children who are looked after in public care or adopted (Anglin 2002; Schofield and Beek 2006), but are relevant in many other contexts where children have experienced abuse or significant problems in their early care.

Ideas about resilience developed out of attachment theory, in part as a counterbalance to emphasis on the negative long-term consequences that often arise from early adversity and abuse. Chapter 19 observes that resilience has been influential particularly in schools, child psychiatry and social work, but has many similarities with desistance thinking in relation to crime, addiction and other problematic behaviours. The former deals with factors and processes involved in overcoming difficult early childhood environments – the latter is concerned with factors and processes that promote reduction or cessation of negative behaviour or lifestyles. Hill suggests that recognising the crossovers between resilience and desistance can provide commonalities not only among professionals working with children, but also between adult and children's services.

Finally Chapter 20 reviews ideas about transition as they apply to young people with learning disabilities. Two main kinds of transition may be recognised. The first is the psycho-social transition, which involves going through a major life event such as birth of a sibling, separation from family members, death of a loved one and marriage. The timing of psycho-social transitions is variable and some may be experienced at any age. The events tend to be mainly positive or mainly negative, but even the more extreme experiences usually have both aspects. Marriage is normally a very happy event but also entails some stress, whereas bereavement is, of course, normally very distressing, but nevertheless offers opportunities to build coping skills and connectedness with others in the same position.

The second type is a life-stage transition, which most or all people typically go through at roughly similar ages. Life-stage transitions may be divided into those with a direct biological basis (puberty, the menopause, old age) and those which relate to social institutions (starting and leaving school, retiring). The online *International Journal of Transitions in Childhood* contains a range of relevant articles. Like psycho-social transitions, life-stage transitions provide losses, challenges and opportunities as in the move from childhood to adulthood, which represents a blend of the biological and social. Macintyre describes how this particular transition is negotiated by young people generally in the UK. Then she shows that this can be especially problematic for young people with learning disabilities.[1] This arises partly because their assumption of independence may be delayed, and partly as a result of discontinuities and gaps in support involved in the change from children's to adult services involved with different dimensions of their lives like education and health. Thus, this final chapter links to the theme of inter-professional cooperation, explored further in Part IV.

Reflective exercise

In relation to a children's problem or issue you are interested in, review how different theories affect the ways the problem/issue is framed and how that affects policy and professional responses. What kind of research findings about the causes, processes and consequences could help guide responses?

---

[1] Readers interested in the experiences and transitions of younger disabled children may wish to consult Robinson and Stalker (1999) and Connors and Stalker (2002).

Chapter 15

Understanding different kinds of family in context

Lynn Jamieson

Summary points

- Family relationships, particularly between main carer(s) and child, remain fundamental to children's acquisition of a sense of self, their place in the world and the values orienting their conduct.
- Family forms are diverse and the boundaries around families are often fuzzy.
- Normative ideals of traditional family life persist, but the quality of relationships are nowadays generally seen as more important than formal roles.
- Friendships are important complements and sometimes alternatives to the support and care provided by close family.
- Disruptions to family households sometimes also disrupt care networks when they are particularly needed.
- The combination of dual-earning family household and heightened expectations of intensely intimate relationships creates inevitable time pressures and tensions.
- Differences in access to resources, connections and knowledge through families and their networks reproduce social divisions of social class and ethnicity.

Introduction

Nearly all children grow up in families of one kind or another. Family relationships influence every aspect of their lives and crucially influence their life chances and trajectories. Social research on families and personal relationships offers insight into the diversity of family lives as they are lived and into how social change in families and personal life impact on children and young people. The research evidence includes a growing body of work directly mapping how children and young people themselves experience and perceive family dynamics and family change. Some of the academic work in this topic area addresses concerns that are both more theoretical and more wide-ranging than those normally addressed by professional practitioners or policy makers. It includes, for example, understanding how personal life adapts to long-term social change and attempts to evaluate common beliefs such as the idea that people are becoming more individualistic and less socially integrated. This chapter offers some engagement with such wider issues and with more focused research on the family lives of children and young people.

Professionals seeking to be collaborative change agents need to have an informed view of family diversity to guard against inappropriately treating one model of family life as normative and inadvertently creating exclusion or harm. They also require understanding of the interrelationship between people's conduct of their personal lives and the family (and wider) contexts that shape individuals' room for manoeuvre. Otherwise, efforts might be misdirected to changing individual behaviour without consideration of how significant relationships may work against such change. Similarly, interventions directed at collaboratively modifying wider contexts in which families operate in order to enhance the lives of children and young people require a shared sense of what is amenable to professional intervention and its likely impact. The sketch offered here of how diversity and social change in families impact on children and young people offers insight into a range of academic literature that professionals can then combine with the specific knowledge they draw from their own practice.

Definitions and concepts: family practices and informal networks of care

The conceptual apparatus used by academics to describe families has modified in response to the diversity of family forms and the fuzziness of boundaries around what is and is not family. While family relationships can be formally defined in terms of biologically and legally constituted relationships, in reality families and households have never been confined to married parents and children or even to extended kin. For example, in preceding centuries with higher rates of mortality, there were many instances not only of relatives substituting for dead parents and bringing up nephews, nieces and grandchildren, but also of informal fostering and adoption arrangements by non-kin without the sanction of law. Over the past 100 years or so, high rates of couple dissolution have replaced death as the most common reason for reconfiguration of children's family households and parenting arrangements. In the late twentieth and twenty-first centuries various forms of donor-assisted conception and surrogacy create new biological complexities. Neither the legal recognition of arrangements as 'real' family nor everyday naming conventions have kept up fully with changing patterns of family lives. In the UK half of children are now born to parents who are not legally married. In most cases unmarried parents are living together, but the law has only very recently extended legal parental responsibilities and rights to unmarried fathers registering their child's birth (2003 in England and Wales, 2006 in Scotland). Labels such as in-laws and step-parent seem less successful when cohabiting birth parents are not married, and serial cohabitation is more common than marriage, divorce and remarriage. Social researchers have moved away from preconceived definitions of 'the family' to an analysis of 'families' or 'family life' and, more recently, 'family practices' as lived, experienced and defined by those who are studied. 'Family practices', (Morgan 1996, 2011) side-steps the issue of providing a definition of the family in terms of a particular household structure or composition of types of relationships; rather, it focuses on the process of how people themselves conceptualise and construct their family.

In terms of many people's ideal view of how families should be, family life remains about practically caring *for* people and caring *about* them (love). Children's decisions about who is a member of their family usually depend on experiences of both being cared for and being cared about (O'Connor et al. 2004; Pryor 2006). Children with neglectful, alcohol-abusing parents may forgive lapses in practical acts of care if they feel they have other routine evidence of their parent's love. However, some children respond to social ideals by expressing loyalty even to parents who have been extremely neglectful (Backett-Milburn et al. 2008). Children who have never even met their father can cherish hopes that one day they will have a relationship with him (Highet and Jamieson 2007).

Understanding the extent to which people, children or adults, are cared about and the potential of their intimate personal ties to deliver care for them requires understanding of the nature and quality of the whole constellation of a person's close social network that acts as an informal system of emotional and practical support (see Chapter 9). Children's parents, particularly mothers, typically loom large as significant supports in their lives, but so typically do friends and sometimes siblings and other kin – a grandparent, an aunt or uncle or cousin. Friends are preferred over parents as confidantes for some kinds of information and support (Dunn 2004; Morrow 2004). Some academic analysts of personal life have argued that friendships rather than family relationships are on the ascendant as the ideal-typical intimate relationships of adulthood and that for growing numbers of people friends are key sources of emotional and practical support (Spencer and Pahl 2006; Jamieson et al. 2006). Research has shown considerable similarities in the repertoire of support and intimacy that family and friends perform, though practical acts of care and emotional caring are usually strongest in familial relationships, especially in the child–parent–grandparent line.

A number of academic studies of children's families suggest that the care and support children receive from parents and in families should be seen as embedded in wider informal networks of care, if the strength and resilience of children's support systems are to be fully understood (Hansen 2005; Widmer and Jallinoja 2008). Personal networks have been conceptualised in terms of the access they provide to economic capital (money and material resources), social capital (social connections) and cultural capital (socially valued knowledge) (Gillies and Edwards 2006, Holland 2009). Social class and ethnic differences in children's access to resources through their networks contribute to the reproduction of inequalities. The degree of interconnection between and multiplicity of sources of support within a network also vary with differential consequences for the resilience of the network in the face of disruption. Some children and their families are embedded in close-knit social networks which are supportive, but also bind them to a disadvantageous context with no connections to more advantaged worlds beyond the local and familiar (MacDonald and Marsh 2005). For ethnic minority families, the widespread experience of racism also inhibits connections beyond the ethnic minority community. The networks of families and their access to economic and cultural capital through a local community and/or transnational kinship ties cannot always be predicted by social class or ethnicity – the idea that ethnic minority communities always 'look after their own' has been critiqued as a stereotype (Chattoo et al. 2004; Becher 2008).

Intimacy can be intensified by privacy and exclusion, the active creation of boundaries keeping others at a distance. The creation of boundaries requires acts of imagination and acts of commission – for example, limits in access to the time of family members, to the place of the family home and to family resources (Jamieson 2005). Boundaries around and within personal relationships are not always created mutually or to enhance intimacy, but sometimes to protect and sometimes to ensure control and domination. In status-conscious societies, fear of being judged makes those with little to show off more likely to restrict access to their home. In violent relationships abusers typically work to socially isolate and emotionally entrap the abused. Families and family households vary in the extent to which members actively and consciously create boundaries between those designated as close family and others and in the extent to which alliances and divisions are formed within families. Caring activities and ways of spending time are not always exclusive, dyadic or 'family only' projects. Sometimes coordinated boundary work is a response to a hostile environment – for example, to protect members from racism or the stigmatising response experienced by people with disability. Sometimes children seek to create boundaries between friends and family, because they experience their family as stigmatising. Children with drug or alcohol abusing parents often adopt a strategy of never bringing friends home to ensure they do not see domestic chaos or strange behaviour by their parents (Bancroft et al. 2002). Understanding the state of play with respect to boundary work for a particular family household member can be very helpful for any agency seeking to work closely with a young person and their family.

The changed and changing context of family life

Many of the causes of change in family life are global, although their specific effects vary considerably by national and regional context and the associated costs and benefits are felt unequally (see Chapter 6). The dual-earner family-household as the ideal-typical family was prompted and made possible by the cultural, economic, social and political changes which underpin the combined advanced development of democratic welfare states and global capitalism with associated high levels of consumption. Most men and women in rich capitalist countries now take for granted state-sanctioned gender equality in education and employment, although women's rights were relatively recently hard won and elements of gender equality remain elusive. Both young women and men seek security of income through employment to achieve their desired standard of living, and, in most cases, as a precursor to having a family. The overwhelming majority still seek long-term partnerships and children, albeit not all in the context of marriage or a heterosexual relationship (Sobotka and Toulemon 2008).

A significant social change in personal life discussed by academics since the mid-twentieth century has been a shift in normative emphasis from 'institution' to 'relationship' – that is, a shift from celebrating marriage and the family as conventional, legally and religiously sanctioned institutions to celebrating intimate relationships (Smart 2007). While marriage remains an alliance between families and religious duty for many British Asian families (Shaw 2004; Becher 2008), for most white British couples the act of marriage lacks moral weight, but is simply about celebrating their relationship. The majority of British couples have lived together before marriage and, while some see marriage as the final step in commitment, many say it makes no difference (Jamieson et al. 2002; Wu Musick 2008). Moreover, for the majority of couples wishing to have children together, this is not taken for granted as an outcome of their union but sought for the quality of the parent–child relationship. Arguably intimacy, the quality of closeness and connection in relationships, has become more important than 'the family' as such, although some minorities continue to place cultural emphasis on traditional gender and generational hierarchies (Lee et al. 2002).

Patterns of demographic change in rates of fertility and mortality also follow a dominant pattern globally of declining fertility, smaller family sizes and improving mortality as standards of living rise, leading to ageing populations (Harris 2006). As in most of northern Europe, the typical pattern of family formation in the UK no longer follows a traditional sequence of marriage, setting up a household and then having children. The majority of couples who form legal partnerships have lived together prior to marriage and half of children are born to unmarried parents. Average family sizes among white British families have shrunk such that many children grow up with only one sibling or no siblings at all. The average age of becoming a parent has increased, particularly among educated middle-class parents, although rates of teenage motherhood remain higher in the UK than in the rest of Europe. Late childbearing increases the proportion of parents combing childcare with care of older relatives. While many children grow up with two parents, high rates of couple dissolution mean a significant minority proportion of children live in post-divorce/separation arrangements: lone-parent households, households with one parent and the parent's partner and/ or moving between households of a mother and father. Rates of divorce are much lower among some ethnic minorities where divorce continues to carry a strong stigma. Post-'divorce' arrangements can disrupt children's relationship with their father and his kin, and when parental separation also triggers moving home and school then children's informal networks of care may be significantly damaged or cease to function, thus enhancing their vulnerability. However, children usually adapt to such changes with at least some degree of success (see Example 15.1).

Example 15.1 Loss of a parent from the family home

Danny lived with his mother, who had a non-resident boyfriend. Danny's account of the situation indicated that his mother slowed the pace of her boyfriend's involvement to avoid complicating parenting arrangements. Danny and his siblings made weekend visits to his father's household, shared with a stepmother and her two daughters. When interviewed at age 11, he claimed not to like his step-mum and said he did not get enough time alone with his father. His mother encouraged him to persist and a girl at school with separated parents also advised he would get through it. When interviewed again about six months later, he had become reconciled to the visits, acknowledging that 'because I kept going, even though I didn't want to, that it made me like it'.

Susie was very unhappy following the death of her mother, who she regarded as her best friend. This loss was compounded by disappointment in her father, who was immersed in work. Also, support from wider

▶

kin was limited, because it has been her mother who organised contact with her grandparents, aunts and uncles. By contrast, Rebecca appeared to have adapted as well as could be expected to the death of her father when she was age seven. This had been helped by her mother's extensive careful preparation for her father's death including a long family holiday together when her father was still able to travel.

(Highet and Jamieson 2007 © CRFR)

These brief case studies illustrate the importance of informal networks of care continuing to provide support at times of family disruption and their vulnerability. Although contact with paternal grandparents is often reduced when a father leaves home, a prior good relationship with a grandparent is likely to persist and offer continued support (Hawthorne et al. 2003; Ferguson et al. 2004). When a parent dies, the response of the surviving parent is crucial, especially as bereaved children may become more isolated from friends and family. Only rarely do they receive professional help (Ribbens McCarthy 2006).

In the UK, as in most of the world, the main burden of domestic work continues to be carried by women in the majority of households, despite the explicit acknowledgement by the majority of both British men and women that domestic tasks should be shared equally by dual full-time-worker couples. Working mothers have the most acute experience of time poverty – the experience of tension created by the gap between expectations of gender equality and realities is most likely in their households (Crompton 2006; Wajcman 2008). Fathers as full-time carers remain a relative rarity. When gender role reversal has taken place, it is sometimes an unsought consequence of men's unemployment rather than a chosen strategy (Charles and James 2005), although Brannen and Nilsen (2006) suggest that exceptionally family-oriented men may seek under-employment. Statistical analysis of the time employed fathers spend looking after their children indicates higher average times among high earners working shorter hours (Koslowski 2010). Although there is evidence of more widespread intimacy between fathers and children than in the past, the majority of children still have a sense of a closer tie to their mothers than their fathers (Pike et al. 2006).

The combination of dual-earning and heightened expectations of 'quality time' creates significant pressures. Children sometimes crave time unstructured and unsupervised by adults, while parents seek 'quality time' with their children (Christensen 2002). The literature discusses the extent to which intimacy requires equality and democracy in order to flourish, both between genders and across generations. This includes debate over whether the tendency for parents to want to be more friend-like with their children, that became common in the late twentieth century, meant a loss of parental authority and inevitable tension between parental desire for intimacy and control (Brannen et al. 2004). In the UK there have been a number of studies noting that parent–teenage talk claimed as evidence of intimacy by parents can be seen as surveillance by the child (Solomon et al. 2002). The work suggests that children's experience of their parent's mobile phone calls is often in terms of surveillance and control, though this can be interpreted as positive concern (Ling and Yttri 2006; Hill et al. 2006).

Family households are key sites of consumption of the technologies of globalised capitalist markets. Children have themselves become consumers and 'a market', as recipients of an ever expanding repertoire of aggressively marketed toys and services of 'normal' childhood (Schor 2004). The digital technologies of the internet, the mobile phone and rapid transport technologies that are the socio-technical aspect of 'globalisation' are not available in the poorest family households of the rich world (Livingstone 2009), just as they are not available in much of the majority poor world. The car has become an aspect of how the majority of families live their lives and a way of ensuring children's safety in transit outside the home in many households. Its ubiquity has profound consequences for the freedom of all childhoods. The steep social-class gradient in collisions between cars and children as pedestrians (Grayling et al. 2002) reflects differences in the use of walking for travel, children from poorer families being less likely to have access to a car, and differences in access to safe play space and proximity of busy roads.

Although the significance of social class may have diminished as a marker of identity in the UK, and class boundaries have blurred, cultural legacies of periods of starker class differences persist which are more than simply matter of economic advantage. Class differences in parents' orientations to their children's education often communicate different philosophies – white middle-class parents with professional and managerial experience are more likely to communicate a sense of their child's uniqueness and entitlement to special treatment, while working-class parents are more likely to encourage their children to 'fit in' and be part of the crowd (Gillies 2007). Some aspects of class difference have all but disappeared, such as working-class expectations that children and young people contribute to the household economy by their early teens (Jamieson 1987), but differences in expectations of achieving early independence persist. It is working-class young people who are more likely to make early transitions to adulthood through unplanned pregnancy and early exit from education, albeit often in spite of intentions (Henderson et al. 2007; Jones 2009). Irwin (2009) found that, although the emotional support young people get from their family has a positive effect on their academic motivation, and working-class young people were as supported as their middle-class peers, social class remained a strong influences on expectations of getting to university. Some educationally motivated, working-class young people were not anticipating university, whereas some middle-class unmotivated young people were.

Ethnic minority and transnational families

The UK has always contained transnational families, both white British families with active ties to relatives who have emigrated and immigrant ethnic minority families with ties to their original homeland. Immigrant and ethnic minority families are a growing, albeit still quite small, proportion of the total population (Hill 2009a). British official statistics, including the Census, have adopted a classification of ethnicity using a white/ethnic minority, non-white classification, further broken down by national and global-regional labels. Ten per cent of UK family-households with dependent children have mothers defining themselves as from an ethnic minority group – 5 per cent Asian (Indian, Pakistani, Bangladeshi or Asian British), 2 per cent Black (African, Caribbean or Black British) and 3 per cent a range of other ethnic groups including Chinese (Maplethorpe et al. 2009). In 2007 white non-British groups, white Europeans, Irish and other white groups, outnumbered the combined total of Indian and Pakistani background (ONS 2009).

Studies of the personal lives of second- and third-generation migrants and long-established, once-migrant, ethnic minority communities in the UK have typically found transnational and multi-local families embedded in continuing ties and caring relationships across kin separated by national boundaries and continents (e.g. Goulbourne et al. 2010). In the UK many ethnic minority families from the Indian subcontinent are part of established migrant communities with continued links with their place of origin; use of extended kin connections (*biradari*) for arranged marriages helps to maintain cultural conventions of respect for gender roles and generational hierarchy (Yeoh et al. 2005; Shaw 2004) although with the variation of bringing husbands to bride's families as well as the conventional arrangement of wives living with husband's families (Charsley 2005). However, there is considerable variation among ethnic minority families both in cultural and religious views, and some have lost their sense of connection with wider kindred. Also tradition should not be seen as only passed down the generations. Becher (2008) suggests that in some British households religious knowledge was being passed 'upwards' with children acting as 're-instaters of tradition', since they had access to the formal religious education that their parents lacked.

The term global 'care chains' was coined (Ehrenreich and Hochschild 2003) to describe a relatively new pattern of migration whereby women from poor countries are employed in rich countries for care work, replacing women's 'family care' and sending remittances back for the care and education of their own children and/or the care of their own parents. In some cases pioneer migrants pay a high price. For example, traditional views of appropriate gender roles stigmatise Philippine migrant mothers despite their strenuous efforts to remain good mothers, actively playing a part in the lives of their children though constant flows of communication (Parreñas 2005). Another form of migration results from asylum seekers, who experience major disruption of their supportive ties and identities – see Example 15.2. Unaccompanied child asylum seekers and refugees are particularly bereft of family and other supports, so that they require help from a range of agencies, first to meet their immediate needs and then gradually to build up new social resources (Kohli and Mitchell 2007).

Example 15.2 Migration

Serila arrived in the UK aged 8 as part of an asylum-seeking family with her younger brother, sister, mother and father. They all had previously lived with Serila's paternal grandparents in Turkey. Serila described her prolonged sadness at the sudden loss of daily access to her grandparents, friends and other kin, the place she felt was home, freedom to play outside, her possessions and the currency of her language. By age 13 she was fluent in English and happy at school, but her life was otherwise mainly home-based out of school hours because of parents' fears for her safety and sense of propriety. Her support beyond her parents came from two friends, Turkish girls in similar uncertain circumstances whom she feared losing.

(Highet and Jamieson 2007 © CRFR)

Conclusions and implications

Families are normally the main providers of practical care of children and emotional care about them (see also Chapters 17 and 18). They can also generate problems when there is conflict or loss as a result of death, separation or movement, which may bring them to the attention of official services. In many contexts, working with children entails working with families. Hence, professionals who work with children require an understanding of family dynamics and critical awareness of how family life is shaped by wider social norms and ideals.

Understanding social and family change involves scrutiny of the interaction between the common 'generational' or cohort experience of those at a particular age in a particular historical context – e.g. 'baby-boomers', 'Thatcher's children' – and how people work individually and collaboratively with the specific constraining and enabling circumstances of their own biographies. Widespread patterns of demographic, economic and cultural change are associated with radical change in the rhythms of age-and-stage transitions of family life and typical family trajectories (Henderson et al. 2007; Hobcraft 2009). They have also modified inequalities and social division between genders, social class, religious and ethnic groups, but such inequalities persist and continue to be reproduced as well as further modified by families and their informal networks of care. State policies and interventions in education, training, housing, employment and welfare are elements of that wider context. Children, young people and families are agents of social change and have no choice but to manoeuvre within the affordances of their time and place. All of the evidence reviewed indicates that family relationships, and particularly the part played by a child's main carer or carers, remain crucial to a child's acquisition of a sense of self and their place in the world. That includes their participation in social differentiation. The family home is where differences of gender, generation and other distinctions which underpin social divisions are first learned, resisted and enacted.

The contemporary emphasis on the quality of 'relationships' should not mask the endurance of the practices that made families worthy of being conceptualised as 'institutions', bringing up children, transmitting values, bestowing and maintaining identities and providing care across generations. The overwhelming majority of children are cared for and feel cared about within families, and the few who are neglected give up very reluctantly on their family. However, what 'a family' is cannot be taken for granted as having a particular structure or constituents, but rather is what people experience it to be. Effective support for families will typically require an understanding of what families and their wider informal networks of support look like to their members and neutrality concerning the nature of 'family'.

The boundary between care provided by family and friends is often fluid, and children's carers typically draw on wider informal networks of support, grandparents, other kin and friends to deliver their care. Transnational families providing care across national boundaries are increasingly common and testimony to the resilience of kin relationships. Unfortunately, when family relationships are disrupted, as they commonly are by the dissolution of the parenting couple or, in some cases, by migration or death, then the informal networks that provide children with care are sometimes also damaged. This may be a point where professional intervention might be particularly valuable either substituting for absent informal ties or helping to rebuild them.

Exercise

If possible, speak with a child known to you about his/her family (or consider your own situation as a child). Who counts as part of the family and why? How is caring for and caring about the child distributed among family members and others? How has the family been affected by losses of members and by moves? In what ways is social and technological change affecting relationships and communication within the family. Think about how answers to such questions may assist you in your current or planned work with children.

Recommended reading

Highet and Jamieson (2007) discuss responses to family and social change from young people's perspectives.

Edwards, R., Hadfield, L. and Mauthner, M. (2005) *Children's Understandings of Their Sibling Relationships*, London: National Children's Bureau/Joseph Rowntree Foundation. Considers sibling relationships from young people's perspectives.

Ribbens McCarthy, J. (2006) reviews young people's experiences of loss and bereavement.

Twine, F. W. (2010) *A White Side of Black Britain: Interracial Intimacy and Racial Literacy.* Duke University Press, North Carolina.

Provides insights into the struggle of young people and their parents against racism.

Chapter 16

Protective and risk factors in child health

Helen Roberts

Summary points

- A child born into poverty is more likely than the better-off baby in the next cot to die in the first year of life, be born small or early or both, become overweight or die from accidental injury in childhood.
- Inequalities in child health result largely from social inequalities. Risks are unevenly distributed.
- The health gap between the most and least disadvantaged children in the UK remains wide, and for some health outcomes it may be widening.
- Parents, usually mothers, are the main providers of healthcare for their children. Most do this well, even in difficult circumstances. Policy and practice messages that parenting needs to be 'fixed' can be undermining.
- Children and parents are an important source of lay expertise. This expertise can be tapped to inform and underpin successful policy and practice development.
- Important sources of support for practice and policy development in health and social care are provided by organisations such as NICE, which provide research evidence including 'user' expertise and analyse costs in relation to benefits.
- The health service on its own cannot tackle inequalities in child health. A secure family income, a good education, living in a safe environment and good, affordable childcare are essential for promoting child health and eradicating inequalities in health. Parents, teachers and a whole range of professionals beyond healthcare play an important part in addressing health risks to children.

Introduction

Although the National Health Service tends to be seen largely in terms of dealing with illness, health is, of course, a broad concept. The WHO definition, in force since 1948, is that 'Health is a state of complete physical, mental and social well-being and not merely the absence of disease or infirmity' (WHO 1948). All the key people in a child's life contribute to this – teachers, neighbours, health professionals and, where appropriate, other professionals including those in social care.

The majority of health care is done in the home, usually by mothers, most of whom do a good job. However, it is ill-health that tends to hit the headlines. Child and infant mortality are often taken as proxies for the general state of a nation's health and commitment to the well-being of its citizens. Every country, and many international agencies, give a degree of priority to child health. We know that many child illnesses are preventable, and that insults to health and well-being in childhood cast a long shadow forward into adult life – a problem in both human and economic terms. On the more positive side, there is good evidence that many of these problems are far from intractable. There have been substantial improvements to child health over the last century and a steady drop in deaths in childhood. Deaths from measles, diphtheria and other former killers in childhood have been virtually eradicated with the introduction of vaccines. New problems are a matter of concern – for instance, those relating to childhood obesity, its determinants and its consequences – but there is every reason for optimism in relation to child health in affluent societies such as our own. The early years remains high on the policy agenda in the UK, as the 2010 report on child poverty (Field 2010) and 2011 report on early years intervention (Allen 2011) demonstrate. Only time will tell whether the rhetoric of these reports will translate well into the reality of children's lives.

The risks that remain to child health are not evenly distributed. The health of those who are already better off tends to improve faster than those who start life at a disadvantage, often because of access to services or the means of improving health, most notably a good general education – health education of the old-fashioned tying a message to a brick type has a more mixed effect. Some people believe that a trade-off must be had between improving a nation's health overall (where the gap between the best off and worst off is likely to widen) or narrowing the gap and reducing the steep social class gradient. However, it has been plausibly argued (Wilkinson 1994; Wilkinson and Pickett 2009) that it is not only the poorest who are at risk as a result of inequality. It also has a corrosive effect on the better-off, meaning that the more equal societies do better all round in terms of health and other indicators of well-being than the most unequal. In the United States, where mean living standards are high, the infant mortality rate, for instance, is greater than that in most other developed countries, and appears to be worsening. In 2004 the United States tied with Poland and Slovakia, ranked at 29th in the world in infant mortality.

This chapter focuses on some of the structural, family and individual factors that influence children's current health and well-being, and their future health prospects. Much of what can usefully be done lies beyond the NHS. Many people, including parents, teachers and a range of professionals in social care, have a crucial part to play in promoting health and reducing inequalities. Most children in the UK have good access to primary, secondary and tertiary medical care. The focus here is largely on what can be done beyond the surgery, A&E department or hospital ward. It provides examples from some of the health-damaging determinants of health (e.g. poor housing, cars and roads) and health-enhancing factors (education, decent housing, employment, adequate income), as well as specific conditions and problems including obesity and unintentional injury. The chapter brings together evidence on risks to child health, the state of knowledge on improving child health in the UK, and policies and programmes designed to promote health and well-being and reduce inequalities in health and life chances.

What do we know about major risks, and protective and risk factors?

Epidemiological and cohort studies and the good sources of statistical data available in the UK referred to in the resources section at the end of this chapter enable us to have a reasonable grasp of the major health risks in childhood. The factors likely to have the strongest effect, such as an adequate income, good education, good housing and good transport policies, are amendable to intervention at the policy level and practitioners may influence these through research-informed advocacy. Behavioural interventions play an important part, particularly if they are directed towards the behaviour of decision-makers, educators, planners and policy makers (such as the move to abolish corporal punishment in schools and elsewhere – an important factor in keeping children safe). However, behaviour change is more frequently directed towards children crossing roads rather than towards drivers; towards children eating the wrong kinds of food and being sedentary rather than towards those who market food or sell from school or public playgrounds or sports fields.

An independent review into the most effective evidence-based strategies to reduce health inequalities in England was published in 2010 (Marmot 2010). The recommendations below, summarised from the report, are strongly focused on children and families and emphasise the importance of prevention – i.e. the fence at the top of the cliff rather than the ambulance below.

Example 16.1 Recommendations of Fair Society, Healthy Lives: a strategic review of health inequalities in England post-2010
www.marmotreview.org

- **Giving every child the best start in life (highest priority recommendation)** – what happens during early years (starting in the womb) has lifelong effects on many aspects of health and well-being – from obesity, heart disease and mental health to educational achievement and economic status. Later interventions, although important, are considerably less effective where good early foundations are lacking. The review proposed a rebalancing of public spending towards the early years, more parenting support programmes, a well-trained early years workforce and high-quality early years care.

    Enabling all children, young people and adults to maximise their capabilities and have control over their lives, educational achievement brings with it a whole range of achievements, including better employment, income and physical and mental health. Building closer links between schools, the family and the local community are important to reducing educational inequalities.

- **Creating fair employment and good work for all** – being in employment is protective of health; conversely unemployment contributes to poor health. Jobs need to offer a decent living wage, opportunities for in-work development, good management practices, the flexibility to enable people to balance work and family life and protection from adverse working conditions that can damage health.

- **Ensuring a healthy standard of living for all** – having insufficient money to lead a healthy life is a highly significant cause of health inequalities. Standards for a minimum income for healthy living need to be developed and implemented – the calculation includes the level of income needed for adequate nutrition, physical activity, housing, individual and community interactions, transport, medical care and hygiene.

- **Creating and developing sustainable places and communities** – many policies that would help mitigate climate change would also help reduce health inequalities – for instance, more walking, cycling and green spaces. Good-quality neighbourhoods can make a significant difference to quality of life and health – this relates both to the physical environment and to the social environment.

Reducing inequalities is important because risks are unevenly distributed. The general conclusions of the Marmot Report on family and household health are mirrored and developed when the focus is narrowed onto the health of children.

Table 16.1 illustrates some of the major health risks and risk factors for child health in the UK, together with some of the protective factors for reducing or eliminating risk amenable to intervention.

Table 16.1 Risks, risk factors and protective factors

Health risk	Risk factors	Protective factors
Infants and children aged 0–4		
Death at or around the time of birth	Low socio-economic status; prematurity; low birth weight; maternal health; smoking	Adequate income; good prenatal and intra and post partum care; smoking cessation
Unintentional injury	Poor housing; overcrowding; low socio-economic status	Warm, affordable, adequate housing; some safety equipment including working smoke alarms; high-quality daycare,
Respiratory illness	Environmental factors including poor housing and air pollution	Clean air legislation; warm dry housing; good evidence-based primary and secondary care
Primary school children		
Unintentional injury	Poverty; overcrowded housing; being a boy; low socio-economic status; living near a road; being a pedestrian	Enforcement of speed limits; traffic calming measures; working smoke alarms; effective parenting support; building on the ways in which parents keep their children safe in unsafe environments
Overweight and obesity	Genetics; more energy in than out; poor diet; low socio-economic status	Breastfeeding in infancy; reduced use of cars; increased exercise; healthier diet
Teenagers and adolescents		
Unintentional injury/violence	Male gender; car use; alcohol and substance use; low socio-economic status	Safe affordable public transport; learning the skills to recognise and walk away from risky situations
Substance abuse (tobacco, alcohol, illegal drugs)	Familial factors; lack of connectedness including being brought up in the care system; early initiation, peer use of substances	Acquisition of skills by young people and by those who want to help them; promoting social inclusion; employment/education
Being overweight or obese	Genetics; poor diet; insufficient exercise; low socio-economic status	Walking to school and for leisure activities; exercise and sport; more energy out than energy in; friendship networks that encourage activity
Sexual health problems including unintended or unwanted pregnancy	Alcohol and substance misuse; lack of knowledge/information; being brought up in the care system	Good general education; high self-esteem; protective friendship networks; access to contraception; condom use
Suicide and deliberate self-harm	Male (suicide), female (self-harm); self-harm a significant risk factor for later suicide; death by suicide of someone close; being brought up in the care system	Identification and treatment of depression; restricting access to lethal methods of self-harm

Health problems hitting the headlines

The kinds of child health problems that hit the headlines are normally hospital based, including in recent years heart surgery, the provision of special care cots for premature babies and unusual presentations such as the separation of conjoined twins. However, obesity, alcohol and sexual health also catch the media imagination. Creating a moral panic, as sociologists have long argued, is unlikely to be helpful, and by demonising young people and their parents may do the reverse. Alarmism can both obscure the actual distribution of risk, making policy response more difficult, and exacerbate harm. In the case of reporting of, or dramatic depiction of, suicide in the print or broadcast media there is some evidence of a copycat effect (Hawton and Williams 2002), as a result of which guidelines urging caution have been developed for the media (Samaritans 2008).

The evidence of what works (or helps)

In addressing health risks for children, the use of research evidence is not the only source of knowledge, but it is an important one. The desire to 'do the right thing' to help, and to prefer action to inaction while springing from the best of motives, can do harm. For instance, well-meaning campaigns teaching children to cross roads in the right kind of way – not crossing between cars or if they can see a car coming – are less likely to save lives than addressing those who speed, or creating environments that make it possible to cross a road safely. Clearly, safe road crossing is an essential life skill, but providing these skills should be seen as an unfortunate necessity – it should not divert attention from the source of the problem. As one Scottish safety campaigner remarked of efforts of this kind: 'It's like teaching your kids to swim in a pool full of alligators'.

Lessons from clinical research can be extended to the wider contexts and causes of ill-health. The introduction of evidence-informed medicine has greatly reduced the number of unnecessary tonsil and adenoid operations, and the use of data on sudden infant death demonstrated that Dr Spock's advice on putting an infant to sleep on her front was mistaken.

However, even good science cannot resolve all issues, or provide a sufficient basis for decisions which draw on cultural or moral values and judgements. The most important outcomes for children may reveal differences between the child or parent's view and that of the professionals. Occasionally, children and their parents may take a different view on potentially life-saving surgery or chemotherapy; clinicians and parents may take different views on whether keeping a very sick or disabled child alive promotes or undermines human rights. In terms of other kinds of risks, however, differences between children and parents, or children, parents and professionals (see exercise later) may be more of a problem, if less dramatic. Scientific research evidence cannot answer social value-judgement questions such as these, although techniques including young people's consultations may inform them.

Even where the appropriate resources for developing effective policy appear to be predominantly or wholly scientific rather than cultural or moral, analysis and hence prescription can be difficult. In trying to understand what works, we are naturally tempted to look at other countries. Much of the more robust and accessible evidence comes from the USA, but we need to bear in mind that many of their outcomes for children and young people are less good than ours. Finland consistently has the best school results, and education more than any other factor is closely linked to good health across the life course. The Finns claim not to know what is behind this success, though it can be observed that there is little independent schooling, not much homework, children don't start school until seven and there are no league tables for schools. Other Nordic countries have very low rates of child injury on the roads, which may be explained by the separation of children and traffic. Their child health and well-being is exceptionally good, at the cost of high (or as many in the Nordic countries would have it, appropriate) taxation. In the Netherlands, on the other hand, teenage pregnancy rates are the lowest in Europe. This has been attributed to the Dutch being more open in their attitudes towards sex, and more willing for there to be discussion with children and young people. However, replicating policies in different contexts may well not have the same result – context matters, and correlation and cause are very different. With an inadequate evidence base, researchers and, on occasions, policy makers are inclined to say 'more research is needed.' This is difficult in the case of problems where a solution is viewed as urgent or where a commonsense solution, irrespective of whether it is the correct one, has strong face validity. Two examples discussed below (obesity, unintentional injury) are public-health problems where the media both shape the agenda, and suggest possible – not always evidence-informed – solutions.

Obesity

A health issue which has recently received wide public and media attention is obesity, and this illustrates both the problems of analysing and the possibilities of addressing health problems among children. Headlines such as the 'Fat Kid Crisis' (*Scottish Sun* 2010) and 'Now Britain is the fattest country in Europe' (*Daily Mail* 2010) are a reminder that whereas in most of the world having sufficient nutrition is the issue, the wealthier world has different problems (OECD 2010). Notwithstanding some young people in the UK (usually but not always young women) having eating disorders such as anorexia nervosa and bulimia, at a population level the major food-related problem is that many of children in the UK are or are at risk of becoming unhealthily overweight. Compared to their peers with healthy weight, obese children have a higher risk of a range of problems including fatty liver disease, diabetes, low self-esteem and being bullied (Butland et al. 2007). The prevalence and consequences of childhood overweight and obesity tend to be underestimated by parents, either as a result of optimism (they'll grow out of it) or denial of a stigmatising problem. Like many health problems in childhood, obesity casts a shadow forward into adulthood, and is associated over the life course with an increased risk of premature death. Obesity in childhood is also projected to have significant future cost implications both inside and outside the NHS. The societal costs of obesity are projected to be £49.9 billion in 2050 (NICE 2006).

In terms of dealing with the problem, the National Institute for Health and Clinical Excellence (NICE) provides guidance based on systematic reviews, among other evidence, on the prevention, identification, assessment and management of overweight and obesity for staff and managers in local authorities, schools and early years providers, workplaces and for the public, and includes advice on how to put the guideline's recommendations into practice. Much of the legitimacy of evidence depends on how it is produced and by whom. In this case, the guidance producers worked with a group of professionals from local authorities, education, employers and the NHS, consumer representatives and technical staff to review the evidence and draft the recommendations.

Measures that NICE (2006) suggests to address the social determinants of overweight and obesity include:

- **Local authorities** should work with local partners to create and manage more safe spaces for incidental and planned physical activity by providing facilities and schemes such as cycling and walking routes, cycle parking, area maps and safe play areas. Other measures include making streets cleaner and safer, traffic calming, congestion charging, pedestrian crossings, cycle routes, lighting and walking schemes.

- **Nurseries and other childcare facilities** should minimise sedentary activities during play time, and provide regular opportunities for enjoyable active play and structured physical activity sessions. They should also implement guidance on food procurement and healthy catering.

- **Headteachers and chairs of governors** in collaboration with parents and pupils should assess the whole school environment and ensure that the ethos of all school policies helps children and young people to maintain a healthy weight, eat a healthy diet and be physically active, in line with existing standards and guidance. This includes policies relating to building lay-out and recreational spaces, catering (including vending machines) and the food and drink children bring into school, the taught curriculum (including PE), school travel plans and provision for cycling, and policies relating to the National Healthy Schools Programme and extended schools.

A systematic review of children's views of body size, shape and weight (Rees et al. 2009) found no research that explicitly asked children what they thought might help them to achieve or maintain a healthy weight. However, they found studies that showed very overweight children experiencing body size as a problem and unhelpful responses to their own body size from other children, as well as adults. Fat-related name-calling and bullying was a normal occurrence. They also reported that children in general are acutely aware of body size and our society's attitudes towards it. They are conscious of the size of their bodies and judgements about its acceptability. Many are dissatisfied and some feel anxious despite having a healthy body size. Many girls want to be leaner, regardless of their size. Many boys and girls aspire to very lean body shapes that are unattainable and likely to be unhealthy.

Despite social pressures to be slim, obesity is on the increase as a result of the increasing imbalance between energy in (food) and energy out (exercise). Children are becoming more sedentary – few schools now have the cycle racks that they had in the post-war years of the last century – and food advertising increases the pressure to eat high-energy products.

The example of obesity illustrates how policy priorities may be influenced by public discussion and media attention. A range of responses to action have included accusations of 'nanny state' if there are suggestions to regulate food sales or advertising, parent-blaming if children eat the wrong kind of food and hurtful media representations of overweight children. It illustrates, too, the complexities of both cause and remedy and the need for informed, complex and pragmatic action in responding to health issues. Such responses would not rule out, for instance, bariatric surgery in complex medical cases, are sensitive to the dangers of emphasising weight in a way that leads to excessive weight loss in normal-weight children and strongly emphasise dealing with some of the determinants of being overweight.

Unintentional injury

While the consequences of obesity for health, both short term and long term, are alarming, the major cause of death in childhood in the UK (and most of the richer world) is unintentional injury. Unintentional injury has the steepest social class gradient of any cause of death. In the UK, for instance, a child in a family living in poverty is 15 times more likely to die in a house fire than a child in a well-off family. Road injury, particularly to pedestrians, shows a similar pattern.

Children are unlikely to resist road safety messages (nor should they), but many road users resist attempts to change their behaviour through regulation, traffic calming or surveillance. Although many child deaths on the road make local headlines (often accompanied by an explanation of mothers identifying the location as a dangerous crossing some time ago), nationally drivers are better represented as an interest group. A headline in the *Daily Telegraph* (2010) suggests that roads have not been made safer by the 20mph speed limit – though much further into the story the data are described as flawed. Similar stories have appeared about traffic cameras. The Coalition government, elected in the UK in 2010, has declared an end to 'war on the motorist', suggesting that in the field of infringement of traffic laws, motorists and others are insufficiently aware of the consequences of their actions.

Most accidents occur in hazardous environments. Spatial and socio-economic differences in accident rates are a reflection of differences in the location of risky environments. Effective reduction of risk and accident prevention is concerned as much with environmental change as with behaviour modification. Road traffic accidents, as the Nordic countries have demonstrated, can be 'planned out' of urban areas by the use of road lay-out, traffic calming and off-street parking or restrictions on parking and car use in new developments. In practice, between a third and a half of accidents to children may be preventable through engineering, environmental or legislative measures (Stone 1993).

Among the effective interventions to reduce unintentional injury are listening to parents and children and acting on what they say. People who live in unsafe environments are well placed to inform effective solutions. Prevention policies need to explore the ways in which safety behaviours are integrated into everyday life and the trade-off between one risk and another (do I take my children down two flights of stone stairs to hang out my washing, or take them with me while carrying the laundry?) (Roberts et al. 1995).

Public debate frequently concentrates on individual responsibility and choice, as if this were both the principal cause of any outcome and a matter of free, unfettered individual resolution. Public policy, by contrast, can be most effective when it concentrates on the contexts within which such choice is facilitated, encouraged or circumscribed. A recent systematic review (Thomas et al. 2007) challenges the idea of 'risk-taking' as a helpful umbrella term. The review assesses the extent to which risk-taking contributes to accidental injury. The authors conclude that, while young people undoubtedly undertake actions that result in injury, a move away from individual behavioural explanations towards a focus on structures and material resources is likely to be a more productive approach to understanding overall patterns of accidental injury.

While a significant investment in accident prevention is through the education of parents and children, evidence of effectiveness for written or pictorial information about dangers is poor, changing knowledge in the short term but leaving behaviours largely unaltered. Parents have described such leaflets as raising levels of anxiety without addressing the causes – one Scottish mother suggested that leaflets could be best used if turned into papier mâché road humps.

In terms of data, at present, most of it used by those trying to prevent child accidents are insufficiently localised and detailed. In effect, they tend to be data on injuries rather than accidents, describing the consequences to the body of the accident rather than the accident itself and the antecedents. People living with risks will often find ways of avoiding them most of the time – they know what they are: the broken fence by the railway line, the cars that don't stop even when the green man is showing. Children as young as seven are able to identify these kinds of risks, though they may be less good than adults at avoiding them. Although some of these issues may be picked up by coroners' courts or the procurator fiscal, slow progress in addressing localised dangers suggest that a different approach may be needed.

Example 16.2 Managing risk: health and safety, injury and obesity

In July 2010 a London couple were widely reported in the UK press for letting their children, aged eight and five, cycle a mile to school unsupervised. It was reported at the time that the parents had met the headmaster and were told that, unless they supervised the journey in both directions, they would be referred to children's services. Since the major cause of death and serious injury in the UK is from traffic injuries (Edwards et al. 2006), there is indeed a risk. At the same time, children getting to school under their own steam has hugely declined over the last generation (Hillman et al. 1991; Hillman 2006), and many children are taken to school by car, which increases the injury risk to children outside the car – pedestrians and cyclists. Few schools now have bike racks and obesity is becoming a serious problem in childhood. This is why making local policy in a way that involves parents, children and planners is important.

Conclusions and implications

'Resilience' is sometimes suggested as a way of combating risk (see Chapter 12), and there is something moving and heart-warming about the resilience of people enduring hardship, as the Chilean miners trapped and then released in 2010 showed. However, the fact that we can learn from resilience does not mean that this is the best or the right way to address health risk.

For those researchers, practitioners, policy people or planners wanting to 'do something' about health risks to children, the wish to act rather than wait for the evidence tends to be strong. It is easier for most front-line professionals to act on individual behaviours of those who are subject to health insults. It is as well to remember, as Stone (1989) has pointed out, that intervening at this end of the chain is cheap, generally uncontroversial and safe. If it works the politicians take the credit, and if it does not the target population takes the blame.

In countries such as the UK, where austerity budgets are likely to be in place for some time to come, child health, at least in relation to the NHS, is in the relatively fortunate position that it is likely to have a measure of protection from direct cutbacks. The same cannot be said of the factors that influence risks to health. Cuts which will affect the determinants of health – housing, schools, transport and employment – may well lead to the kinds of low-level health deficits that will not send a child to her death, A&E or a hospital ward, but which, given what we know about health and illness across the life course, will affect health adversely in the longer term.

On the more positive side, austerity budgets may mean that research evidence could play a stronger part in developing policy. The history of policy-making, however, suggests that lobbying plays the more important part. Smoking reduction in Australia demonstrates the importance of slowly accumulating research and practice evidence so that, when the opportunity arises, serious lobbying can be well informed (Chapman 2007). There is an increasing evidence base for addressing the health risks faced by children and young people by addressing the social determinants, which can be found in the resources section under Marmot 2010.

The need to use evidence and combine a passion to change things with a readiness to engage with policy and practice represents an opportunity for both researchers and those delivering services. Workforce development for those working with children is still failing in many cases to deliver interventions based on sound evidence, or offering the opportunity to those working most closely with children to contribute effectively to this evidence.

Exercise

Using Example 16.2, discuss the perspective(s), evidence and arguments you would bring to the discussion if you were:

■ the parents;

■ the headteacher;

- the older child;
- the younger child;
- the head of child protection in the locality;
- the director of public health;
- a spokesperson for the Child Accident Prevention Trust;
- a local authority planner.

Recommended reading

http://www.statistics.gov.uk/hub/children-education-skills

Some of the important data, particularly on the early years from the Office for National Statistics (ONS) can be found here.

http://www.cpag.org.uk/povertyfacts/index.htm

The Child Poverty Action group produces a summary of facts and figures on children and poverty.

http://www.evidence.nhs.uk/default.aspx

Provides a sound source of evidence in health and social care. It ranks search results according to relevance and quality, and through My Evidence – users can personalise searches.

http://www.scie.org.uk/children/index.asp

It includes research briefings, reports, government documents, journal articles, events and websites.

http://www.ucl.ac.uk/gheg/marmotreview

Fair Society, Healthy Lives: A Strategic Review of Health Inequalities in England Post-2010 (also known as Marmot 2010)

This website provides good research evidence, and now has advice on implementation and examples of good practice.

http://www.foresight.gov.uk/OurWork/ActiveProjects/Obesity/Obesity.asp

Tackling obesities – future choices.

Petticrew, M. and Roberts, H. (2003) 'Evidence, hierarchies and typologies: Horses for Courses' *Journal of Epidemiology and Community Health*, 57: pp. 527–9.

This article sets out the contributions different kinds of studies – including trials, qualitative work, cohort studies and reviews – bring.

Spencer, N. (2000) *Poverty and Child Health*, Abingdon: Radcliffe Medical Press.

This book brings together historical and current evidence, and considers the practical implications for health and social policy.

Chapter 17

Infant mental health

Christine Puckering

Summary points

- Infant mental health is a holistic construct referring to the social, emotional, cultural and developmental well-being of very young children.

- Environmental experiences in pregnancy and the early years shape the development and functioning of the infant brain.

- The brain structures laid down at this time have lifelong effects and become increasingly difficult to change. Hence, it is vital to try to ensure that the early environment is favourable and, where there are problems, to intervene as soon as possible.

- Interventions to promote good infant health should focus on promoting the infant's relationships with a small number of consistent and responsive caregivers.

- Simple, universal, public-health measures, such as backward-facing buggies and baby slings are effective in ensuring that babies get the face-to-face interaction and close contact best suited to their needs.

- Effective interventions for families with additional needs focus on interaction and may use video feedback as a tool.

- Multidisciplinary and multi-agency training are essential for the recognition of families with additional needs and the delivery of effective interventions.

Introduction

The term 'infant mental health' still meets a sceptical response in some quarters. If mental health were to be equated with mental illness, it would indeed seem preposterous to apply this label to infants. Mental health is not the same as mental illness, however, nor does it even denote an absence of mental illness. Rather, it is a more holistic concept which covers the social, emotional, cultural and developmental well-being of the person. Positive infant mental health is important, not only in its own right, but because it lays the foundations for future well-being.

The effects of early experiences on later development

There is an apparent paradox. How can it be that things that happen in the period before we have any conscious memories have long-term effects? Surely babies do not remember what happened to them; they 'just forget'. Growing evidence suggests, however, that infancy has profound and long-term effects on all aspects of life, with effects that last well into adulthood. Furthermore, recent research on young children's brains has shown that they evolve in response to environmental influences and in ways that are much harder to modify later. The manner in which the brain develops in early life in turn has a major influence on how individuals function, currently and in the future.

With the increasingly sophisticated development of brain-scanning techniques, the reasons for the long-term importance of early brain development are becoming clearer. Infants are born with around 100 billion brain cells or neurons, almost the full number they will ever have, though recent evidence has shown that some new nerve cells are produced even into adult life. Each neuron has a cell body with a number of branches or dendrites, which *receive* incoming electrical charges from other cells. Each cell body also has an axon, which *sends* outgoing electrical charges to other cells (see Figure 17.1). Thus dendrites and axons act as communication links between cells.

At birth, the brain is largely unspecialised, except for the previously myelinated areas controlling basic biological functions. Over time, connections are made and pathways build up with specific areas becoming specialised for particular functions. This is highly dependent on what the child experiences. The main brain parts and respective functions are shown in Figure 17.2.

Figure 17.1

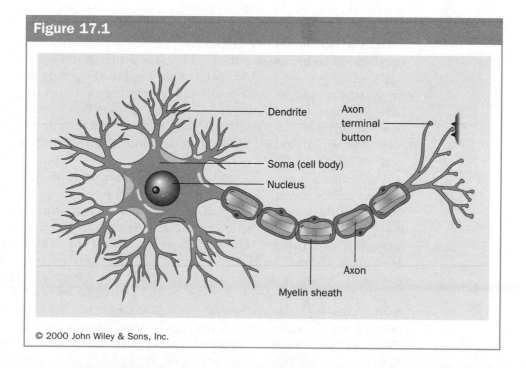

© 2000 John Wiley & Sons, Inc.

Figure 17.2

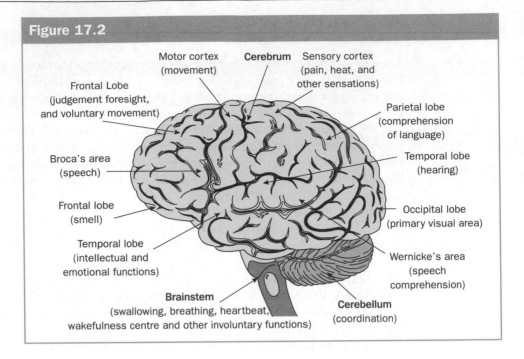

Brain development begins shortly after conception and continues until early adult life, but the most rapid periods of development are during pregnancy and in the first three years of life. Two processes shape the development of the brain. The first is myelinisation, which is the growth of a fatty insulating sheath around the axon. The development of myelin increases the rate of transmission of electrical impulses down the axon and the effectiveness of connections. The back of the brain, which controls involuntary functions like breathing and heart rate, is already myelinated at birth, as is the motor and sensory cortex (Figure 17.2). So, the baby can feel sensation and move, but as yet has no conscious control over this. Over time, the cortex becomes myelinated, with different functions developing at different rates. The sensitive period for social and emotional development is in the first two years of life.

The second process is the production and pruning of the interlacing connections between cells (synapses). These processes are driven by gene activity and the environment so, although no experiences are remembered from this time, these forces are shaping pathways in the brain. The development of connections between cells (synaptogenesis) happens rapidly and initially without any pattern, so that a dense network of connections begins to form. However, only pathways that are used repeatedly become established and 'hard-wired'. The rest are pruned away. Motor control and language develop systematically across the early years, but the pre-frontal areas of the brain, where decision-making, planning and higher levels of thinking are controlled, do not begin to be myelinated and fully connected until about one year of age. Development is not complete until late adolescence. Common sense shows that very young children cannot plan ahead or make anything more than simple decisions. However, by adolescence young people are making career choices, finding romantic partners and managing their future. The underpinning of the growth in these capacities lies in the wiring of the brain.

The development of PET (positron emission tomography) scans, which map brain activity, has confirmed these developing changes in the child brain in the first few years of life. Molecular genetics can take the story even further back. A review by Tremblay (2010), led to his conclusion that even prenatal environmental factors influence the potential development of the infant and later adult. This includes physical health as well as emotional well-being. So, even in the womb the environment provided by the mother starts to shape the baby's brain and physiology. The environment may be one in which the foetus is well nourished and protected from adverse influences, By contrast, the nourishment is sub-optimal when, for instance, the foetus is exposed to alcohol or drugs in the mother's body. Maternal stress leads to an increase in the cortisol hormone, which is known to cross the placenta, so this too can affect the baby in the womb. Research has shown that babies whose mothers experience high levels of anxiety and depression in pregnancy have higher levels of emotional and behavioural disorders at age five, even allowing for the effects of later post-natal maternal depression (Glover and O'Connor 2002). This applies particularly to those who experience low levels of social support or domestic violence. It is clear, therefore, that, where there is any risk to the baby, the earlier intervention begins the better the outcome is likely to be.

What do babies need to thrive?

At birth, the human infant is very immature when compared with other species. The baby cannot keep itself warm, clean, fed or even alive without the care of a mature carer. However, the human infant is uniquely prepared for social interaction. Within minutes of birth, the baby shows a preference for face-like visual stimuli. They are especially attracted by human eyes or images that resemble them. Babies will turn their heads to a face-like configuration in preference to the same marks distributed at random. A human infant turns preferentially to the voice of his or her own mother and to the smell of her breast milk. These stimuli are those that have been available for the previous nine months *in utero*. The baby can also imitate accurately facial expressions such as tongue thrusting. There is no suggestion that this imitation is conscious, rather that the brain is uniquely configured, even at birth, to respond to social stimuli.

Apart from the biological needs for food, cleaning and physical care, the baby needs above all the regular care of a small number of carers who will learn to read and respond to the baby's social signals. Without the availability of regular and predictable carers who provide contingent stimulation, the baby will not develop secure attachment relationships, with the net result that the child will not learn, grow and make sound relationships in the future (see Chapter 18). The good attachment figure provides not only physical nurturance, but also helps the child regulate arousal. The baby needs a carer to nurture and soothe when

Figure 17.3 The Circle of Security

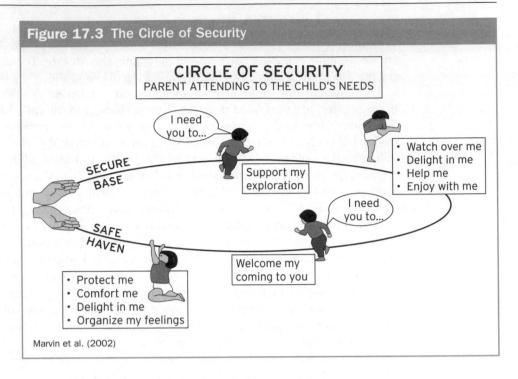

CIRCLE OF SECURITY
PARENT ATTENDING TO THE CHILD'S NEEDS

I need you to...

SECURE BASE

Support my exploration

• Watch over me
• Delight in me
• Help me
• Enjoy with me

SAFE HAVEN

I need you to...

• Protect me
• Comfort me
• Delight in me
• Organize my feelings

Welcome my coming to you

Marvin et al. (2002)

arousal is too high, due to pain, hunger or fear. The carer also raises arousal through playfulness and stimulation when the baby is comfortable and open to learning. The baby's state will vary from sleepy and under-aroused to hungry, frightened or in pain – that is, over-aroused. Only when the parent/carer is able to help the baby to regulate his or her arousal to a comfortable level is the baby able to be social, interact and learn. The parent/carer needs to be alert to the baby's state to help in sensitive regulation and be ready to respond socially at the time the baby is ready to interact. These periods of quiet alertness will be short initially, but will lengthen as the baby matures.

The Circle of Security, shown in Figure 17.3, summarises how young children have different needs, depending on their state of security and arousal. At certain times, as when waking up or being frightened, babies need nurturance and soothing. Once they feel more secure, they will require support to be active, explore and learn. Consequently, parents and carers should be able to recognise the child's position in the cycle, be sensitive to the associated needs and respond accordingly. Professionals working closely with families should in turn be equipped to identify when parents or carers lack the skills, motivation or confidence to act in this way, whether due to lack of experience or support, addiction, mental health issues or some other reason. Then, access to guidance is important and in more serious cases of insensitivity to the child's needs, more focused intervention. Examples of ways to help with early parenting, and hence promote infant mental health, are described in the remainder of this chapter.

Interventions to support infant mental health

For most babies, there is no need for any specialist intervention to provide a good environment for growth and learning. The availability of a small number of warm and responsive adults who take a personal interest and delight in the child will provide exactly the best possible conditions for optimal social and emotional development, as well as a secure base from which the child can explore and learn. However, some simple lessons can be implemented, given that the mental health of babies may not be the first thought in the mind of the parent.

Public health measures

There are some powerful and easy to implement aids to early parenting that could have an impact in the public-health arena. Research has identified a range of measures that are effective in promoting emotional closeness and opportunities for learning. They include communication tools like *Bookstart* (Wade and Moore 1998) and *Talk to your Baby* (Clark and Hawkins 2010). The way in which young children are carried and transported has been shown to affect interaction – thus, backward-facing buggies are helpful as they allow the infant to see the mother's face (Zeedyk 2008), while baby slings give the mother (or father) and baby the best chance to make and maintain a close bond (Anisfield et al. 1990). There is little doubt that the tendency to keep babies in car seats, baby carriers and forward-facing buggies distance the baby from close human contact just at the time it is most crucial. Of course, there may be times, for example when in a moving car, that it is important for the baby to be protected by a hard seat, but it is antithetical to some of the fundamental needs of babies for this to be the baby's most common environment.

Universal services

Almost all women seek antenatal care during their pregnancy, but the universal services, such as GPs, midwives and obstetricians, rarely recognise the potential role they can play in facilitating infant mental health. To date, few psychosocial interventions have been show to be effective during pregnancy, although programmes are in development by the Solihull Approach, Triple P and Mellow Babies.

Postnatally the range of options proven to be helpful is growing. To date, the Solihull Approach (Milford et al. 2006), Brazelton Neonatal Assessment Scale (Nugent and Brazelton 2006) and baby massage (Onozawa et al. 2001) have been shown by systematic research to be helpful at the universal level.

Families with additional needs

A number of formal programmes have been developed to address infant mental health needs in families with additional and complex needs. These have mostly been initiated and applied by different professionals working together, typically psychologists, nurses, doctors and/or social workers. Strong evidence exists of what is helpful in such programmes (Bakermans-Kranenberg et al. 2003). The characteristics seen to promote improvement in parent child sensitivity and attachment were:

- focus on parent/carer sensitivity rather than general support or maternal mental health;
- 5–16 sessions;
- use of video feedback.

The same factors increased paternal sensitivity, though the effects were attenuated if mothers and fathers were seen together. So far, research has not demonstrated benefits from antenatal intervention, though it could be hypothesised that for vulnerable families, engagement early might lead to better take up of later services. The Nurse–Family Partnership offered to young first-time mothers, starting in pregnancy and lasting for three years, has shown long-lasting beneficial effects for both mothers and children with good retention in the programme as long as the home visitor is a nurse and maintains an unbroken relationship with the family (Olds et al. 1998).

Three programmes that meet the criteria for success suggested above will now be discussed more fully.

Video interaction guidance (VIG)

VIG is based on the principles of good communication. From this theoretical base a system of individual feedback has developed, in which the guider replays to the parent edited clips of their interaction with their own baby, choosing those which illustrate effective communication skills. By providing only positive feedback, and also using the principles of attuned interaction in the relationship between the guider and the family as well as the parent and child, it is expected that such positive interaction will increase. Juffer et al. (2008) have shown that VIG enhances communication between parents and children, leading to increased sensitivity in parents and more secure attachment relationships.

Circle of Security

The Circle of Security programme is offered either individually or in groups and similarly uses video feedback to examine the interaction between the parent and their own child (Marvin et al. 2002). Edited video feedback helps to identify which part of the circle the child is in (Fig. 17.3). Does the child at a given moment need nurture and comforting or, alternatively, stimulation and encouragement to explore? The capacity of the parent to detect those messages depends to some extent on the clarity of the child's message and to some extent on the sensitivity of the parent and his or her capacity to accept the child's needs. Some parents may find it difficult to allow a child to move away to explore, whereas others will be relieved to keep the child at a distance while tending to avoid intimacy and nurturance. The child's needs will be inaccurately interpreted by the parent if they challenge what the parent is able to tolerate. The child quickly learns to mute the messages the parent cannot accept.

During the programme, caregivers are encouraged to increase their sensitivity and appropriate responsiveness to the child's signals of the need to explore or alternatively comfort and soothing. The programme also aims to increase the caregivers' ability to reflect on their own and the child's behaviour, thoughts and feelings. Their own experiences are examined in the context of this useful model, with the opportunity to override their own default response and react to the child's needs. Hoffman et al. (2006) have demonstrated how this programme enables toddler and preschool children to move to a more secure attachment pattern. Cassidy et al. (2010) have shown that the programme has remarkably powerful effects even in a prison population, whose own attachment histories were very troubled.

Attachment and bio-behavioural catch up (ABC)

Mary Dozier's ABC programme was developed to help foster carers make secure relationships with children who have a previous history of abuse and neglect. The ABC programme uses videos of children displaying various attachment styles (see Chapter 18), to help foster carers recognise the child's need for nurturance and how the foster parent's responses, as in Circle of Security, may be partly conditioned by their experiences. As the children had previously been abused or neglected, they had already developed an attachment style, which means they are mistrustful and so may spurn efforts by carers to get close. Resistance or even anger by the child towards carers' attempts to show affection can be discouraging since the superficial message from the child is that love is not needed. Therefore, carers are helped to learn the importance of persisting with their nurturing approach, even when the child appears to be signalling avoidance, and are supported to do so. Experience shows that given time and patience, the children will usually become more trusting and responsive. The programme also explores the foster carers' own experiences of being nurtured and promotes attuned interaction through live feedback and video review. The delivery of the programme is tailored according to the parents' or foster carers' experiences based on their own attachment styles. The programme uses live practice, video feedback, psycho-educational material and discussion to raise parents' awareness of attachment relationships and their impact.

The initial success of the programme in normalising the abnormal patterns of diurnal cortisol in abused children under two years of age led to the programme being offered to high-risk birth families in Baltimore (Fisher et al. 2006; Dozier et al. 2008; Dozier et al. 2009). A case study of the first use of ABC in the UK is shown in Example 17.1 (Puckering et al. 2011).

Example 17.1 ABC programme

Mrs S had no intention of having children, as a result of her own poor experiences as a child brought up by very young parents who had little time for her. When she found herself pregnant, she did not wish to continue with the pregnancy, but her very warm and loving partner was keen to have a child. When the baby was born, the health visitor noted that Mrs S was very detached from him and neither looked at him nor spoke to him. Mrs S agreed to take part in the ABC programme over ten weeks. On the first visit she had been ringing day nurseries to try to find one that would take a child as young as eight weeks. By the end of the programme she was enjoying the baby's company so much that she made a positive choice to take a longer maternity leave and postponed use of the nursery.

Mellow babies programme

Originally Mellow Parenting was designed for families with a child under-five. When it became clear from emerging research that there was a need for a programme for under one-year-olds, the Mellow Babies programme was developed using the same underlying structure.

Both Mellow Parenting and Mellow Babies were based on understandings from attachment theory (see Chapter 18) and research showing that the very common experience of parental postnatal depression in the first year of a child's life had long-term implications for the child's sub-optimal development in emotional, cognitive and language areas (Hay et al. 2001). Treatment of the maternal depression alone is not enough to improve the outcome for the child (Murray et al. 2003).

The aim of Mellow Babies groups is to support and address the mothers' well-being, support the fathers of the babies if they are still in contact, and to develop sensitive attunement between parents and babies, the mechanism by which babies develop a strong sense of security from which to learn and develop good relationships. Two strands were developed in parallel to meet the needs of two different types of family. The first was for families where there were child-protection concerns and the second a group of mothers who had a high risk of postnatal depression, as indicated by high scores on the Edinburgh Postnatal Depression Scale, EPDS (Cox et al. 1986). The two strands were subsequently merged, giving trained practitioners the option to choose workshops appropriate to the needs of the group of parents with whom they were working.

The blended programme ran one day a week for fourteen weeks and included opportunities for mothers to explore their own background, current relationships and mental health. Workshops were offered to invite reflection on past and current relationships as well as on depression, anger management, assertiveness, anxiety and relaxation using a framework broadly based on principles of cognitive behavioural treatment (CBT). This helps modify beliefs, expectations and attributions so that participants think and act more positively.

The second component of the group, the parenting workshop, was based on individual video feedback to the mother on her own interaction with her baby.

Mothers gained greatly from seeing positive examples of mother–child interaction and in supporting each other in problem-solving. The parenting workshops also used psycho-educational videos such as on postnatal depression. The Social Baby video (Murray and Andrews 2005) highlights the competencies babies typically display in social interaction.

A third component of the day was a joint lunchtime with staff, babies and mothers to promote playful and enjoyable activities. These were reinforced by 'Have a go' tasks, to practice the baby-centred activities at home, or CBT worksheets.

A series of three partners' evening were set up which were very well attended. Fathers in the postnatal depression group were clearly hungry for information about postnatal depression and what they might do to help. The evening activities replicated in brief many of the mother's group activities with psycho-educational video, parent–child activities and some work on how best to support partners.

The attendance at the groups was very high. A small randomised controlled trial showed that compared with a waiting-list group, the mothers in the Mellow Babies group showed improved mood as measured by the EPDS. The interaction of the mothers in the Mellow Babies group became more positive over the course of the group, whereas the waiting last control group showed an increase in negative interaction. The salutary and sobering message was that interaction deteriorated if intervention was delayed even by four months (Puckering et al. 2010).

Example 17.2 Mellow Babies

Ms C had a lifelong history of difficulties including physical and sexual abuse by her father, leading to her moving to foster homes in her teens, where her behaviour became increasingly troublesome. After a period under heavy medication in a psychiatric hospital, she was discharged but became homeless and was involved with drug and alcohol abuse. She had been diagnosed with a hereditary sensorimotor neuropathy, as had her mother before.

After the birth of her son, Thomas, he was placed on the child-protection register on the grounds of physical abuse and neglect. A team of carers assisted with his daily care as Ms C was not able to bathe him safely alone. She was referred to the Mellow Babies group by her social worker and health visitor.

By the end of the group, Ms C was able to respond positively to Thomas' needs, and had changed her behaviour towards him, having seen other mothers playing and talking to their babies, something she had not thought to do herself. Her need for support with Thomas' care continued, but her engagement with health and social work services had become more open and accepting. She agreed to start attending the local parent and toddler group in the company of another mother from the group.

Conclusions and implications

The evidence of the importance of the very earliest periods in a child's life, pregnancy and infancy has become steadily stronger as the understanding of the development of the child's brain has developed. Far from being an irrelevant and quickly forgotten period of life, the influence of pathways laid down in infancy has proven to be long lasting and widespread across all aspects of health, social and cognitive development and mental health.

The implications for services and agencies are widespread. Almost all women seek antenatal care, providing a window of opportunity for recognition of needs and intervention. Those involved at the universal level, GPs, obstetricians and midwives, need the understanding and tools to recognise families with additional needs. However, it is unrealistic for them to offer support outside the antenatal and perinatal period. Multidisciplinary and multi-agency working with health visitors, early years services and social work have the best chance of supporting families and infants in the earliest period of their lives. This requires these practitioners to recognise the need for services, but also to develop high levels of therapeutic skills in delivering effective interventions, particularly for the neediest families. Few practitioners of any discipline gain this level of skill in their basic training, and there is an urgent need for the skills of all practitioners who might come in contact with families with young infants to be enhanced by specific infant mental-health training. Of particular concern is the paucity of such awareness and training in those who work with adults having substance abuse or mental-health problems and who may consider the needs of the unborn child or the infant too late in the day or outside their agenda.

Exercise

1. What are the most salient facts that all professionals working with young children need to know about infant mental health?

2. Which professions or agencies would you want to involve in designing a model infant mental-health service??

3. How can the key messages about infant mental health best be delivered to all parents?

Recommended reading

http://booktrustadmin.kentlyons.com/downloads/NationalImpactEvaluation09.pdf.

Bookstart evaluation

www.headsupscotland.co.uk/.../Infant%20Mental%20Health%20-%20Good%20Practice%20Guide%20-%20Final%20Edit.pdf.

Scottish Government Infant Mental Health Good Practice Guide

http://www.dailymotion.com/video/xdcm59_neonatal-imitation_people.

Neo natal imitation video

Barlow, J. and Svanberg, P. O. (2009) *Keeping the baby in Mind. Infant Mental Health in Practice*, London: Routledge.

Shonkoff, J. P. and Phillips, D. A. (eds) (2000) *From neurons to neighbourhoods: the science of early child development*, Washington DC: National Academy Press.

Zeanah, C. H. (ed.) (2009) *Handbook of Infant Mental Health*, 3rd edition, NY/London: Guilford Press.

Chapter 18

Attachment and loss in childhood and beyond

Helen Minnis and Graham Bryce

Summary points

- Attachment is a powerful instinct that, when it works well, brings infants and caregivers close.
- An understanding of attachment theory is helpful in working with children and families.
- Secure and insecure attachment patterns describe relationships, not individuals.
- Children who have experienced significant losses and traumas in early life may not go to adults for care or problem-solving when stressed or hurt. 'Gentle challenge' may be required in order that fresh attachments can blossom.
- A shared language based in attachment theory can facilitate effective inter-agency working.

Introduction

> In the home for abandoned children they become sad and may die of sadness.
> (1760, from the diary of a Spanish bishop, cited in Spitz 1945)

This quote, from 250 years ago, reminds us that growing up bathed in the safe care of adults who consider us special is essential for life. We hope, in this chapter, to give the reader an overview of how attachment impacts on relationships across the lifespan. We will start with some detail about what attachment is and how it is measured. This will include a discussion of the range of attachment patterns and problems. We will touch on the way that attachment interacts with development and we will complete the circle by discussing how adult attachment styles impact on parenting. But what of children and families in which there are attachment difficulties? Children who have had difficult early attachment experiences may give confusing signals to caregivers and professionals. We will discuss ways that this can be overcome, including the part child and adolescent mental health services can play.

An overview of attachment theory

We have known for centuries that children need close relationships with caring adults in order to survive and thrive. Concerned that existing theories did not adequately explain the impact of early adversity on how children's lives developed, J. Bowlby, a British psychiatrist and psychoanalyst, took time out of his clinical practice to study ethology – the study of animal behaviour. This experience allowed him to develop attachment theory (Bowlby 1982) in which he described how young infants across species, when stressed, seek closeness with adult caregivers or 'attachment figures'. This is not simply to find food or warmth, but is a protective strategy – young infants separated from the herd are likely to be picked off by predators (Blaffer-Hrdy 1999). Stressed infants achieve proximity with caregivers by exhibiting 'attachment behaviours' – signals to their caring adults to 'come close – I need protection and soothing' and Bowlby suggested that this was a powerful instinct. In human infants attachment behaviours include crying and, later in development, reaching out to be picked up or, once mobile, following a caregiver. Some of these attachment behaviours are present from birth, a fact to which any parent who has heard their newborn baby crying on that first night will attest. Early in life, infants are reasonably comfortable being comforted by any adult. However, at the age of around six months, selective attachment begins to develop (Bowlby 1982). For example, the tiny baby at a christening will be happy to be passed around family and friends who all want to welcome the new arrival, but an older sister or brother will tend to stay close to the small group of adults – mother, father, grandparents – who are already known and trusted, and will protest if picked up by someone else. Again, this is an important protective mechanism, determined by evolution, for staying safe and feeling comfortable in the known world.

Attachment patterns

Ainsworth (1979), a psychologist and student of Bowlby's, put attachment theory on a research footing by developing the Strange Situation Procedure (SSP), described as 'a drama in eight episodes' during which a young infant, aged 12–18 months, experiences a series of separations and reunions with his/her parent and a stranger. The beauty of the SSP is that any child, anywhere in the world, who goes through this procedure will experience a similar level of stress, so results can be compared internationally. Across hundreds of studies in many countries, it has been demonstrated that child–parent pairs (known as dyads) from the general population can be categorised into four 'attachment patterns'. Attachment patterns are not descriptions of individual children, but of relationships. Children can have different attachment patterns with different adults.

Around 60–70 per cent of infant–parent dyads can be described as 'securely attached'. This proportion is remarkably stable across cultures. During play, the infant uses the parent as 'a secure base from which to explore' – safe in the knowledge that the parent is going to be available when needed, the infant can investigate the environment and maximise their learning. Around 30–40 per cent of infants will exhibit less optimal attachment behaviour in the SSP and there are three types of 'insecure attachment': *insecure avoidant*; *insecure resistant-ambivalent* and *insecure disorganised-disorientated*. Each of these insecure patterns is present in around 10–15 per cent of dyads with some variation across cultures. Infants in insecure avoidant dyads appear calm and relaxed in the SSP. When the parent leaves the room, they carry on playing as if unperturbed and, when the parent returns show little sign that the reunion is of any importance. Research has however shown, using heart-rate monitoring, that these infants are stressed but, for reasons we will touch on in a moment, fail to show this (Zelenko et al. 2005). In contrast, infants in insecure resistant-ambivalent dyads do seek closeness with the parent on reunion in the SSP, but this closeness does not help the child to calm down. These infants continue to whine and fuss and have less time to explore through play. And finally, infants in insecure disorganised-disorientated dyads are characterised by unusual behaviour in the SSP (Main and Solomon 1986). In disorganised-disorientated attachment, it is as if the infants have no strategy for dealing with the stress of separation and reunion. When the parent returns they display odd, contradictory behaviour – for example, running towards the parent and then pulling away when picked up or veering away at the last minute.

It is important to remember that insecure attachment is not only expressed via emotions, but also through behaviour and capacity to learn, so relationship problems at home may first become apparent through issues arising in nursery or school.

SSP is a relatively expensive and time-consuming procedure, and unfortunately no similarly robust but simpler measure of attachment exists (Lim et al. 2010). It is challenging for practitioners to judge the quality of attachment relationships in fieldwork situations because, if sufficiently stressed, most children will exhibit many of the 'insecure' behaviours seen in the SSP. For example, almost any child will act like a whiny, hard-to-comfort, resistant-ambivalent infant if pushed around on a supermarket trolley for two hours, so it is important not to make assumptions about the attachment pattern of a particular infant–parent dyad in the absence of robust tools like the SSP.

On the other hand, an attachment framework can be a useful way to help parents and carers think about the behaviour of young children, and this can be done without making strong pronouncements about the existence of particular patterns. Such a framework can also be helpful as a common language that can aid inter-agency working and can be helpful when considering whether or not to refer a child on to child and adolescent mental health services.

A particular challenge in the attachment field is how to measure attachment patterns beyond infancy. Toddlers act out their inner feelings in a way that is usually obvious. For example, an infant who, in the SSP, goes to the door her parent has just exited and cries 'mummy mummy' is obviously feeling distress and wants her back. Older children may keep these feelings inside. A mother of a teenager described how her daughter had acted responsibly in calling an ambulance for a sick friend. When asked how she knew what to do, her daughter said 'I just thought of what you would have done Mum'. In other words, she was using her mother as a secure base from which to explore, but in a way that could not have been measured using an observational test. Techniques have been developed using play to tap into the way children think about their attachment relationships. For example, the Manchester Child Attachment Story Task (MCAST) described by Green et al. (2000) explores children's internal working models of attachment by offering the beginnings of attachment-related stories that children are asked to complete using a doll's house. Hodges et al. (2003) developed a similar set of story stems that are particularly appropriate for use with looked-after and accommodated children.

The role of the caregiver

Although the attachment instinct is powerfully present in all young infants, what happens when a child exhibits attachment behaviours seems to be determined, to a large extent, by the way the parent responds. Parents who are *sensitive* – i.e. who are able to respond quickly and warmly to the child's expressions of need during stressful situations on most occasions – are likely to develop secure attachment relationships with their children, and their children are likely to go on to develop optimal functioning in future relationships (Ainsworth 1979). In contrast, parents who consistently fail to respond to their infant's expressions of distress tend to have insecure avoidant relationships with their children, and parents who are very inconsistent in their responses are likely to have insecure resistant-ambivalent patterns of interaction in the SSP. Finally, parents who respond in a frightening way during attachment episodes, perhaps as a reflection of abuse or trauma in their own lives, are likely to have insecure disorganised-disorientated attachment relationships with their children. Children whose early experience is of insecure attachment are more likely than securely attached children to have difficulties in their family, school and peer relationships (Ainsworth 1979).

It is important to remember that attachment patterns are features of a specific *relationship* and not of a particular child. This means that it is possible to have an insecure attachment relationship with one parent, but a secure relationship with another parent, grandparent or other adult. This may be why some children who have had insecure attachments in infancy are resilient and do not have future problems with relationships or mental health. Attachment patterns tend to be stable across time, unless external circumstances change significantly (Sroufe 2005). Bowlby suggested that by middle childhood children have developed 'internal working models' of relationships that reflect their predominant experience in early life. These internal working models act as templates for future relationships. So, for example, if a child has had mainly secure attachment relationships, he will arrive at primary school expecting that the adults he meets will be sensitive and will provide warm comfort when he is stressed. In contrast, a child who has not had attachment needs met in early life will expect no more from the other adults they meet. However, these are *working* models – i.e. are not written in stone and are amenable to change. If a young child who has experienced nothing but rejection and fear in early life is placed with a loving, sensitive caregiver who is committed to that child, secure attachment can blossom within weeks (Dozier et al. 2001; Stovall-McClough and Dozier 2004).

Adult attachment

By late adolescence and adulthood, internal working models can be explored through language. In the Adult Attachment Interview (AAI) developed by Main, an adult is asked to give five adjectives to describe his/her own parent. Most of the rest of the interview is concerned with asking for specific examples from early childhood to back up the adjectives that came to mind. The analysis of the transcribed interview is based not on the content, but on the form of the interview – i.e. not on *what* the adult said about early childhood, but on the *way* they said it. 'Autonomous' adults are those who give a concise, coherent, consistent account of early childhood, even if their experiences were not positive ones. Research has show that when these adults have their own children they are more likely to develop secure attachment relationships with them (Fonagy et al. 1991). 'Dismissing' adults act during the AAI as though early attachment experiences are not important to them. They may deny memories of early childhood, give a thin account devoid of detail or use idealised adjectives that they fail to back up with biographical detail. These adults are more likely to develop insecure avoidant attachments with their children. 'Preoccupied' adults give long but woolly accounts of early childhood and are more likely to have insecure resistant-ambivalent relationships with their children. Finally, a minority of AAIs are classified as 'unresolved' – in other words, there is evidence that the adult has not come to terms with grief or trauma from early life. These adults are more likely to have insecure disorganised relationships with their children. The mechanisms are intriguing – some disorganised attachment relationships appear to be rooted in maltreatment. When the infant is stressed it has the instinct to approach the caregiver, but if that caregiver is likely to be abusive then the infant will not know whether to approach or avoid – hence the contradictory behaviours seen in the SSP. The other route into disorganised behaviour seems to be parental dissociation on being faced with a stressed child. From the child's point of view, a stressful situation results in the instinct to approach the parent, but a dissociating parent is scary so the child doesn't know whether to approach or avoid.

Separation and loss

After describing attachment theory, Bowlby went on to detail how children respond to separation from a loved one (Bowlby 1973) and loss of a parent or carer by death or permanent separation (Bowlby 1980). Reactions include showing despair, distrust or anger, and in extreme cases detachment. Some of Bowlby's conclusions about the effects of short-term separations have not been supported by subsequent research, but the usually negative impacts of bereavement or long-term separation have largely confirmed, though the quality of care and support provided by alternative attachment figures is a crucial mitigating factor. Reactions to the loss of an abusing or neglectful caregiver can be just as intense, because children can still be attached to maltreating adults when they lack substitutes (Baer and Martinez 2006).

How can we best help children recover from loss and grief? Research has now demonstrated that 'traumatic debriefing' by therapists who are effectively strangers can actually do harm (Bisson et al. 1997). In contrast, safe nurturing care from a primary caregiver can effect rapid and apparently complete recovery – if this is achieved early enough in life. A child experiencing loss of one parent may be greatly comforted by living with another attachment figure, e.g. parent or grandparent. For this reason, recent work in areas experiencing disaster has placed more emphasis on reuniting family and friends than engaging therapists.

Dozier and colleagues have conducted a series of landmark studies that illustrate this remarkable phenomenon. Young infants can form secure attachments with foster carers very quickly, despite having previously experienced very severe abuse. If the foster carer is a sensitive, secure individual, a previously maltreated infant can begin to show secure attachment behaviours within two weeks (Stovall-McClough and Dozier 2004).

However, as many adoptive parents and foster carers have already discovered, for some maltreated children love is not enough. The children's early negative experiences have left them with a tendency not to go to adults for care or problem-solving when stressed or hurt. A carer who is simply sensitive will take the child's lead and this will result in no comfort being offered. Dozier has described how important it is that foster carers are 'gently challenging' – offering care even when it is not being sought and does not appear to be needed by a maltreated child (Dozier 2003). As Cairns (2003) describes, children with attachment difficulties can give out confusing signals and evoke negative emotions in professionals too, and they may find these hard to cope with unless they understand the reasons.

How can an understanding of attachment inform day-to-day work with children?

In many parts of the world Bowlby's work has had a substantial impact on the way that children are cared for. We have described how the relationships between a child and a caregiver can be reliably characterised as secure or insecure, with subcategories. But specialised and time-consuming investigations are seldom going to play a part in informing practitioners working day-to-day with children in schools, in playgroups, in youth work and elsewhere.

One particularly simple but comprehensive way of distilling attachment theory into thinking about the care of young children is the Circle of Security (Hoffman et al. 2006; see Chapter 17). This indicates that children need both to explore their world and at other times seek safety, and highlights that caregivers need to be able to provide both a 'secure base' for exploration and a 'safe haven' into which to retreat. Different parent or carer activities go along with exploration, such as watching, helping and taking delight, while others constitute the safe haven, such as protecting, comforting and, most important, helping to organise feelings.

So, let's turn our attention now to considering how ordinary challenges of life unfold in the light of our understanding of attachment theory. We'll begin with an example of a parent responding to a child's experience of loss. For many children and families the process of grieving loss is an ordinary, though often difficult, part of everyday life. A sensitively attuned parent tolerates their six-year-old having a toddler-quality tantrum in the days after the guinea pig has died. They might spend some extra time that evening over a bedtime story, give some extra cuddles over the next few days, expect the odd slip-up on the independence front for a while.

This parent knows that being reasonably consistent in their approach to their child is important, but also realises that it can be wise to be a bit more flexible for the time being, because the child is grieving. Some writers refer to this process as 'grief work' because it demands energy and time to complete the task. Nonetheless, the important thing is that, given time and the opportunity to work through the loss, we can anticipate the resumption of normal service – i.e. developmentally appropriate functioning from both child and parent.

This is usually the way that things unfold where a child has experienced 'good enough' early care and has had the opportunity to develop a secure attachment relationship with their primary caregiver; but a child who has an insecure attachment with their parent may well behave differently when faced with a stress like this – although distressed they may struggle to accept comfort and soothing. This may, in turn, produce a dilemma for the parent who feels, on one hand, concerned about the child's distress while, on the other, frustrated by the child's difficulty in accepting comfort. We can see here the potential for the dynamic of insecure attachment reasserting and maintaining itself. Dozier's work suggests that, certainly with younger children, the parent is well-advised to 'respond to the need not the behavior'. In other words, this is a time for persevering with comforting and helping the child to tolerate their conflicting feelings in the knowledge that such an approach will tend to help the child become better regulated emotionally.

However, those working with children – for example, in schools and nurseries – come across children from time to time who behave in more unusual ways. Some, for example, appear fearful of the adults in stressful situations. These situations can wrong-foot even experienced workers but, thanks to our understanding of attachment theory, we can now recognise these behaviours as being like a flashing road traffic sign that reads: 'Warning! Internal working model at work!' So what is going on? This child, unwittingly, is 'casting' the adult in a role that, although unfamiliar to the adult, is familiar to the child. While such an experience can be quite discomfiting, the adult does well to consider the significance of this experience since it may well be an indication that this child's experience has taught them to *protect themselves* from adults. The adult has to approach the child in ways that will allow the child to find them to be reliable (a secure base) and trustworthy (a safe haven). While such an approach may not come naturally to the adult, this is exactly the 'gentle challenge' that Dozier was referring to, and persisting with such an approach is likely to help the task in hand, be it childcare, teaching or everyday family life.

What are the contributing factors affecting loss and recovery?

There are five key ingredients to consider in relation to loss and recovery: the child, the parent, their relationship, the wider context and the nature of the loss.

Children whose development is not running smoothly are at much greater risk of encountering difficulty when ordinary but challenging tasks, such as coping with loss, come along. Personal temperament also plays a part in these matters, and there has long been evidence that some temperamental differences, especially tendencies toward restlessness/overactivity and towards rigidity/inflexibility, are 'hard-wired', i.e. substantially genetically determined (Chess and Thomas 1991; Plomin 1995). This can come into sharp focus at a time of stress, when a child who tends towards inflexibility is likely to find it difficult to adapt to the changes that a loss can bring.

A parent who is attuned to their child can make a sensitive response to the child's grief-related coping difficulties. But it is not difficult to imagine circumstances in which a parent may struggle to react in such a constructive fashion. A parent may be stressed or preoccupied by issues unrelated to the child's dilemmas, but nonetheless find that those issues impinge on their ability to think and act in a child-focused fashion. This commonly arises where a parent is depressed (Murray et al. 1993). Furthermore, where one partner is depressed the likelihood of conflict between partners is significantly increased, with consequent impact on the child who witnesses this (Hibel et al. 2009). Substance abuse can have a similar impact, effectively preoccupying the parent and deflecting them from their caregiving role (Barnard and McKeganey 2004). The social context of substance abuse is often such that additional factors coexist and contribute to the impact on the child.

The parent's own experience of parental care, particularly where that has included significant loss or where they have themselves experienced neglect or abuse in childhood, is very likely to shape the way that they conduct themselves in similar situations with their own children, and in turn the quality of the attachment style of the caregiving relationship. In turn, the attachment relationship will, depending on its nature, support or undermine the child's recovery from loss.

It will be easier for a child to recover from loss if the wider context in which they live is supportive. Unfortunately, some children are born into situations where negative life events seems to follow on from others, especially where major problems like parental substance misuse lead to a chaotic lifestyle in which the child is poorly supervised.

Finally, the nature of the loss itself will have an impact – greater losses (e.g. a parent dying) usually have a greater impact than smaller ones (e.g. a friend moving away). However, a supportive attachment relationship can help ameliorate even the most traumatic of losses and may be at the root of what we often refer to as 'resilience'.

Working with loss and grief

For some very traumatised children, the process of recovering from past hurts and forming new relationships can be extremely challenging. The habit of not expressing hurt can become entrenched and carers – often as a direct result of their sensitivity – can respond in kind by withdrawing. The result can be an interactional desert where no one knows how to express care for the other. A psychologist from the USA has developed a relationship-based treatment programme called Dynamic Developmental Psychotherapy (DDP) aimed specifically at helping such children integrate into 'new' families (Hughes 2007). The approach taken is called 'PACE'

– playfulness, attunement, curiosity and empathy – and aims to help parents and carers gently challenge the child using methods appropriate for older children.

What part do child and adolescent mental health services play?

Where children already have serious established attachment difficulties, child and adolescent mental health services (CAMHS) may have a useful consultative role in supporting those caring for the child. We conducted some recent research with residential workers about their knowledge of attachment difficulties. The city in which our participants worked had had an 'attachment-promoting policy' in residential care for the past decade and that had included greater involvement of a specialist CAMHS team for looked-after and accommodated children in the units. It was clear that the residential workers had learned a great deal from regular discussions about children with CAMHS workers, not only about the kinds of difficulties these children could suffer from, but also about which problems they should involve CAMHS colleagues in addressing and which they could reasonably manage themselves (Ferguson et al. 2010).

There is a great deal of confusion among professionals about the difference between insecure attachment and mental-health problems. Just to reiterate, insecure attachment is a feature of a *relationship* not of an individual, and since 30–40 per cent of us will have had an insecure attachment pattern in infancy with one or other of our parents, it is clearly too common to be a disorder.

Example 18.1

Rachel was an 8-year-old girl who was seen in CAMHS with her mother, who had been a chaotic drug user during her infancy but was now stable on methadone. In early life Rachel was neglected by her mother and witnessed violence associated with her mother's chaotic lifestyle. When assessed in CAMHS, she had attention deficit hyperactivity disorder (ADHD), which is more common in children who have experienced early neglect (Stevens et al. 2008), and she also had more specific psychiatric symptoms associated with neglect, such as indiscriminate friendliness. Her attachment pattern with her mother was assessed using the MCAST and found to be secure. This impression was strengthened by the observation that when she trapped her finger in one of our toys, she immediately went to her Mum for a cuddle – so she was using her mother appropriately in stressful situations. Our thoughts were that since her mother's lifestyle had settled down, they had been able to develop a warm and secure attachment relationship. Sadly this had not cured the mental-health problems that had probably grown out of her early neglect.

The helping services have a critical part to play in the lives of vulnerable children like Rachel, and it will help us understand the role of CAMHS if we can locate it in that wider context. As attachment theory reminds us, children need the protection of adults in order to survive and attuned care from sensitive caregivers to thrive. Where the care available does not meet those standards, the child's development is at risk. Where the care is significantly out of phase with the child's needs, the child is in danger. Everyone who works with children has the responsibility of alerting child protection services where they think a child may be at risk. Children's services and social work services, in particular, have the critical responsibility for assessing that risk and deciding on the steps that are necessary to protect those children. In some cases, safe care is not available to the child in their home setting and the social worker must then seek an alternative arrangement where the child will be safe. That intervention will often require the use of compulsory measures of care, and the legal system becomes involved in adjudicating on whether or not the measures proposed are reasonable and appropriate.

CAMHS can and should work with vulnerable children and high risk families, but that work should *not* take place where children are at risk of continuing harm from their carer. Clinical experience indicates that behaviours which have led to a referral to CAMHS are not infrequently symptomatic of the child's fearful response to a dangerous caregiving situation. Similarly, when children who are in need of *protection* from their parents are moved into safe settings, it is not unusual that earlier concerns diminish dramatically indicating, as attachment theory has taught us to expect, the direct relationship between safe care and healthy development. In the context of safe care it becomes possible to consider working with children and their families to investigate the feasibility of those parents ever resuming the care of their children – Zeanah and his colleagues (2001) in New Orleans have developed a model for such work.

Conclusions and implications

Attachment theory has lifelong implications for relationships. When children have experienced difficult early attachment relationships, they may have difficulties expressing their need for nurture, so that it is difficult for the parent or carer to know how and when to be soothing. For these children, a 'gently challenging' approach can be very helpful. There are some new therapeutic techniques, such as Circle of Security, Attachment and Bio-behavioural Catchup and Dyadic Developmental Psychotherapy that help parents and carers understand attachment and use gentle challenge when appropriate.

For professionals, understanding attachment theory can provide both a better understanding of individual children and families, and a common language to share with other professionals. An understanding of attachment theory can assist in a variety of contexts – for example:

- in assessment when making connections between relationship, behaviour and learning;
- directly helping children;
- supporting parents and carers;
- seeking help to deal with practitioners' own feelings and thoughts provoked by attachment difficulties;
- knowing when to refer to specialists.

Exercise

- Outline how disorganised attachment might manifest itself in a setting in which you work with children.
- Discuss how you could adapt your approach in order to help a child and parent facing this issue to gain more from contact with your service.

Recommended reading

Cairns, K. (2003) *Attachment, trauma and resilience: therapeutic caring for children*, London: BAAF.

Holmes, J. (1993) *John Bowlby & Attachment Theory*, London and New York: Routledge.

Howe, D. (2011) *Attachment Across the Life Course*, Basingstoke: Palgrave Macmillan.

Perry, B. and Szalavitz, M. (2006) *The Boy who was Raised as a Dog*, New York: Basic.

Chapter 19

Accentuating the positive: resilience and desistance approaches to children's needs and behaviour

Malcolm Hill

Summary points

- Ideas about resilience and desistance have developed in different domains, but reached similar conclusions. Both help professionals to support informal coping and recovery processes.

- 'Resilience' means doing well despite adverse or high-risk circumstances. 'Desistance' refers to cessation or substantial lessening of problematic behaviour.

- Research on resilience and desistance has shown that positive results occur when there is a combination of individual characteristics, preparedness to change, social support and access to relevant resources and opportunities.

- Assessments and interventions based on resilience or desistance highlight the identification and promotion of strengths as much as responding to needs and risks.

- The two approaches have much to offer as a means of reformulating and re-energising services and professional activities, though there are dangers to be avoided.

Introduction

Collaborative work requires cross-fertilisation of theories and evidence underpinning practice. As an example, this chapter will provide a sympathetically critical review of two examples of approaches to service intervention for children and families – namely, resilience and desistance. The research and theorising related to each have emerged in different fields but have much in common, so they can reinforce and enhance each other. They both emphasise that, wherever possible, anyone working with children should attempt to understand and work with the grain of positive qualities in a child, family or community. Positive resources can be identified and brought to bear on learning, health, behaviour or self-esteem.

In this context *resilience* refers to the factors and processes that enable individuals, families or communities to overcome serious adversity or high risk. It has a more specific sense than general robustness in the face of everyday challenges. *Desistance* refers to those influences that enable an individual or family to give up a socially disapproved behaviour, such as offending, drug misuse and self-harm. Both concepts are concerned with successful outcomes despite difficulties. They are applied mainly to individuals who are vulnerable, challenging or both, which means they have mainly been used in specialist contexts, but they also have relevance for children using general and universal services.

Resilience and desistance compared

Writings about these two phenomena have been hitherto largely segregated. Resilience ideas have their roots in developmental psychology and epidemiology, and have been refined through application mainly in child and adolescent psychiatry and social work, though also in some educational and care settings. Thinking about desistance originates in criminology and sociology, and has been mainly applied in probation with adults and in relation to youth justice and substance misuse.

Superficially, resilience and desistance apply to very different kinds of difficulty. Resilience ideas help to understand children brought up in adverse circumstances which can result in major care and safeguarding needs. Desistance applies to young people (or their parents) who engage in illegal and other problematic behaviour. Yet research has shown that these two types of situation have similar causal factors. Furthermore, many young people and adults who commit crimes or become addicted were known to services when young for child-protection reasons (Hill et al. 2007a).

Resilience and desistance thinking share many themes despite the differing origins and focus. The research base for both evolved from investigations of how people get over or out of difficulties. Studies revealed the impact of informal supports and processes and external events, which often had as much impact as official interventions or more. The emphasis on how problems are overcome embodies a belief that individuals are not necessarily trapped by their circumstances or history. A related strand is that the kinds of processes that help a person or family get over a problem may be different from those that caused the problem in the first place. A child's unhappiness may have resulted from negative parenting that is difficult to alter, but can be alleviated by a caring neighbour or teacher, success at school or good friendships (Bukowski 2003). Another shared assumption is that lessons learned from those who succeed in overcoming problems can be applied to those who are still struggling, though the transfer of lessons may not be straightforward.

Both stress the role of individual agency, while also recognising the importance of social context. They are future-oriented and contrast with risk-based methods, which focus largely on past or present vulnerability factors and then seek to tackle them. Encouragement is offered to professionals by highlighting that outcomes can be good, even from very unfavourable beginnings. A classic American long-term study by Werner and Smith (1992) followed up a sample of children whose early lives were characterised by poverty, family problems and often abuse. In later childhood, about one-third were doing well, while by the time they reached early adulthood a majority were functioning satisfactorily.

Factors and processes affecting resilience and desistance

Much research on resilience and desistance has produced a long list of diverse factors, which provide useful pointers to the kinds of action that can be helpful. For instance, resilience has been shown to be helped by self-belief, humour, access to a supporter or champion and involvement in organised activities, which are all things that a professional can seek to develop (Gilligan 2001; Daniel and Wassell 2002). It is common to group factors into three levels (Olsson et al. 2003):

1. Individual – e.g. talents and interests;
2. Family – e.g. extent of caring support;
3. Community and societal – e.g. neighbourhood and school environments.

It is generally recognised, though, that piecemeal attention to individual factors in isolation is inadequate. To overcome severe adversity or behaviour problems usually requires an interaction of external resources and opportunities on one hand, with internal capacities and readiness to make use of these on the other. Moreover, progress is often uneven with positive periods giving way at times to lapses in coping or resumptions of negative behaviour (McNeill and Maruna 2007).

Self-concepts, motivation and cognitive change

Resilience research shows that key personal qualities of individuals who cope better are self-confidence and a sense of efficacy – i.e. a belief that you can influence events in your life. Finding positive meaning in seemingly negative circumstances is also helpful (Bayat 2007).

Giordano et al. (2002) regard cognitive transformations as crucial in desistance, though these interact with external circumstances. They identified four main elements:

- openness to change;
- 'hooks for change' or turning points;
- envisioning a new kind of self;
- transformation in the view of past behaviour.

These can be seen as including processes that occur as a result of naturally occurring agency (free will), as well as orientations and skills that can be taught. Young people who have ceased to self-harm state that the main reason for this has been a growing realisation of the pointlessness and hurt. Only a minority attribute cessation to family or friends, with few having told a professional, let alone given up as a result of such contact (Young et al. 2007).

Close relationships

One of the most consistent findings of research on desistance is that giving up a criminal lifestyle is often prompted by a new or revived close relationship with someone, usually a family member or partner, who offers alternative sources of satisfaction and incentives to adopt a more law-abiding life (McDonald and Marsh 2005). According to Barry (2006) this is connected to social recognition – i.e. being valued by someone or a group for reasons other than antisocial activities and associated bravado. In order to give up a lifestyle based on criminality, gang activity or addiction, it is important to distance oneself from others engaging in that behaviour. That is difficult to do unless access can be made to an alternative peer group or partner, possibly through links outside the area (McIntosh and McKeganey 2001: Bannister et al. 2010).

Similarly, the support of family, friends or others is crucial to managing and overcoming difficult circumstances or life events. Not uncommonly, a source of support and help may be someone who may not be obvious or known to a professional. This is usually a person trusted by the child or young person and with the capacity to help them, even though not necessarily having a connection or expertise in relation to the problem at hand (e.g. school janitor, friend or parents' friend). Research on children in public care who have done well educationally highlights the importance of 'a special person in my life to back me up' like a teacher, mentor or social worker (Martin and Jackson 2002, p. 128).

While attention has mostly been given to individual coping, some investigations have taken place of family resilience in response to different kinds of crisis, ranging from bereavement to environmental disasters. Unsurprisingly, a general conclusion is that families whose members cooperate well tend to cope with external threats best – they communicate openly and constructively; pool resources; support individual and collective change (Walsh 2003; Benzies and Mychasiuk 2009). This usually reflects longstanding emotionally closeness, based on shared beliefs and meanings, spending a lot of time together and having common celebrations and routines (McCubbin et al. 1996).

Activities, skills and opportunities

Children with unsatisfactory family or care situations can be helped to develop self-esteem and skills that will help their education and employability though involvement in a range of 'recreational' activities, such as sport, drama and music. These may build on or initiate interests and talents in the child. They also provide access to supportive peer and adult relationships (Gilligan 2001). Organised leisure pursuits can also be transforming for children living in poverty by widening their horizons and supporting their development of both human and social capital (Wager et al. 2009).

Example 19.1

Here is an instance of an individual helped to overcome family difficulties and modify his behaviour.

Alan is a young man with a history of aggression, especially towards females, and of placements away from his birth family. After moving to a new foster home aged 15, he got on well with his foster father, who encouraged Alan to join him on fishing trips. This provided a break from tensions at home and an opportunity to talk over relationships with mother-figures. In the longer run, Alan made friends with a shared interest in angling and chose to dissociate from a gang with whom he had repeatedly been in trouble.

Schools can aid resilience for children with psycho-social problems in a variety of ways (e.g. Howard and Johnson 2000):

- opportunities for sense of achievement and status;
- support and guidance from teachers and/or other staff;
- supportive peer relationships;
- opportunity for a positive identity;
- skills and knowledge development to increase options for lifestyle choices.

Identity

The interplay of personal and interpersonal processes in resilience and desistance is often linked to a person's perceptions of who they are. People who demonstrate resilience tend to have a strong sense of themselves as competent people. Those who have experienced trauma can overcome the worst effects when they are able to put their past history into a new perspective and shape a new future, perhaps assisted by counselling (Newman and Blackburn 2002).

Likewise young people who turn away from crime and addiction often need to change their ideas about who they are and what they can become by reviewing the narratives of their past lives and potential futures (McNeill and Maruna 2007). For this to happen, opportunities for more conventional practices and the availability of models and routines about how to perform them have to coincide with a capacity to make an identity shift (Rumgay 2004). For young women who become pregnant, concern for their child along with the new identity associated with motherhood are prominent in accounts of desistance (Barry 2006). In relation to drug misuse, cessation is often gradual as the perceived costs and benefits alter and an alternative identity becomes available through a partner, parenthood or employment, though it can also occur suddenly in response to a tragic loss (McIntosh and McKeganey 2001).

Social and neighbourhood issues

Resilience and desistance processes seem to be fairly similar for males and females, and for different ethnic groups in the UK, but gender and ethnicity play a part in how and when they operate (Hill et al. 2007a; McIvor 2010; Weaver and McNeill 2010). The nature of the neighbourhood and local peer associations in particular affect in major ways the manner and ease or difficulty of taking advantage of resources and opportunities (Webster et al. 2006; Wager et al. 2009). Economic and social policies on such matters as education, employment and housing crucially affect the amount and types of opportunities available, constraining or supporting the scope for individual agency (Farrall et al. 2010).

Implications for service delivery and practice

Resilience/desistance approaches entail recognising and promoting competencies, skills, resources and opportunities for personal improvement, in individuals or families and their social networks, taking into consideration preparedness to change (Farrall and Maruna 2004; Raby and Raby 2008). Most applications adopt an empowerment stance, with children and parents fully involved in discussions and decisions and identifying their priorities, so they exercise and develop their sense of personal control (Fraser 2004). Modification of feelings, modes of thinking and behaviour will often form part of the work, but there is a wider goal to strengthen inclusion in supportive and pro-social networks and activities that will help sustain improvements as well as provide broader social benefits (McNeill 2004).

Such ideas have proved applicable to a range of settings and methods (with groups and individuals; short-term and long-term work) (Newman 2004), though it might also be regarded as a weakness that the central ideas are adaptable because fairly generalised. Some organisations have adopted resilience (less commonly desistance) as the rationale underpinning the whole agency aims and ethos, whereas in others the principles are used in a more targeted way for direct work with children and families. A comparative study of children's social work agencies found that in the UK a resilience approach focused on enhancing individual skills and self-esteem, whereas in Australia there was more emphasis on building on parental and network resources (Daniel et al. 2009).

Assessment

Assessment frameworks tend to be based largely on ideas about need and risk, with a number of standard risk-assessment tools being widely used in the fields of safeguarding children and youth justice e.g. YLS, ASSET (Stephenson et al. 2007). Important as these are, resilience and desistance models give weight to assessing strengths and resources, actual and potential, formal and informal. This requires identification of positive characteristics of the individual and mapping network relationships, contacts and activities. Ideally this should be done in dialogue so that the assessment not only informs professional decisions, but the child or parent concerned also weighs up the positive and negative influences in their lives in order to seek ways of altering the balance (Hill 2002; also Chapter 9).

Strength-based assessments help to identify personal or social resources that can assist in overcoming the problems at hand; skills or interests to be developed partly to compensate for deficiencies in other aspects of a child's life; to recognise where official help is required to make up for gaps in informal support. A crucial component is to identify and benefit from input by members of informal social networks who can assist in one or more ways (e.g. as supporter, confidant, carer, role model, tutor, provider of material resources, facilitator of links to formal services). Assessments should not be blind to negatives requiring attention too. Care should be taken to assess situations where individuals are superficially resilient or desistant, but an underlying hurt or continued propensity towards negative behaviour persists. Otherwise their needs will be overlooked (Hill et al. 2007b; Murray 2009).

The drug-misuse literature emphasises the importance of assessing people's readiness to change and its converse, resistance to treatment (Prochaska et al. 1992). When individuals lack motivation to cooperate then the focus of professional action should be on understanding and addressing the reasons for this, otherwise clients/patients will simply not attend or respond. Some writers have recognised a cycle of motivation, in which people move from hostility or indifference, via guarded interest, to genuine willingness to change. Intermediate stages in the cycle can be deceptive, as individuals make small or token steps towards modifying their attitudes or behaviour, but often slip back into familiar patterns. While the image of a regular cycle with a fixed order of stages does not represent many situations accurately (Barber 2003), the broad notion of identifying degrees of preparedness to change and adapting strategies to take account of this can be generalised to a range of problems.

Professional roles

The approaches described in this chapter do not require professionals to abandon their customary methods of work. Rather, they encourage an orientation that is geared to working with existing restorative forces and to promoting personal and network resources. Sometimes this will be the primary focus of work; sometimes it will be secondary to more specific actions, to teach, attend to an illness, give advice etc. Children and young people particularly value professionals who go beyond their immediate role, provided this is experienced as caring and not intrusive (see Chapter 2).

The resilience model has been used in schools and teacher training – for instance, to increase children's sense of mastery, problem-solving, optimistic outlook and access to external resources. Specific educational resources have been developed to aid class work (Greeff 2005). Teaching about resilience and emotional intelligence can help self-awareness and coping for children with significant difficulties, while enhancing empathy and responsiveness among potential peer helpers.

Key components of desistance- and resilience-based work with individuals and families include:

- identifying with children what their capacities and priorities are;
- modifying attitudes, feelings and understandings;
- promoting practical and social skills;
- helping the development of a coherent narrative for oneself and others to make sense of past hurts, both received and given;
- supporting interactions with positive role models and informal supporters;
- encouraging appropriate new links – for instance, by introduction to a club, activity or agency or by the allocation of a volunteer supporter, befriender or advocate;
- helping to take advantage of educational, recreational and employment opportunities;
- facilitating stability of accommodation;
- developing activities and social associations that promote responsibility towards others and pro-social identity.

Paper and on-line charts and templates or board games can be used with children individually or in groups to promote discussion of problems, aspirations, risks and resources. Family group conferences with professional facilitators are an increasingly common means of seeking to capitalise on family resilience and to enhance it.

McNeill (2009a) emphasises the crucial significance of the subjective meanings that individuals attach to opportunities to change behaviour. Workers can help individuals and families see opportunities as relevant to their priorities and offering positive attractions. People with a negative self-image are often fatalistic about their ability to change. Porporino (2010) draws on positive psychology to emphasise how practitioners can assist such individuals by enhancing self-esteem, self-efficacy, coherent meaning in life and a sense of continuity.

A further implication of desistance thinking is the need for professionals to facilitate the development of generativity – i.e. making a positive contribution to others (McNeill and Maruna 2007). This is in keeping with, but broader than, victim awareness and empathy-raising programmes (see Chapter 10).

Much work with troubled children and families consists of formalised programmes, often with components that evaluative studies have shown to be effective in reducing offences or improving parenting, for example. These programmes have a part to play but it has been argued that in the youth justice field in particular this model has been applied too inflexibly. Services should be able to adapt to and support individuals' change processes rather than expecting everyone to respond in the same way to pre-ordained models (McNeill and Whyte 2007).

Transformative activities and mentoring

Evidence about both resilience and desistance highlight the significance of leisure activities, not simply for their intrinsic merits but for crucial additional qualities. Recreational services are rarely invited to join inter-agency groups and meetings but can make a vital contribution.

Particularly for young people with personal or family difficulties and those living in disadvantaged households and areas, access to recreational activities can provide vital opportunities to develop skills and thereby increase their self-esteem, as well as to establish links with pro-social peers and supportive adults. Involvement in organised activities at school and elsewhere helps reduce exposure to risk of bullying, harassment or engagement in crime. Families living in poverty have fewer facilities in the areas they live in and usually can ill-afford costs of travel, entrance or the equipment and clothing associated with certain activities like music and dance. Hence the importance for them of low-cost local provision and assistance with indirect costs (Wager et al. 2009).

Formal mentoring services have become increasingly common that link young people to adults previously unknown to them, and who are usually lay people given some introductory training. These have been shown to be helpful in relation to both educational achievements and socio-emotional issues (Rhodes and Love 2008; Erickson et al. 2009), though vagueness and uncertainty about roles are common (Colley 2003). However, young people often prefer to obtain help from people they already know and trust, rather than from an official befriending project (Philip

2008). HomeStart and similar services offer similar kinds of support to parents, particularly those with young children.

The timing and nature of intervention

Understandings about desistance indicate that the nature of work undertaken should be adapted to fluctuations in openness to change and variations in the processes likely to affect change at different times (Rumgay 2004). Involvement of resistant individuals in formalised programmes, whether focused on behaviour change, education or support, may need to wait until they are more open, as otherwise non-attendance or drop-out are likely. Similarly, helping access a new job, network or other opportunity will often only succeed when a person has reached a readiness to take advantage (Porporino 2010). Heightened openness might result from a change in circumstances, self-evaluation, persuasion or legal pressures (a court appearance or legal order). Thus, early contacts with unmotivated people may need to involve unthreatening relationship-building, consciousness raising and/or the enlisting of other service users to help engagement. Only later are more specific methods deployed to help change (e.g. anger management, empathy development, increasing awareness of consequences). Development of trusting relationships with professionals is often a prerequisite for the emergence of a strong wish to change (McNeill and Whyte 2007). For example, one voluntary agency working with challenging young people provided frequent, informal and accepting contacts with staff in order to build trust, before introducing targeted methods to modify behaviour (Robertson et al. 2006). In the mental-health field it has been found that young people who are resistant to cognitive-behavioural methods can respond better to relationship-based and network-support approaches (Kingdon et al. 2007).

For entrenched problems like addictions and sexual abuse, a third stage after engagement and change-oriented work is relapse prevention, which recognises that desistance from addiction, crime or abusive behaviour is rarely sudden or complete (Lerpiniere 1999; Barber 2003). Methods include detailed discussion of risks and temptations, along with monitoring arrangements and coping strategies. Anticipating future problems and planning how to deal with them is also important – e.g. for those children with care or mental-health problems (Friesen 2007; Hawkins-Rodgers 2007). Once contact with a service ends it is easy to slip back, so that for some people follow-up is necessary.

Both resilience and desistance thinking highlight the need to take into account age and life-stage. For instance, in relation to offending there is evidence that in the early teens formal processes may be counterproductive in reinforcing criminal peer associations, status and identity. By contrast for young people in their late teens, fear of legal sanctions or weariness with police and court involvements can be significant factors in decisions to alter behaviour, especially if combined with other relationship changes like commitment to a partner or child (Smith 2006).

Writers on resilience have described how important life transitions can provide a good opportunity to help achieve substantial change, as there is generally more openness (Newman and Blackburn 2002). Most major changes and new experiences engender a mix of anxiety and anticipation. The widespread development of transition programmes to help children adjust to moves into primary and secondary school demonstrate how information, support and careful preparation can help ensure that usually the positives of new academic and social opportunities outweigh problems of discontinuity and unfamiliarity.

A concept shared by resilience and desistance writings is that of 'turning point'. This signifies an occasion when an event or decision opens the possibility of a significant change, which can then have cumulative benefits if a reformed status or identity is reinforced. Services can help to recognise, create and capitalise on such turning points.

Implications for interprofessional working

Resilience advocates see interprofessional work as key to this model, in recognition of evidence that the ability to cope effectively with or recover from serious adversity usually requires attention to interacting influences in different life domains and at different levels (individuals, family, community) (Luthar 2003). In the field of foster care, programmes have been developed, some explicitly labelled multi-systemic, which involve collaboration among several key agencies to optimise children's opportunities to overcome difficulties across a range of care, education, health and behaviour issues.

Example 19.2

Some agencies have committed themselves to a strengths- or resilience-based ethos, blending the skills of different professions. Brownrigg et al. (2004) described a family resilience service with social work and nursing staff, working with depressed parents and their children to help each acknowledge and build on their skills and external resources and to improve family communication. Family meetings assessed roles, rules, boundaries and networks of support. An evaluation of the project showed increases in children's engagement with peers and social activities.

Formal legal measures can reinforce criminal identities, so that diversion from formal processes is often helpful. This requires police, legal system gatekeepers and service providers to confer, act flexibly and provide positive informal alternatives (McAra and McVie 2010).

Critical review

Resilience and desistance models fit well with other frameworks that focus on building up positives alongside, or even instead of, seeking to rectify negatives. These include:

- competence-based work;
- solution therapies;

- health promotion;
- mental health recovery;
- strengths approaches;
- positive psychology.

What these all have in common is a commitment to seeing people with problems in a rounded way, as having capacities and abilities as well as difficulties. Furthermore, these positive qualities can, when worked with, help overcome, alleviate or distract from negatives.

Some positive frameworks have set themselves firmly in opposition to more traditional ways of working, which are seen as aiming to correct defects or deficits in individuals, families or communities in a very top-down manner. For instance, one exponent of strengths-based work strongly criticised conventional practices, especially those that rely on diagnostic categories (Saleeby 2002). He claims these result in professionals treating people largely in terms of labels like 'young offender' or 'attention deficit and hyperactivity disorder' rather than as whole individuals whose complex social contexts require understanding and action (see also Lloyd et al. 2006). This critique may be based to some extent on caricature, but evaluations of strengths-based work have indicated that practitioners can be energised and service users feel more respected and engaged. Similar results have been found with respect to resilience- and desistance-oriented practice (McNeill 2004; Daniel et al. 2009).

Usually it is more useful to see resilience and desistance ideas as correctives to previous methods rather than total replacements. This was reflected, for example, in attempts by Antonovsky (1996) and others to widen the horizons of clinicians from dealing exclusively with illness to promoting positive health, which has indeed become a much more central feature in health settings and schools over the past few decades.

While this chapter has pointed to merits of resilience/desistance thinking within a wider spectrum of positive frameworks, it is important to recognise potential drawbacks. It is essential to avoid an apple-pie approach, which sees only the good in people and situations. A number of child-abuse enquiries have shown that optimistic evaluations of parents have repeatedly led professionals to overlook or underestimate ill-treatment of children, so it is vital to remain alert to warning signs of risks to children's safety and welfare. Similarly, it is important that a focus on overcoming risks and adversity does not divert energies from tackling the causes of families' and children's difficulties, including poverty and inadequate preparedness for parenting.

A further danger is that services and, indeed, the wider public come to expect that overcoming difficulties is easy and to blame or give up on the 'non-resilient' and 'non-desistant'. This is not the purpose of these frameworks – rather the aim is to help children and families struggling to cope increase their resources for doing so.

Conclusions and implications

Many academic and professional theories applied to different areas of work develop in isolation. Identifying crossovers can help people work together better.

This chapter has reviewed evidence about the many similarities in processes and influences that help individuals and families overcome adversity (resilience) or move away from negative behaviour (desistance). Research and theorising in these two fields have developed independently and differ in detail, but have reached broadly similar conclusions about the importance of informal support, changes in thinking and taking opportunities to pursue new or modified life-paths and identities. Considering resilience and desistance together can provide a framework that bridges different children's services. It also identifies commonalities in change processes relevant to both children's services and agencies working with parents and other adults. These often need to cooperate to deal with family problems.

Of course, adversities and risk factors should be reduced whenever possible, but often these are in the past or intractable, so may be hard to modify. In such circumstances, resilience and desistance approaches show that change can still come about. An essential part of the work of professionals, whether working alone or collaboratively, should be to understand and work with basic coping and change processes that children and parents typically deploy to deal with everyday challenges and more serious circumstances and life events. Successful overcoming of severe difficulties usually requires deployment of a combination of individual, family and wider processes and resources, so that it can be vital for different professionals to work together to identify and promote those aspects and strengths that each is best equipped to help develop (Schoon 2006).

Exercise

Consider ways in which a service known to you could improve the ways it assesses, takes account of and works with resilience or desistance processes and factors. Also review the limitations of such an approach.

Recommended reading

Daniel, B. and Wassell, S. (2002) discuss many key ideas, practice aids and learning resources in three user-friendly volumes about resilience in the early years, school years and adolescence. The application of their approach in a children's home is described by Houston (2010).

The Scottish Government website section on *Getting it Right for Every Child* describes a resilience matrix for use in child assessments.

Porporino (2010) gives a critical overview of the application of desistance ideas to practice with offenders.

Barry (2006) discusses varied pathways taken by young people who commit crimes and shows how changes in behaviour interact with social identity, recognition and social capital.

Chapter 20

Working together at the transition to adulthood: services for young people with learning disabilities

Gillian MacIntyre

Summary points

- The transition from childhood to adulthood for all young people has become increasingly complex.
- Young people with learning disabilities face a range of additional barriers and are likely to experience delays in attaining conventional 'markers' of adulthood such as paid employment, living independently and having children.
- Parents of young people with learning disabilities face challenges in preparing for the time of transition and may need support during this period of adjustment. They are often excluded from the interprofessional discussions.
- The transition period has been increasingly identified as a problematic time by policy-makers. As a result a range of guidelines has been developed in order to promote more seamless transition pathways for young people. A personalised approach is helpful.
- A number of barriers remain, which include deficiencies in joint working. Greater clarity is needed about agency responsibilities during transition.

Introduction

The transition from childhood to adulthood should be a time of excitement and opportunity for young people. Yet increasingly, the nature of transition is changing and young people are faced with a number of challenges in terms of finding employment and living independently. This is particularly so during times of economic crisis, and such times of uncertainty are likely to be felt particularly keenly by young people with learning disabilities. This chapter will explore the transition from childhood to adulthood for this group of young people. It begins by outlining the main issues for young people in the general population making the transition before looking in more detail at the experiences of young people with learning disabilities. The chapter will then look in detail at the role of professionals in terms of supporting young people at the time of transition. Relevant policy guidance and legislation will be discussed before highlighting some of the barriers faced by professionals in terms of working collaboratively to support this group of young people.

The transition from childhood to adulthood

The transition from childhood to adulthood has become increasingly complex in recent years for all young people. This is the result of a range of factors including the collapse of the youth labour market and the resultant increase in participation in further and higher education among young people, changing family composition and a lack of affordable housing (Jones 2002; Furlong et al. 2003). Nowadays the transition typically involves three main aspects:

- leaving school and engaging in further education, training or employment;
- leaving the family home and moving to a home of one's own;
- leaving the family of origin and establishing a family of one's own.

Although cultural and individual variations exist, academics have recognised a common expectation that making a 'successful' transition to adulthood requires achieving these markers of adult status (e.g. Jones 2002). Yet young people may find that focusing on one of these areas creates difficulties in other areas. For example moving on to Higher Education might impact negatively on a young person's ability to move to a home of their own. Indeed, as the sections below illustrate, the nature of the transition from childhood to adulthood has changed to make management of the adjustments increasingly complex. This is particularly true for young people with learning disabilities for whom the conventional markers of adult status are difficult to achieve. If a person fails to achieve these transition goals, it does not necessarily mean not reaching adulthood. 'Childhood', 'adulthood' and the transition between both states are socially constructed – i.e. expectations around what it means to gain adult status vary across time and place.

Research has suggested that the transition from childhood to adulthood has grown increasingly protracted, complex and unstable (Johnston et al. 2000). Pias (2000) referred to this as the 'yo-yo-isation of the transition to adulthood' (p. 220). Young people leaving school today face greater uncertainty in terms of finding and keeping a job. Government responses over many years have been a host of training schemes for young people in order to avoid large-scale youth unemployment. A parallel development has been to encourage young people to stay in full-time education for as long as possible, thus deferring their entry into the labour market and economic independence (Jones 2002). An unintended consequence has been that the advantages for some young people of staying on in education are less than previously (McDonald and Marsh 2005).

This increasingly protracted and complex transition from school to further education, training and employment has a knock-on effect on the other areas of transition. Young people are increasingly staying in the family home for longer and achieve financial independence from their parents later. In addition, the route out of the family home is increasingly complex and many young people experience cycles of leaving home and returning.

Of particular concern is the growing number of young people not in further education, employment or training. Those young people most at risk of this are early school leavers with low levels of attainment. Howison (2003) found that young people who left school early were less likely to get a job if one or more parents were unemployed. Other risk factors include deprivation, financial exclusion, low attainment, weak family and other support networks, stigma and debt adversity (Scottish Executive 2005c).

Raffe (2003) has pointed out that for many young people, being without education, training or employment is part of a wider pattern of disadvantage and powerlessness that may need to be tackled on a broader front. One research study found that: despite continued commitment to finding and keeping a job, most [of the sample] were still experiencing poor, low-waged, intermittent work at the bottom of the labour market . . . after obtaining poor school qualifications, further poor training and education had not improved their employment prospects . . . this had ramifications in other aspects of their lives, resulting in social exclusion (Webster et al. 2004: V).

It would seem therefore that those young people who have experienced difficulties in making transitions at an earlier age are likely to experience future disadvantage. Perhaps most worrying is an increasing polarisation between young people who experience extended transitions and those who make accelerated transitions, between the rich and the poor and between those with qualifications and those without (Jones 2002). More and more young people are taking longer paths into the labour market, which were previously associated with the educated middle class in Britain. However, there is an identifiable disadvantaged group of young people who are missing out on the extension and expansion of education, who are making accelerated transitions by, for example, leaving the family home or having a child of their own at an early age.

In a society of declining employment opportunities for young people and increasingly high demands for qualifications, the future prospects for young people with learning disabilities looks worrying. Not all young people are able to negotiate transitions in the same way. Brannen and Nilsen (2002) argue that current economic trends suggest that only the best-qualified young people will have the opportunity to make plans for the future. They argue that only certain groups – the relatively privileged young whose education is likely to lead to better career opportunities – are really free to make choices. Berzins (2010) suggests that factors including personal agency, future outlook, intellectual ability and positive relationships with parents relate to successful transitions. The implications of this for young people with learning disabilities are considerable. Young people with learning disabilities are likely to be among the most marginalised of young people who find it difficult to negotiate risk and manage their transition to adulthood.

Specific transitional needs of young people with learning disabilities and their families

Young people with disabilities generally have expectations of adult life that are similar to those of young people in the general population. A study by Tarleton et al. (2006) found that young people with learning disabilities expected to work, go to college, have a social life, continue their leisure pursuits, make friends and have relationships. Yet, according to Bignall et al. (2000), although there has been a great deal of rhetoric about opening up choices to young disabled people, in practice the structures of education and training channel them down particular and narrow routes that may not reflect their own aspirations.

The transitional process for young people with learning disabilities can be problematic, with their moves towards independence tending to last longer and be more limited, with some barely taking on adult responsibilities at all (Hudson 2006; Blomquist 2007). Young people with moderate learning disabilities experience transition in ways and at a pace more similar to the experiences of other disadvantaged young people than those of young people in the general population (Caton and Kagan 2007). This appears to be the case regardless of the *type* of disability, while those with more complex needs are likely to be further disadvantaged. Young disabled people are more likely to experience social isolation and many have severely restricted social networks (Hudson 2003; MacIntyre 2008).

Young disabled people continue to experience segregation within further education. Negative attitudes, low expectations and a lack of appropriate support services mean that employment is not considered a viable option in every case. Findings from a national study conducted between 2004 and 2007 found a clear bias towards moving young people with learning disabilities into further education college after they left school. Indeed 60 per cent of those carers questioned in the study reported that schools had failed to mention employment as an option (Beyer 2008). MacIntyre (2007) found that despite an increasing range of options in relation to education, training and employment young people remained in a marginalised position. They were more likely, for example, to be over-represented in the group of young people who were not in education, employment or training. Although most young people are experiencing extended transitions with a range of choices and opportunities, the *experiences* of that delayed transition are very different. For young people with disabilities, the transitional experience is likely to be less fulfilling and less optimistic (Caton and Kagan 2007). They often view the extended periods that they are likely to spend in education or training negatively. Parents are often anxious to minimise risk, and activities such as accessing money and choosing friends are areas where they feel it is legitimate to intervene (Shepperdson 2001).

It is unsurprising that these negative experiences are further exacerbated for young people with more severe or profound disabilities. For this group of young people, leaving home is likely to take place later, and young people will not gain legal independence if they are not deemed to have capacity. Young people with complex needs are also less likely to have an independent social life as a result of a lack of accessible transport, communication issues, adult surveillance and lack of access to a peer group.

The experience of transition for parents

The transition from childhood to adulthood can also be a difficult time for parents. They can find themselves facing a range of stressful situations, many of which are not faced by parents of children without disabilities (Ytterhus et al. 2008). A study of parents of young people with autistic spectrum disorder in the United States (Graetz 2010) found that they worried about the future of their young person, particularly as they grew older themselves. At the time of transition they may find themselves excluded from planning and decision-making after many years of acting as an advocate on their child's behalf. Thorin and colleagues (1996) have suggested that this is a time when parental involvement and control is expected to diminish, yet the reality suggests a greater reliance than ever on parental resources and support by service providers. Yet tensions become apparent when professionals (and often young people themselves) perceive parents to be overstepping boundaries (Iles and Lowton 2010). It would appear that there is a need for a delicate balancing act for professionals between encouraging parental involvement and at the same time enabling young people to move towards independence.

Professional support at transition

A number of agencies are involved in supporting young people at the time of transition. Some support *all* young people including:

- schools;
- careers service (Connexions in England and Wales, Careers Scotland in Scotland);
- JobCentre Plus;
- local authority housing departments and housing associations;
- voluntary organisations that provide a range of training opportunities for young people.

Young people with learning disabilities are also likely to receive services from these organisations, but might also receive additional support from:

- social work departments;
- post-school psychological services;
- health professionals (including mental health services);
- specialist key workers.

Some of this support will be available on a time-limited basis. Riddell et al. (2001) have suggested that this might lead to confusion and an overlap in service provision. Devolution complicates matters further. Employment, for example, remains a reserved area controlled by the Westminster government, while in Scotland Lifelong Learning and Enterprise is the responsibility of the Scottish government. Specialist transition services might be particularly valuable in terms of assisting young people with learning disabilities to navigate their way through the complex maze of service provision. Specialist teams have been established in some local authority areas, but this has not developed in a uniform way across the country in the way that Throughcare teams have developed to ease the process of transition for young people leaving care.

Policy measures to support young people with learning disabilities at the time of transition

The difficulties associated with the transition from childhood to adulthood have been recognised by policy-makers, and the transition has been highlighted as a priority in a number of different policy and guidance documents. In 2001, objective 2 of *Valuing People* stated that measures needed to be taken to ensure that:

> As young people with learning disabilities move into adulthood to ensure continuity of care and support for the young person and their family and to provide equality of opportunity in order to enable as many disabled people as possible to participate in education, training or employment.
>
> (Department of Health 2001a)

Similarly, the National Service Framework for Children and Young People pointed out that:

> Disabled young people need high quality, multi-agency support to allow them to have choice and control over life decisions and to be aware of what opportunities are open to them and the range of support they may need to access services.
>
> (Department of Health 2004)

To this end, a number of changes were introduced. These changes recognised the importance of various agencies and professionals working together to improve transition pathways for young disabled people. Learning Disability Partnership Boards were introduced in all local authorities in England and Wales in October 2001. These boards were responsible for adult-learning disability services, and it was envisaged that they would ensure arrangements were in place to ensure a smooth transition to adult life for young people. In recognition of the need for information about the issues and services involved in transition, an information network was established. This disseminated advice produced by the Department for Education and Skills (subsequently renamed) for young people with learning disabilities making the transition from school.

Despite these measures and a plethora of good practice guidelines (see e.g. Department of Health 2008), the government recognised that implementation of transition planning had been patchy and inconsistent and, as such, planning for transitions remained a high priority. This was illustrated in a consultation paper stating that:

> Young people in transition should always be a focus and target for early action when developing strategies to support people into paid work, access ordinary housing, introduce individual budgets and undertake comprehensive health checks.
>
> (Department of Health 2007)

The policy goal was introduced that every young person with a disability in England and Wales will have a plan that will be written in Year 9, to be reviewed annually from the age of 14 to 19. The plans and reviews should be person-centred – i.e. should involve the young person and be based on their individual wishes.

A range of initiatives have sought to encourage and help young disabled people to progress into the labour market, such as the New Deal for Disabled People.

Similarly, it has come to be expected that more will take up individual budgets and direct payments. A transition support programme was established, including funds to promote these person-centred approaches to transition. An aim is for all young people with learning disabilities to be provided with an information pack and have access to an advisor and advocacy service. In addition, the *Getting a Life* programme brought together funding and assessment systems for young people going through transition, with the aim of getting a job, an education and a social life (Department of Health 2007; Liveability 2008).

As noted above, much of the guidance outlined here is based on the concept of person-centred planning. Person-centred planning was developed over a period of 30 years in the United States and is based on a number of key components (Mansell and Beadle-Brown 2005). It should take account of the unique circumstances of the individual and should take account of their aspirations and capabilities. It should also include the person's family and wider social networks. It ought to be person-led rather than service-led.

Effectiveness of transition planning

It is perhaps too early to evaluate the effectiveness of this raft of measures, and there is limited evidence to suggest what works in terms of ensuring smooth transitions between services and positive outcomes for young people (Beresford 2004). Hudson (2006) has suggested that initially a lack of resources and clear targets were not been helpful in terms of moving things forward. Research evidence illustrates the difficulties that young people making transitions continue to face. It would appear that planning for transition still occurs too late, and parents and young people still experience gaps in information and advice (Tarleton and Ward 2005). Osgood and colleagues (2010) identified particular problems relating to eligibility criteria, inadequate funding for transition services, a lack of coordination across service systems and a lack of adequate training on developmental issues for professionals.

MacIntyre (2007) found that most providers felt that, while there were some positive features of their current transitional arrangements, much could be done to improve things. In particular a need for earlier intervention and better sharing of information were identified in line with the policy developments outlined above. The transfer arrangements from education services, or children and families social work services, on to adult services was perceived to be particularly problematic. A representative from social work services suggested that:

> We need to improve the interface and steps have been made to do that . . . but I don't think it's as good as it should be . . . what you really want is the adult services involved in the planning at an earlier stage. But sometimes . . . it's not an unwillingness to do that but often it's also because of just the numbers of people. It's something that we know that if we're going to actually have a seamless service for people then we need to get earlier.
>
> (MacIntyre 2007)

The transition to adult services is characterised by uncertainty. Kirk (2008) found that young people needed to adapt to different cultures and ways of working and at times expressed a sense of loss in terms of their changed relationships with professionals.

Inter-agency working

There is a lack of clarity concerning who should take responsibility for transitions, with different agencies taking responsibility for children and young people at different ages and stages. This can create further confusion. According to Riddell et al. (2001), the area of further education, training and employment for people with disabilities is a crowded one without much coherence:

> Welfare policy for disabled people is currently influenced and delivered by a bewildering array of agencies including the Benefits Agency, the Employment Service, Further Education Colleges, Adult and Continuing Education Departments, Local Enterprise Councils, social work departments, housing services, NHS Primary Care Trusts and voluntary organisations.
>
> (pp. 256–7)

MacIntyre (2007) found that taking responsibility for the needs of young people with disabilities making transitions was often seen as problematic. Confusion and tension were identified around which agencies should be taking responsibility at certain times. This ambiguity was recognised by the Scottish Executive who published a guidance document *Partnership Matters* (Scottish Executive 2005b) in order to provide clarity on the roles and responsibilities of each agency within the field of further education. Daniels and colleagues (2007) have suggested a need to recognise and access expertise across professional boundaries. Further confusion arises about when responsibility should end. Within local authority education departments, this was previously seen as straightforwardly determined by school-leaving age, but policy changes such as the introduction of post-school psychological services may mean that education departments now have responsibility for young people with additional support needs after that date.

Joint working or inter-agency working has taken on increasing significance in recent years. Riddell and Tett (2001) suggest that the partnership between public, private and voluntary sector agencies, individual service users and communities is seen as an important way of promoting social capital. Stewart et al. (2003) meanwhile argue that:

> Integrated working irrespective of the organisational structure will increasingly become mandatory rather than permissive. The debate will not be whether but how, and the spotlight will be on the detail for attaining the process of integrated working.
>
> (p. 349)

In relation to transitions for young disabled people there is a need to strengthen the traditional partnerships between health and housing, which has been good, though not as strong as with other service-user groups such as older people (Stewart et al. 2003). Moreover, the service network should be extended to include employment and training providers, benefits offices and voluntary organisations. Joint working in these remains problematic (Riddell et al. 2003). Yet, MacIntyre (2007) found a commitment to increase joint working among research respondents. Developments in Scotland, such as the establishment of Inclusiveness Projects to assist disadvantaged young people making transitions from school, helped to bring joint working into sharper focus. Key workers acted as a signpost to help guide young people through the various services. To do this effectively they attempted to bring partners from various agencies on board to share information and provide training in order that all services working in the sector had a greater awareness of what others are doing.

A number of barriers to joint working remain. Working with young people who have a wide variety of needs is complex and involves a large number of agencies at different times and stages of a young person's life. Bringing different agencies together with their different ways of working and different priorities alongside issues of information sharing and confidentiality limit inter-agency working, and such barriers have been well documented elsewhere (Stewart et al. 2003; Hudson 2003; Petch 2008). In addition, different types of eligibility criteria and different levels of funding available for children's and adult services mean the nature and extent of services available at transition are likely to change. For example, families previously entitled to short break or respite provision may find that this is no longer the case (CSCI, 2007). Singh et al. (2008) have documented similar issues in relation to the transition from child and adolescent mental health services (CAMHS) to adult mental health services (AMHS).

Despite the barriers identified in this chapter, there is scope for optimism and examples of good practice in relation to collaboration exist. Successful collaboration involves making greater use of person-centred planning. The increased use of direct payments alongside the introduction of individualised budgets may assist in shifting the focus of intervention to outcomes identified by the service user (MacKay and MacIntyre, forthcoming). These developments offer an important means of achieving a range of opportunities for young people with learning disabilities. Yet shifting the balance of control to young people and their families will only be effective if appropriate planning measures and services are available. Local commissioners will have an important role to play in terms of ensuring that the full range of services needed by young people with learning disabilities are available as they make the transition from childhood to adulthood (Liveability 2008).

Example 20.1 Debbie

Debbie is 15 years old. She has a moderate learning disability that was diagnosed by psychological services when she was seven years old. She attends a mainstream school where she has received additional support from a classroom assistant. Debbie is often bullied by her classmates and does not enjoy her time at school. She has difficulties with reading and writing and would like to leave school as soon as the law permits because she does not see its relevance. Her mother has difficulties with alcohol misuse and Debbie has no contact with her father or siblings. Currently Debbie has support from an educational psychologist, a social worker and an advocate from a voluntary organisation.

What opportunities are there to support Debbie at the point of her transition from school?

Example 20.2 Sean

Sean is 19 years old. He lives with his parents in a fairly affluent area. He has a learning disability and high support needs. Sean attends college three days a week during which time he is accompanied by a personal assistant. He has intimated to his personal assistant that he would like to move into his own flat. Sean's social worker has discussed this with his parents, who are reluctant for Sean to leave home. They are worried that his needs will not be met elsewhere. This has created tension between all members of the family, including Sean's older brother and sister. The social work department have raised some concerns about the potential costs of any future care package. The local housing association have confirmed that there is currently no suitable accommodation close to Sean's family home.

How might a personalised planning process help Sean's transition to his own home?

Conclusions and implications

This chapter has outlined the extent to which young people with learning disabilities face difficulties as they make the transition from childhood to adulthood. Young people with disabilities have a range of options available to them in terms of further education, training and employment, but are less likely to attain positive outcomes in comparison with young people in the general population. Overall, their transitional experiences more closely mirror those of other marginalised and disadvantaged young people such as those leaving care or with experience of the criminal justice system. Certain markers of adult status, such as living independently and experiencing adult relationships, remain difficult for young people with learning disabilities to attain. In addition, they are more likely to experience social isolation and have limited social networks.

Alongside these issues, young people with disabilities often have to negotiate the *transitional process* of moving from children's to adult services. This creates a further layer of complexity for young people, their families and professionals to manage. Policy-makers have recognised the importance of smooth transitions for young people with learning disabilities in order to achieve more successful outcomes in adulthood, and the chapter has outlined some of the most significant guidance in this area. Despite the increased emphasis on transition, a number of barriers remain. These relate to poor transition planning, uncertainty around professional roles and responsibilities as well as the barriers that exist around joint-working more generally.

Successful transitional experiences for young people with disabilities should not rely on the goodwill of individual professionals. Instead, a partnership approach must be utilised, and good practice has emerged in this area. Where partnerships work well, they do not only exist between professionals but also between young people and their families. Young people should be at the centre and should be viewed as active participants in the process. Professionals need to ensure that parents are involved in the process while at the same time enabling young people to maximise their independence. Adopting a person-centred approach to transitional planning at an early stage will assist professionals to identify the most appropriate services to meet young people's needs. If such services are unavailable locally, this must be identified at an early enough stage to enable alternatives to be sought. This will help to guard against young people falling between the remit of different services, and will allow greater opportunity for professionals to work with young people to prepare them for what can be an unsettling yet ultimately fulfilling experience.

Exercise

Thinking about a young person that you are currently working with, or using one of the case examples above:

- List the issues you might need to consider when planning for the young person's transition.
- Which other professionals should be involved?
- What barriers might you come across when working together?

Recommended reading

http://www.scld.org.uk

The Scottish Consortium for Learning Disability offers a range of useful resources for young people and professionals.

http://www.jitscotland.org.uk/

The Joint Improvement Team provide guidance on joint working and offer examples of good practice in relation to collaboration.

Meads, G., Ashcroft, J. and Barr, H. (2005) *The case for inter-professional collaboration in health and social care*. Oxford: Wiley Blackwell.

Provides a useful overview of the need for collaborative working with a range of good practice examples.

The *Journal of Inter-professional Care* is a good source of relevant journal articles.

Petch, A. (ed.) (2009) *Managing transitions: support for individuals at key points of change*, Bristol: Policy Press.

Discusses issues relating to transition for a range of service user groups.

Part IV

WORKING TOGETHER: CHALLENGES AND OPPORTUNITIES

Collaborative working with other professionals involves a great deal of energy and activity to ensure that differences in values, approach and skills enrich services that are being provided to children, young people and their families. In this final part we explore the challenges and opportunities that working together presents.

Quite commonly more than one type of agency or professional is involved with the same situation. For example, where child abuse or neglect occurs or is suspected then typically a GP, health visitor, hospital doctor, social worker and police officer will have parts to play in assessment and action, usually along with school or nursery staff. Serious cases will require the intervention of legal representatives and decision-makers. Similarly, parent–child difficulties, behaviour or attendance problems at school, criminal activity, health issues and financial pressures are often present in the same family and neighbourhood, resulting in actions by a wide range of official agencies. Unless some degree of coordination takes place, different professional and agency requirements may hinder or duplicate each other. Parents and children often find it confusing to interact with many different professionals on the same issues.

Much of the impetus for closer working, 'integration' or 'partnership' has come from government, as noted in Chapter 1. There has, though, also been a bottom-up process whereby practitioners have recognised that children's lives are not neatly divided into segments that correspond with agency or professional identities, so a holistic approach that starts with children requires multidisciplinary inputs (Foley and Rixon 2008).

It is not easy, though, to achieve effective and satisfying collaboration among a wide range of individuals and organisations, each with their own distinct functions, expectations, resources and preferred modes of working. Moreover, time spent communicating, meeting and perhaps working jointly with others takes time away from each professional's key role, so a balance needs to be kept. Hence, it is necessary to understand not only the benefits of cooperation and suitable ways of working together well, but also the challenges, limitations and unintended consequences.

In Chapter 22, Hill discusses different types and extents of cooperation, along with factors that help or hinder. Effective collaboration can serve to enhance the identity and autonomy of individual professionals, a point which is reinforced in Chapter 25 by Kuenssberg, Reid and Taylor in their examination of interprofessional learning. Practical examples of effective and non-effective intervention with children who are looked after are provided in Chapter 24. Dougall shows that children living away from their parents often have greater health needs than others, which are also closely linked to educational and personal support issues. Hence, this population highlights the importance of all professionals, whatever their primary functions, recognising how they can make contributions to improving health and well-being.

In this final part we also explore theoretical insights into collaborative working in Chapter 22 where Forbes and McCartney argue that social capital theory, which focuses on human relations, provides a productive framework for examining co-working and emphasises the importance of developing trust between professionals. They analyse different kinds of contact between professionals in terms of bonding, bridging and linking social capital. The chapter illustrates the application of these ideas, particularly to relationships between teachers and speech and language specialists, but shows their relevance to collaboration more widely.

In Chapter 23, Head argues that the function of schools is not only about academic achievement, important though that is for children's life-chances and the good of society, but also about belonging and inclusion. This means that a range of professionals should work together with teachers to promote enhanced learning – for example, as regards empathy or human rights. This point highlights the fact that theories about learning are not simply essential for educationalists, but relevant to other professionals too, and outside school contexts. In relation to schools and other contexts like hospitals, Head emphasises the need for professionals to learn differently, as well as children. For collaboration to work well, learning from each other produces a form of collective competence.

Many of the programmes deployed in relation to parenting, youth justice and children's mental health are also based, at least in part, on ideas about how people learn and hence change. Many such interventions include an element of behavioural learning, particularly that some kind of reward is helpful in motivating change. However, most now also have cognitive components (e.g. helping people alter negative, fatalistic or egocentric beliefs) or social aspects, such as the importance of positive role models. Cognitive-behavioural and social-learning theories tend to focus on how professionals modify behaviour, but other approaches place more emphasis on people as active learners seeking to make sense of their worlds (Daniels 2001; Jordan et al. 2009). Similarly, concepts about adults as active learners through experience are vital parts of the armoury of people who train professionals. It is helpful for those undergoing training to be aware of them too (see Chapter 25).

Agencies working with children and families differ in the kinds of needs they address and the resources they provide or access from other organisations. The relationship between needs and resources is complex. Here resources may refer to the types of service available or to the amount of financial support for the service. It is quite common for different agencies to pool or contribute resources in kind such as staff or premises, and sometimes staff posts or even whole teams may be jointly funded (notably by health services, education, social services and/or police). More comprehensive sharing of finances has been rare and when it has happened it has sometimes been problematic. Especially when overall funds are limited, agencies understandably wish to retain control of money and allocate it for their own priorities.

Some policy-makers and practitioners have sought to shift from a resource-led service, where people are fitted into the kind of service traditionally provided, to a needs-led service, which is intended to be more flexible and personalised. Particularly in relation to disability, this has often entailed more flexible use of cash and staff than in conventional centres and programmes, with parents and children having more say in how the service is created. Similarly 'wrap-around' services for very vulnerable young people involve individualised packages of support, including 'out-of-hours' and crisis help. Cooperation among social care, education, employment and housing services if often crucial in such cases.

Typically, public agencies are not funded to meet all the needs they address, so some kind of prioritisation occurs, which may be referred to more critically as rationing, or be used as a rationalisation for spending cuts. Assessments of need may be affected by resource constraints, with front-line workers overruled by managers or more subtly influenced to avoid or shorten the use of an expensive facility even if this is thought to suit a child's needs best. One of the reasons why many young people have to leave residential or foster homes at a considerably lower age than their peers leave family homes is the expense of maintaining placements. Organisations like the NHS have developed strategies intended to make prioritisation more explicit and participative, usually by invoking some kind of threshold of eligibility based on assessments of need or risk. Yet, individual staff still often have to make difficult choices about how to allocate their time (Roulstone 2007).

While some agencies are concerned with universal needs of all children, others are targeted on particular needs or groups of children. This includes children and young people who have are looked after or who have a disability as discussed here. The learning of vulnerable groups was for a long time dominated by a needs approach. The designation 'special educational needs' focused on individual deficits and subjective decision-making as the basis for segregating or integrating children. Such labelling, though intended positively to provide additional support for learning, was often stigmatising and could lead to different or lower expectations. More recent thinking and policy has shifted towards the principle of right to inclusion (Head 2007). In practice, though, it is often hard to separate rights from needs, since the basis for a legal or moral right often involves a claim that a need exists and is not being met.

Different professions also use language differently, as is seen in Chapter 25. For example, medical and health professionals typically deploy the idea of diagnosis when assessing need. Diagnostic categories based on physical or behavioural symptoms act both as triggers for action and guides to the appropriate treatment (Anning et al. 2006). Most child psychiatrists support the use of diagnostic classifications, as they are seen to be an economical way of describing clusters of 'symptoms', which can be reliably recognised on the basis of agreed criteria, and can be linked to treatments that have been tested in relation to a specific condition (Salloum and Mezzich 2009). An alternative approach preferred by many psychologists, educationalists and others is 'dimensional'. Problems are seen as spread along a continuum and so can be ranked as more or less serious, whereas diagnoses tend to represent a problem as present or absent, though of course when present can vary in seriousness. Rutter (2011) takes a middle position. He accepts that it is useful to have certain terms that can be applied across many settings, but argues that there are too many diagnostic categories and that some are ill-founded, so concludes that a combination of categorical and dimensional approaches is desirable.

Diagnostic categories have been criticised for pathologising or marginalising those who acquire a diagnostic label and for detaching a 'condition' from its social context (Davis 2006; 2011). Conversely, some children may be denied a service because they do not qualify as having a recognised 'disorder'. There are dangers that the whole child becomes forgotten, as professionals are led to focus the child's primary identity in terms of a diagnosis, such as cerebral palsy or conduct disorder. Communication difficulties and conflict may arise between those who espouse diagnostic, dimensional or non-categorical approaches. This has happened especially in relation to diagnostic labels whose applicability has been contested (e.g. dyslexia) or which some believe have led to stigma or over-medication (e.g. ADHD) (Lloyd et al. 2006; Lindsay 2007).

Davis (2006) argues that it is essential for practitioners to engage children in defining and responding to their problems rather than imposing a label and its associated solution. In relation to disability particularly, he suggests it is vital to include multidisciplinary perspectives that do not negate the biological, but include the social and educational. He also argues that attention and behaviour issues at school need to be placed in the context of the general power relations between teachers or parents and children.

Reflection and thought may help avoid miscommunication and disagreement between professionals. They also have broader aims of improving services and ultimately children's well-being. Rixon (2008b) notes that reflection on how to improve practice is central to relationship-based approaches in social work, the classroom and healthcare. The idea of reflective practice as a desirable process across a range of disciplines was popularised by Schon (1983). The ability and commitment to reflect and learn from daily experience was seen as crucial to improve performance and hence lead to a better service. Arguably, this has become an even more essential quality now that a myriad influences on professionals and children's lives appear to be accelerating. Reflective practice can be seen as a counterbalance to the rationalistic emphasis of outcome driven planning and managerialism (Canavan et al. 2009). Technical, rational knowledge is important, but it can only take you so far (Cooper 2011).

Critical practitioners question assumptions and received wisdom, do not accept things at face value and seek to problematise the situations they face (Davis 2011). Reflection has several components. In an immediate sense it involves questioning of explanations and problem-solving to look for better ways of doing things, especially when the results of professional actions have been disappointing. *Critical reflection* involves examination of typical ways of thinking or working by oneself, one's own profession or another, while *process reflection* attends to the feelings and dynamic interplay of professional practice (Wilson et al. 2008).

Critical reflection should take place within an individual and through discussion with others. Among the practical actions that can assist with deep and regular reflection are discussions with colleagues and supervisors, accessing an external consultant, obtaining feedback on your practice from children and parents, keeping a reflective journal and presentations at clinical case conferences (Hitching 2008; Loewenstein 2011).

Reflexivity is however not confined to awareness of self and evaluation of assessments and treatments, but extends to critical examination of the policy and power contexts which affect children, families and professionals. As Hitching (2008) describes, it involves questioning such matters as the underlying values and hidden agendas in policies or syllabi, the relative status of different kinds of knowledge and the ways that some individuals or groups benefit from particular measures more than others. Critical reflection involves not only scepticism, but also constructive imagining of alternatives.

Reflective exercise

The following questions designed for individual reflection or group discussion will assist you in engaging with the concluding chapters in this book.

1. What are the factors that reduce opportunities to work effectively with colleagues from your own profession or agency? What might be done to improve the current position?

2. How are the skills that are required to work collaboratively with children, young people and their families most effectively gained:

   ■ Through life experience?

   ■ By observing other professionals in their everyday practice?

   ■ From reading and reflection?

   ■ From lectures, workshops and seminars?

3. In your experience are some individuals or professional groups more 'collaborative' than others?

   ■ Which are the most collaborative? Which are the least?

   ■ Why might this be the case – is it to do with status, different approaches to confidentiality, professional autonomy or independence?

Chapter 21

Interprofessional and inter-agency cooperation: the rough and the smooth

Malcolm Hill

Summary points

- Cooperation between services is long-standing. Legislation and policy between 2001 and 2010 promoted 'joint working' and 'integrated services'.
- Cooperation may involve two or more professions and/or two or more agencies.
- The processes and factors affecting relationships between professions differ from those affecting inter-organisational linkages.
- Experience and research has shown that close cooperation can produce benefits, but is hard to achieve.
- When planning to develop better cooperation, policy-makers and managers should be clear about the purpose and degree of closeness required.
- When collaboration works well, the identity and autonomy of particular professionals is not threatened.

A brief history of working together

Cooperation between children's agencies has always happened in practice, but usually in a piecemeal fashion and with respect to only parts of the service system. In the first decade of the twenty-first century, though, government policies advocated 'joint working' and 'integration' across all relevant agencies in service planning, individual assessments and service delivery. This chapter considers the practical and legal basis for cooperation, and then takes a critical look at relevant concepts and evidence.

Substantial moves towards reducing divisions between services and creating inter-disciplinary provision developed early in what used to be called 'pre-school provision'. Separate facilities had been created by education departments (nursery schools and classes) and by health and then social work services (day nurseries) with different ethos and functions, while playgroups were later initiated by self-help efforts and then voluntary and private organisations. Increasingly it was recognised that it was difficult and undesirable to separate facilities or staff dealing with care, education, play and health issues, so that combined children's or family centres have become increasingly common (see Chapter 8).

The idea that primary and secondary schools should work closely with residents and other agencies in their catchment areas is an old one, although their main focus has understandably been on within-school activities. In recent years extended schools and learning communities have been developed to improve access to health and social work professionals and by parents (see Chapter 11).

New Labour strategies for health services across the life span emphasised working in partnership with local authorities and voluntary agencies – for instance, via Health Improvement Programmes and Health Action Zones. Child health programmes reinforced cooperation between health visitors and children's centres (Anning et al. 2006).

Somewhat different processes have been at work in more specialist areas, particularly dealing with problematic behaviour by parents or children. Inquiries and media outcries about the deaths of children killed by family members have repeatedly shown failures in communication and cooperation among social workers, doctors, health visitors and police. Early warning signs were ignored, assessments were partial and attempts to protect the child were ill-coordinated. As a result, mechanisms were introduced aimed at improving communication and planning when dealing with child abuse and neglect cases. These have been modified and renamed over the years, but in essence have comprised:

- Area Child Protection Committees to make and review local strategies (now replaced by Safeguarding Boards in England);
- case conferences (interprofessional meetings to review evidence, assess risk and decide on coordinated actions);
- registers of children with known concerns or risks;
- joint investigations (usually by police and social work);
- lead workers (to reduce duplication and working at cross purposes).

The main members of Safeguarding Boards are from local authorities, health services the police and CAFCASS, but few have representation from GPs, children's centres or impendent schools. About half include representation from adult services (France et al. 2009).

Inter-agency meetings have been a key means of trying to improve planning and cooperative action with regard to a range of other difficulties. Many authorities and schools created inter-agency forums to deal with such matters as disruptive behaviour, actual or potential exclusion from school and truancy (Lloyd et al. 2001). Typically, besides teachers, other people involved include educational psychologists, school nurses and doctors, and social workers.

In relation to youth crime, a significant trend of the 1990s that continued into the next decade was the establishment of Youth Offender Teams (YOTs) in England and Wales. These multidisciplinary teams assess cases referred by the police, make decisions about whether court action should be taken in relation to crime or antisocial behaviour and provides programmes intended to tackle behaviour (Morgan 2009; Chapter 7). Multi-Agency Public Protection Arrangements (MAPPA) have been set up, too, particularly to improve information sharing between the police and other agencies, including YOTs and health services. MAPPA and YOTs have overlapping inter-agency membership, but with somewhat divergent priorities with regard to protecting the public and helping young people (Baker and Sutherland 2009).

In the child and mental-health field, a long-standing model of co-located interprofessional collaboration was developed in child guidance clinics with input from psychiatrists, psychologists, social workers and sometimes specialist family therapists. A number of such clinics still function, though commonly now with a different name like child and family clinic or service. A broader development since the 1990s has been the creation and development of integrated Child and Adolescent Mental Health Services (CAMHS). These have to varying degrees promoted closer relationships with other agencies, in line with somewhat different policy emphases within the four UK jurisdictions (Davren 2007; Lavis 2008).

Example 2.1 gives brief illustrations of how a wide range of different services are now seeking to work well together, at devolved national and local levels.

Example 21.1

The Welsh Assembly provided funds to pioneer an Integrated Family Support Services Model for vulnerable children in families with complex problems (Butler and Drakeford 2010). These services should cooperate closely with local communities and have a holistic and rights-based approach rather than focus narrowly on risk. A distinctive aspect is that the multi-agency component embraces both children's and adult services, particularly to address transition and interface problems related to disability, mental health, domestic violence and substance misuse.

In Devon the County Council and Health Board set up a Joint Agency Team (JAT) for children with 'special needs' (Chugg 2009). The JAT includes occupational therapists, various kinds of nurse, social workers, educational psychologists and paediatricians. Each child and family are allocated a key worker to be the main person in contact with the family. Key workers help the family manage relationships with the whole service network and communicate regularly with teachers.

The legal and policy basis for working together

Specific pieces of legislation have for some time required agencies to work together in relation to particular areas. Both disabled persons' and education legislation require an inter-agency approach for disabled children and their families. Similarly the Childcare Act 2006 stipulated that early childhood services be provided in an integrated manner.

More general measures to promote better cooperation have been prompted particularly by concerns about protecting or safeguarding children. The Children Act 2004 (covering England and Wales) followed recommendations from the inquiry into the death of Victoria Climbié. This Act obliged each authority to appoint a single director and lead councillor responsible for both education and children's social services. It required local authorities to establish Children's Trusts with partner agencies including health services, police, probation, youth offending teams and careers organisations. Children's Trusts vary in form, but are required to have integrated strategy and front-line delivery (Anning et al. 2006), in order to promote children's well-being in line with the *Every Child Matters* indicators. The Apprenticeship, Skills, Children and Learning Act 2009 strengthened obligations to work together in Trusts.

The Scottish government has preferred to be less prescriptive, but its *GIRFEC* programmes have encouraged inter-agency cooperation in assessment, planning and interventions. The Highland Pathfinder has been supported to provide a model for collaboration between the local authority, health service, voluntary sector and other agencies (see Chapter 5).

All agencies in England and Wales must collaborate to produce Children's and Young People's Plans for their local areas, following guidance issues by the Secretary of State (England) and Welsh Assembly (Wales), with the latter placing more emphasis on children's rights. Scotland has similar Integrated Children's Services Plans. Health Boards in Wales are required to integrate their health and well-being strategies with these local plans for children's services (Williams 2008).

Sharing of resources, particularly between local authorities and the NHS, has been seen as a key means of improving services. In practice aligning budgets has been more common than pooling, though this has occurred in some areas, particular with respect to child and adolescent mental health services (Longelly et al. 2009). Most areas have a shared strategy for commissioning services, 'but these lack impact because there is little experience or knowledge of joint commissioning' (Audit Commission 2008, p. 4).

Government finance has been used to promote greater involvement of non-government agencies. The Children's Fund in England, which ran from 2000 to 2008, made funding of local projects contingent on partnership between statutory and voluntary service providers, as did the Changing Children's Services Fund in Scotland. *Every Child Matters* and other polices have encouraged co-location of services whenever possible, both to facilitate cooperation among professionals and to simplify access by children and their families.

Better sharing of information between agencies and the adoption of similar assessment formats has been a policy goal for some time, leading to the Integrated Children's System whereby agencies in England and Wales were to record and share information in a more standard manner. This was intended to improve communication and decision-making for children in need or looked after. Some practitioners thought the system led to better cooperation (Cleaver et al. 2008), but many saw it as top-down, unresponsive to local or practice needs, and unreliable (White et al. 2010). A database (ContactPoint) was developed to hold information on every child to facilitate communication among professionals. This was opposed by many on civil liberties grounds of accuracy and privacy. One of the first acts of the Coalition government in 2010 was to decommission ContactPoint. By contrast, the Scottish multi-agency assessment system has greater flexibility about content to make it more user-friendly and was made available only on a need-to-know basis (Freeman 2009).

Having considered the practice and legal basis, our attention now turns to what can be learned from research and theory about what helps and hinders cooperation.

Understanding interprofessional and inter-agency cooperation

Distinguishing inter-agency, interprofessional and intersectoral

When seeking to understand and improve cooperation, it is helpful to begin by keeping certain distinctions in mind. In particular, different considerations affect inter*professional* and inter-*agency* collaboration. Quite commonly a range of professionals work in the same agency, as in a hospital, health centre or extended school. Here the critical issues relate to differences in training, functions, values, expectations and so on – for instance, between a doctor and a nurse or occupational therapist, a teacher and a psychologist or social worker. When people work in different organisations, then other matters are pertinent, such as the legal remit and goals, structure, management, geographical coverage, financial arrangements and so on. Of course, commonly inter-agency and interprofessional links occur together. Nearly all case conferences involve a mix of both professions and agencies.

A specific form of inter-agency cooperation is inter*sectoral*, when voluntary and/or private organisations are involved with statutory bodies. For example, Barnardo's agreed a protocol with Strathclyde Police and Glasgow Social Work Services to facilitate communication about and support to vulnerable young people living rough or in unsettled accommodation. Intersectoral tensions can arise. A local authority commissioning services from the voluntary or private sector will naturally wish to gain 'value for money'. Independent organisations sometimes claim that financial constraints by the authority not only restrict their income but also adversely affect decisions about individual children – for example, by ending use of their service when the child could have benefited for longer.

Most discussion about agencies working together tends to focus on organisations in the same geographical area with a remit for children, but two other forms of cooperation are important. First, cooperation between children's and adult services can be vital, as when children's safety and development is affected by parental substance misuse. Second, collaboration across different areas can be important – for instance, to safeguard children at risk when families move around or to share resources and expertise.

Levels and extent of cooperation

Cooperation may be initiated and expected to operate at different organisational levels. Commonly, three main levels are recognised:

■ strategic (agency to agency);

■ management (between local units);

■ case (among individual practitioners).

Not surprisingly, collaboration tends to work best when all three levels are involved and committed, as required in Children's Trusts (Audit Commission 2008). Difficulties arise when senior staff fail to support front-line cooperation or staff resist arrangements imposed by management.

Cooperation can occur at many points in a continuum of increasing closeness. Unfortunately the precise terminology and categories used are inconsistent. When policy documents, managers or front-line staff use terms like working together, partnership and integration, it is vital to clarify the degree(s) of jointness envisaged in order to avoid a mismatch in expectations.

At one end of the spectrum are communication and liaison where agencies or individuals work in different ways from separate bases, but keep each other informed and may coordinate what they do. Next comes joint planning, which may result in different professionals working separately, but towards shared goals and with awareness of what the others are doing. Joint working involves acting together, as in a family assessment interview or running a group. Police and social workers nowadays routinely carry out joint assessment interviews when child abuse or neglect is suspected. The ideal is to combine their criminal investigation and safe-guarding children roles, though this has sometimes led to tensions (Garrett 2003).

Organisationally, a further step towards closer collaboration occurs when staff from one agency operate from the premises of another. Specialists may visit one or more other agencies to make an assessment or provide a service to children (e.g. school nurses, speech and language specialists and educational psychologists). Alternatively, consultancy is provided to staff, as by child and adolescent psychiatrists. A more substantial commitment occurs when one or more members of staff are outposted in or hosted by another organisation (for instance, social workers in a school or hospital). A growing number of local authorities have created 'cross-over posts', where a staff member's primary role is to facilitate collaboration between two different services whose remits overlap – for example, children's welfare and parental drug misuse (Sawyer 2009, p. 89).

The 'pinnacle' of cooperation is the integrated team or unit. One classification of multi-disciplinary teams was applied to children's services by Anning et al. (2006):

- *fully managed team* – all staff are accountable to the same manager;
- *coordinated team* – the team manager is responsible for overall work, but some members obtain clinical supervision elsewhere;
- *core and extended team* – most members are fully managed, but some are out-posted from other agencies, which continue to provide management;
- *joint accountability team* – members are accountable to more than one agency, but share management of the day-to-day work of the team;
- *network association* – those involved remain full members of different agencies, but plan and coordinate their work with each other.

Research evidence about the processes and effects of cooperation in children's services

Barriers and facilitators to cooperation

It is common to recognise factors that impede or assist collaboration (Sloper 2004). Research suggests that cooperation is especially difficult when there has been a history of previous conflict; one or more professional group wishes to retain power and its familiar way of working; agency procedures prevent flexibility and creativity (Worrall-Davies and Cottrell 2009). A study of school-based assessment meetings found that 'old loyalties and differences of professionals' judgements were still barriers to effective work' (Lloyd et al. 2001, p. 42). Similarly in YOTs different ideas among police and social workers about the causes of crime and appropriate responses have created tensions (Souhami 2009).

Adequate funding and persistent leadership are important, so problems arise when these are inadequate. The Scottish Community Schools pilot programme was hampered by short-term funding and hence difficulties in recruiting and retaining suitable staff (Sammons et al. 2003). Impact was also limited because joint working was widely seen as an add-on to usual school activities rather than an overarching framework for delivery of education and other children's services (Brown and White 2006). Similarly, CAFCASS has been dogged by problems, partly owing to increased referrals and limited resources, but also to problems in leadership and tensions between bureaucratic procedures and professional autonomy (NAO 2010).

Positive facilitators apply at different levels. They include:

- agencies with common catchment areas; unified and trusted leadership; adequate resources to aid preparation and training;
- outward looking and flexible work group and team attitudes and practices;
- individual factors such as personality, warmth, respect and work motivation (Riddell and Tett 2001; Odegard 2006).

The requirements for successful working together have been well established by research (Catchpole 2008; Anning et al. 2006). They include:

- clear vision and leadership;
- organisational cultures and local attitudes that support cooperation;
- common aims, discussed and reviewed at regular intervals;
- clarity about roles;
- retention of individuals' core professional identity, but with flexibility to adapt to achieve the common enterprise;
- clear procedures;
- adequate and sustained financial resources;
- attention to training and team development.

Mandatory collaboration (i.e. a requirement by government or heads of services to work together) can make a difference in providing leadership and resources, but evidence indicates that genuine commitment cannot be imposed top-down and may have little impact unless local support is already present or is carefully nurtured (Anning et al. 2006). When new forms of collaboration are being introduced it is helpful to have opportunities for structured discussion and reflection, since working across boundaries requires time and effort to build trust and resolve differences (Jelphs and Dickinson 2008).

It is common for professionals to fear that joint working requires loss of identity and status or working beyond familiar areas of competence, but research indicates that blurring roles and responsibilities is not necessary for good collaboration and indeed is often unhelpful. Instead, each profession should continue with its central functions, but with a willingness to modify and align practices with others (Brown and White 2006; Bachman et al. 2009).

It seems, though, that staff who are attracted to joining a multidisciplinary team tend to feel different from their colleagues in their parent profession or agency, and hence are more keen to be allied with a different profession. For instance, some police in YOTs hold values at variance with what they see as typical of the force as a whole (Souhami 2009). More generally, many people involved in multi-agency initiatives have developed a career in comparable settings, leading to the suggestion that comfort with a hybrid identity facilitates joint working (Sloper 2004).

Negative consequences of closer collaboration

Practical experience and research have both demonstrated that interprofessional working is not easy. We consider first the more negative evidence and then point to examples of positive gains.

Efforts to cooperate may reinforce stereotypes, create tensions and aggravate difficulties. The benefits may not justify the time and resources diverted from direct work with children and families. The evaluation of Children's Trust pathfinders found many professionals were stressed by change, unclear about its purposes and worried they were having to carry out tasks for which they lacked knowledge and skills. Although these problems diminished as time went by, traditional and inward-looking practices persisted (Audit Commission 2008; Bachman et al. 2009). Concerns about privacy and loss of autonomy resulted in many professionals being unwilling to share information using the Common Assessment Framework. Similar considerations limited communication within MAPPA, in part reflecting differences in views about how best to protect children (Nash and Walker 2009).

It is not uncommon for research on attempted collaboration to find that one profession regards members of another as being 'uncooperative' or expects to receive information or help while giving little in return. For instance, one study of staff supporting children with renal transplants found examples of good cooperation, but also defensiveness and reluctance to see the others' viewpoints. Some staff were not willing to adapt their educational role to health needs or vice versa (Poursanidou et al. 2008).

The Sure Start programmes reported common difficulties at least in their early stages. These included tensions between different professional practices; workers performing similar work yet not having the same pay and conditions; limited joint training opportunities (Anning et al. 2006). Some extended school programmes experienced major problems as a result of the many differences in priorities and organisational systems, especially when collaboration was imposed (Gelsthorpe 2006).

On occasion, attempted integration may founder. Joint NHS and local authority Community Health and Care Partnerships were established in Glasgow in 2006, but dissolved in 2010. The reasons for the 'divorce' were complex but included cultural clashes, difficulties in agreeing financial allocations and concerns that each party's central focus on health or social care would be lost in the joint enterprise (Samuel 2010).

The evidence about barriers and difficulties has led some people to be sceptical about the value of close collaboration or, more guardedly, to suggest it is not worthwhile if support and resources are limited (Brown and White 2006). It may be fairer to conclude that increased cooperation should only occur when the main parties involved are clear about the aims, extent and nature of closer working together and support exists or can be harnessed from a range of directions and levels. Moreover, there is also much evidence about positive results of joint working to provide encouragement when the circumstances are right.

Benefits from closer collaboration

Most studies of cooperation have concentrated on the processes and benefits identified by staff, with only a few examining directly the effects on children and families. As a result Anning et al. (2006) concluded that 'the jury is still out on the effectiveness of integrated services' (p. 9). Even so, a range of positive consequences has been identified.

Some research shows changes in the services and outputs. The Evaluation of Sure Start in England revealed access to a wider range of responses and interventions, speedier referrals and pooling of expertise (e.g. in running parents' groups) (Malin and Morrow 2008). Attachment of health professionals to schools led to improvements in health education (Sammons et al. 2003). Certain Children's Trusts have provided a wider range of services, easier family access and more appropriate linking of families to the service that suits them best. Involvement by parents and volunteers has increased (Bachman et al. 2009).

A number of studies have found a range of ways in which professionals perceive their work to have got better as a result of closer cooperation (Sloper 2004; Brown and White 2006; Easton et al. 2010). Staff have reported:

- improved communication between agencies;
- more holistic assessment;
- mutual support;
- less duplication;
- increased opportunities for learning and development;
- optimism that children will have better outcomes.

In the study of joint assessment meetings, feedback from professionals indicated that they experienced a more comprehensive understanding of the child's background and life, as well as better understanding of the roles, responsibilities and resources (including resource limitations) of others (Lloyd et al. 2001). YOTs staff report gains in their status, opportunities to innovate and access to a wider range of knowledge and skills (Souhami 2009).

It is not so easy to demonstrate that such apparent improvements in services produce benefits for children. Health gains for children and young people have been identified in some evaluations of multidisciplinary teams in primary health care (Sloper 2004). Multi-agency approaches to education have led to reductions in exclusion from school and improvements in attainment and self-esteem among children (Riddell and Tett, 2001; Gelsthorpe 2006).

There is only limited evidence available on consumer perspectives. Parents have usually said they like being able to see different professionals in a single location or having a key worker, which simplifies communication and reduces anxiety (e.g. Malin and Morrow 2008). An evaluation of the Common Assessment Framework similarly found high levels of parent satisfaction, even though professionals expressed mixed views (Easton et al. 2010).

Theoretical approaches to working together

Various theoretical frameworks have been applied to interprofessional and inter-agency cooperation from diverse sources and some of these are represented in other chapters of this book. Certain theoretical frameworks draw on general under-standings of organisations and organisational change, whereas others are specific to interprofessional collaboration and in recent years some have been developed particularly with children's services in mind. An example of a general approach is to envisage work organisations as whole systems with each part affecting all the others and exchanging material and personal resources (Loxley 2007). A key practical implication of a systems perspective is to encourage members of organisations and collaborative networks to take a step back from their own position to view how the whole enterprise operates, and to understand all the main perspectives of other members. Recommended processes include respecting the expertise of all participants, whatever their status or qualifications, and helping others understand your own aims and reasons for actions (Pratt et al. 1999).

Thomas (2006), writing in the context of integrating primary health care, identified the need for changes at four scales (individual, organisational, inter-organisational, beyond the local) and in five dimensions (experiences, attitudes, skills, knowledge and outcomes). He also advocated the use of a range of group-learning techniques to help develop productive change. They include force-field analysis; brainstorming and rainbowing, vision workshops; fish-bowl discussion and role-play.

Reviewing theoretical approaches more specifically about collaboration, though not confined to children's services, Sullivan and Fletcher (2002) suggested that the benefits of theory are threefold, helping understand:

1. *why* collaboration happens – what are the drivers from policy, organisations and individuals;

2. *the form* it takes – the nature and degree of collaboration;

3. *influences* on the practice of collaboration and the extent to which it is likely to be sustained in the long run.

They recognised the seven types of theory summarised in Table 21.1.

Table 21.1 Theories of collaboration (based on Sullivan and Fletcher 2002)

Type of theory	Main focus	Key ideas
Optimistic		*Emphasise benefits and likely success*
Collaborative empowerment	Why? What form? Which influences?	Shared interest in positive goals prompts working together along a spectrum from *ad hoc* cooperation to full integration. Influences include clear leadership, facilitating and negotiating skills, trust.
Regime	Why? What form?	Governments encourage coalitions and may insist on who is involved.
Exchange	Why?	Each party requires deployment of resources held by others.
Pessimistic		*Emphasise problems*
Resource dependency	Why? What form? Which influences?	Resource-rich organisations exert power over more dependent agencies. Partnership is at least partly imposed. Professionals may feel close association with others threatens their traditional practices and autonomy.
Realistic		*Highlight both difficulties and benefits*
Evolutionary	Why? What form?	Technological and socio-economic change promotes collaboration. If joint networks are seen as successful, they become more embedded.
Policy networks	What form?	A close-knit network occurs when there are strong shared interests and values, with limited opportunities for newcomers to join. Looser issue networks are more diverse and have more open access, but also often less influence.
New institutional	What form?	Norms and 'myths' about how organisations should operate and cooperate are crucial factors.

More recently, three further perspectives have been applied in children's services – social capital, activity theory and appreciative enquiry. In Sullivan and Fletcher's terms they tend to be optimistic and their focus is on how to facilitate cooperation at front-line level, with an emphasis on network relationships and communication.

Social capital was defined by Putnam (2000) as an assemblage of networks, norms and trust that enable people to act effectively to pursue shared objectives. For some time this concept has provided a common approach for understanding and increasing social support and for tackling a range of health, social and educational issues (see Chapter 9). However, social capital concepts are also applicable to interprofessional relationships themselves, because connections and the establishment of trust are at the heart of cooperation (see Chapter 22). People seeking to work together or manage cooperation can be helped by understanding and altering the nature of:

1. *bonding capital* – strong relationships nearby;
2. *bridging capital* – weaker but wider ties;
3. *linking capital* – connections across status and power differentials.

Activity theory has its roots in the child psychology of Vygotsky and his followers, which highlighted the purposeful and active role of children. This viewpoint has been expanded and applied to adult human behaviour and learning. Key elements of activity systems are individuals and their motives; community influences including rules and divisions; and mediating tools and signs (the 'scaffolding' for learning) (Leadbetter et al. 2007; Chapter 4). Applied to inter-agency working this theory involves analysis of the various objectives of participants, roles, commitments and tools as a dynamic activity system. This approach also provides means for assisting organisational learning and change by means of workshops, meetings and other forms of communication that can help professionals understand and improve multi-agency working. A crucial tenet in activity theory is that conflict is inevitable, so needs to be openly addressed and resolved for satisfactory change to occur. Team building is understood to arise from the development of shared practices and discourses, which affect professional identity. Establishing a new multidisciplinary community of practice requires individuals to adapt and develop new shared practices, which is often harder for those who have been long engaged in their previous community (Anning et al. 2006).

Appreciative enquiry adopts a human systems perspective to organisational change. It has been applied in a range of settings including schools and child protection services (Onyett 2009). At its heart is the notion that understanding and communication are crucial, not structures and plans (Cooperrider et al. 2008). This approach builds on aspirations that excite the people involved and seeks to create shared visions and projects (Thomas 2006). It aims to avoid staff becoming bogged down by problems and how to resolve them, instead focusing on positive goals and how they may be achieved, while preserving good things from the past. Like the other methods outlined above, appreciative enquiry is based on open dialogues followed by group discussions to develop common aims and a shared commitment.

Conclusions and implications

It is vital that current and future professionals learn from previous experience and research about the kinds of circumstances and factors that help and hinder collaboration. It is important not to embark on cooperation beyond liaison unless and until aims have been thoroughly discussed and agreed on all sides, along with the degree and kind of cooperation envisaged (Williams and Sullivan 2010). Both managers and front-line staff should be engaged. In multidisciplinary teamwork it is desirable to hold periodic reviews of goals and processes.

Theories of learning and group process can help overcome barriers of understanding and attitude. Some shared modules in initial training and joint courses as part of continuing professional development are desirable (see Chapter 25). A range of group communication formats and exercises are available to assist in understanding differences (in backgrounds, priorities, work patterns, values etc.) and in appreciating and modifying these as appropriate.

Exercise

A youth offender team contains youth justice social workers, police officers, probation officers, a local authority education officer, a nurse and drug worker from the voluntary sector. What expertise does each contribute? Consider what differences in values, remit and home organisational structure are likely to affect working relationships.

Recommended reading

See Anning et al. 2006 for a review of policy developments with regard to interprofessional working and applications in practice.

Davis (2011) provides a critical account of concepts and practices involved when different agencies and professionals work together, with links to changing ideas about children and disability.

The special issue of the journal *Children & Society*, 2009, 23(5) dealt with collaboration.

International Journal of Integrated Care http://www.ijic.org/ and *Journal of Integrated Care* cover cooperation across services and age groups.

Chapter 22

Changing children's services: a social capital analysis

Joan Forbes and Elspeth McCartney

Summary points

- Coprofessional working is expected across all children's services, with anticipated positive impact on children's experiences and outcomes. However, little attention has been paid to how professionals work together.

- Social capital theory, which focuses on relations, offers a productive framework for examining co-working. A multi-level framework for identifying and evaluating social capital is presented describing levels, components and sub-types. This is used to analyse one widespread model of co-working, 'consultancy', illustrated by speech and language therapists and teachers working together.

- This example suggests there can be difficulties concerning relations of knowledge, trust and confidence among professionals. Systematic approaches to recognising and building social capital are needed, and how these might be developed is discussed.

Introduction

Children's public services require professionals to work together to provide timely and 'seamless' services, and to ensure specific expertise is available when required. Extensive policy guidance and advice directs such joint work. Professionals work within a variety of employment structures, from integrated services managing different professions within one organisation, to cooperative approaches where local practitioners agree on joint actions to support an individual child. Some structures designed to support co-professional working have however proved transitory. Scottish examples include rapid policy changes related to multiservice community schools; mergers and demergers of education and social services at local authority level; and continuous reconfigurations of community health services. This chapter is predicated on the assumption that managerial structures will continue to change during many professionals' working lives, and that new structures will not remove all tensions inherent in co-working. Other ways will have to be found to improve the experience, and thereby the practice, of working together.

There has however been relatively little discussion of how professionals actually work together, or of *social capital* – the trust and other social relations involved in working relationships, and in instituting and building new forms of professional networks and norms of practice. This chapter uses social capital theory to question and analyse how professional resources and power are built up and operate in and through practitioners' connections.

Social capital theories have value in analysing many forms of co-working, and the model presented here has general utility. Social capital offers a means of 'bridging' across all the children's professions (such as social work, social care, community education, health and allied health professions, police and youth justice) to learn and exchange knowledge about issues and concerns in joining up policy and practice in the fast-changing children's sector. To focus the chapter, however, we have taken as the main illustration one particular, common, model of co-working between public sector staff – that of consultancy. This model is used by a variety of professions including psychiatrists and educational psychologists, and across many services such as schools, residential homes, youth justice projects and child protection agencies. It should, none-theless, be noted that many alternative models and forms of integrated co-working exist and continue to emerge, such as those relating to school nurse and community police officer roles, school transition programmes and joint assessment teams.

This chapter introduces the concept of social capital and the emergence of social capital theory, with levels, concepts and sub-types explained and modelled. The importance of developing good social capital for child-focused working is discussed, and some differing professional perspectives identified. Suggestions about how practitioners' social capital resources might be reconfigured to better serve children and their families, and some implications for future working practices, are offered.

Social capital

Ideas in social capital theory concerning the economic and social benefits of association and networks have been used in health, social and educational policy discourses globally (World Bank 1999; UK Cabinet Office 2002); and provide a theoretical rationale for a recent raft of integrated children's services policy initiatives in Scotland, other UK countries and elsewhere. Social capital theory has frequently been applied to the social resources available to service users (Morrow 1999; Allan and Smyth 2009). However, it has also offered insights into professional relations (Allan et al. 2009; Arshad et al. 2007; Forbes and Watson 2009). Its conceptual framework can provide specific analytical purchase on the forms and functioning of practitioner inter-relationships, and of the knowledge, skills and other resources that practitioners hold and bring to work relations (Forbes 2006; Forbes and McCartney 2010).

Social capital embodies the notion that social networks are valuable assets for individuals, groups, communities and societies. Examining the inequality and power manifested in the social distinctions in society, Bourdieu (1986) identified three forms of capital – economic cultural and social – viewing social capital as the assets of social elites. Subsequently, social capital has had different emphases in its applications. Bourdieu and Wacquant (1992) recognise the resources that accrue to individuals from network membership including, it is argued in this chapter, those acquired in and through transprofessional group membership. Coleman (1988) concludes that trust and reciprocity, key terms in social capital theory, constitute a key family and community resource. He emphasises the role of social capital in building individuals' human capital – workers' stocks of expertise, for example, their professional knowledge and training. Putnam (1995: 664–5) defines social capital as 'social connections and the attendant norms and trust'; and emphasises social capital as a societal resource underpinned by individuals' active participation in the voluntary and political organisations and networks of civic society (2000).

The chapter makes the explicit assumption that developing positive social capital relationships among co-working professionals is beneficial to the services they offer to children.

Social capital: levels, components and sub-types

Social capital has been categorised in terms of *components* and *sub-types*, which operate at three different levels. Halpern (2005) conceptualises social capital as a multi-level matrix, offering a methodological approach that moves between *macro*, *meso* and *micro* systemic levels. These are the *governance and policy* level; the institutional, inter-professional *service delivery/receipt* level, and the individual or *personal/inter-personal* level, taking account of intra-personal human capital in the form of particular knowledge and skills.

Following Putnam (1993; 2000), Halpern (2005: 10) identifies three basic *components* of social capital, including the form of interest here (work-based social capital): a *network*; a cluster of *norms, values and expectancies* . . . shared by group members; and *sanctions* – punishments and rewards – that help to maintain the norms and network.

Distinguishing the components of social capital, the functioning of networks that are underpinned by shared norms and trust, provides potentially fruitful key concepts in analyses of interpractitioner relations.

Woolcock identifies the effects of *linking* ties for individuals: 'linking them across different institutional realms' (1998: 156). Putnam (2000: 22) added two further *sub-types* of social capital connections – *bonding* (exclusive of others not in the group) and *bridging* (inclusive of non-group others). These three sub-types provide analytical purchase for the examination of types of interprofessional relationships. Ozga and Catts (2004: 2) characterise them in the following terms:

- bonding – characterised by strong bonds among family members: this variety . . . can help people to 'get by' but may also be limiting;
- bridging – is less strong but builds relationships with a wider, more varied set of people, for example workplace or business associates, friends from different ethnic groups: good for 'getting on';
- linking – connects people who occupy different power positions, so works across differences in status.

Applied to professions, these sub-types enable the nature of current work relations and organisation to be identified and measured. Ties of fellowship, trust and regard within professions that consistently manifest relations of reciprocity and care equate most closely with the *bonding* category of social capital. The *linking* category recognises organisational and institutional hierarchies' power differentials and inequalities. It, therefore, offers particular value in examining the operation of relations between and among practitioners from different home agencies. Distinguishing 'getting on' (*bridging*) from vertical and hierarchical (*linking*) power connections provides an analytic to identify how practitioners connect to professionals from other agencies and services.

Understanding *bridging* and *linking* categories, therefore, equips staff to recognise, differentiate and evaluate the types and characteristics of work ties among individuals from different home agencies; how individual professionals currently use the three types of ties; and how they serve as a resource. Analysis of such data offers a means to evaluate the effectiveness of current connections and to identify where, in child-focused services, more productive bonds, bridges and linkages are needed. Analysis can also foreground practical, professional, cultural, leadership, governance and other challenges and barriers to forging more fruitful professional connections.

The 'dark side' of social capital (Field 2003) is explored by a number of theorists. Particularly problematic for some are its potential negative consequences, where close bonds, i.e. strong and exclusive ties within a single professional group, function with discriminatory effects to exclude non-group members (Portes 1998; Fine 2001; Arshad et al. 2007). Fukuyama (2001: 8), for example, warns that 'group solidarity in human communities is often purchased at the price of hostility towards out-group members'.

Thus, resentment and other negative effects of intraprofessional and intra-agency group solidarity have previously been recognised, where overly strong bonds and identifications among groups in the same profession and location encourage mistrust of others and sustain risk aversion, promoting 'playing safe' and 'getting by' and setting low 'horizons for action' (Ecclestone 2001).

Analyses are now needed of how social capital ties within different professional groups may operate in a limiting way to reinforce exclusive intraprofessional norms, knowledge, networks and identities. The bridging and linking ties needed for inter-agency working must be explored. Highlighting the intersections of practitioners' and practitioner groups' bonding, bridging and linking connections with professionals' norms (of values and practice), and trust and sanctions (punishments and rewards) focuses the analysis on practitioner interprofessional level connections.

Using components, sub-types and levels to identify and analyse current connections will provide evidence to support decisions about how work relations might be reformed to better support co-working. For example, the worth of classic professional norms of independence, autonomy and individual responsibility within future children's services might be reappraised. 'Getting right' the bonding, bridging and linking ties appropriate to any interprofessional role, and auditing the connections or 'ties-mix' needed to undertake specific roles and tasks, may prove as valuable as, for example, current audits of 'skills-mix'.

A multilevel framework for identifying and evaluating professional social capital

Identifying components, sub-types, and the three levels (macro–meso–micro) at which social capital operates leads to a conceptual map of social capital. It is possible to analyse and map possible intersections, which might suggest worthwhile questions at each level. Such a conceptual map appears in Forbes and McCartney (2010), and the central, meso, section is set out below.

Figure 22.1 A conceptual map of SLI-education social capital (utilising the multi-level france work of Halpern, 2005, p. 27)

	Bonding	Bridging	Linking	
	Strong (exclusive) home professional trust and recognition	Confidence in the practice of other professional groups	Trust and confidence in other agencies' practice	**Trust/Sanctions**
MESO-LEVEL Co-practice, Service-user, Interprofessional level.	Strong (exclusive) ties to home professional knowledge	Knowledge of others' practice, knowledge and skills	Working with others' practice norms at all levels	**Norms**
	Strong (exclusive) ties within home profession	Interprofessional practice as needed across sites	Practitioner links at all necessary agency levels	**Networks**

The mix of bridging and linking social capital

Each practitioner's stocks of social capital will differ according to their knowledge and skills, the interpersonal resources they have previously built up and the opportunities afforded to develop and use social capital in their current post.

At the micro level some children's service relations may be characterised by limiting bonding ties exclusively within each practitioner's own profession. Such exclusive bonding may be an effect of the limitations of a particular job role or remit; or due to a practitioner's resistance to forming bridging ties of trust and shared knowledge to other professions, and linking ties to other professions' leaders and managers. For example, lack of trust and respect by education managers may inhibit the development of the desired linking ties between health/social services practitioners and education leaders.

Questions may also be mapped at the intersections of categories and key terms at the macro, health-education-social services inter-agency level. For example, at agency level, the norms of disciplinary knowledge acquired in initial professional education and in subsequent professional training may operate restrictively. Thus, strong bonding norms of knowledge-sharing and communication may operate among health networks, but the exchange of information and views with social services or education personnel may be limited – to the disadvantage of service users. Such exclusively bonding networks of trust and confidence may undermine work among agencies.

The focus in this chapter is, however, on meso- or workplace-level interprofessional ties. Therefore, questions mapped at this co-practice level of the matrix relating to bridging and linking ties are analysed in greater detail, to illustrate how productive interprofessional social capital is established and deployed. Attention is also given to instances of exclusive bonding ties indicative of points where bridging and linking breaks down.

From the framework, meso-level questions regarding bridging norms and trust ties are:

■ How may practitioners acquire the necessary knowledge of others' practice knowledge and skills?

■ How may practitioners acquire trust and confidence in the practices of staff from the other professional group?

And the questions regarding linking norms and trust ties are:

■ How may practitioners work with others' practice norms at all levels of institutional hierarchies?

■ How may practitioners acquire trust and confidence in other agencies' knowledge and skills, practices, leadership and management at all levels?

Addressing these four questions should provide fruitful insights into two further meso-level questions regarding professional networks – is interprofessional practice, as needed by service-users, in place across sites? And do practitioners link at all necessary agency levels?

Models of co-practice

A number of models of coprofessional working are used in children's services, and individual practitioners use a variety of models as they work within different professional teams. Models vary in terms of how decisions are made (jointly or separately); who carries out the resulting plans with the child, and managerial relationships within the team (McCartney 2009). The social capital framework outlined above is applied here to one model of co-working: *consultancy*. Here one professional advises another, and the second is responsible for implementing resulting decisions with a child.

To further focus, this chapter considers teachers, employed in the UK by education services, working with speech and language therapists (SLTs), employed by health services, supporting children who require individualised service. Teachers and SLTs aim to enhance communication opportunities and development for a child by sharing their professional skills. Neither is in managerial charge of the other, and cross-sector relationships must be sustained if language and communication support for children is to succeed. The example is relevant both as an instance of cross-sector working, and because large-scale studies suggest consultancy is commonly used in statutory children's services (Law et al. 2002; DCSF 2008b). However, the analysis could equally apply to other professional pairings involved in consultancy approaches and to outcomes other than language.

Consultancy may encompass a broad range of co-working practices (Law et al. 2002: 160), but intrinsically one professional acts as 'consultant', with at least part of their role to give advice and guidance to another. Here, SLTs often advise teachers on how to develop communication-friendly classrooms, and on how to incorporate specific language and communication approaches for individual children into the school curriculum. Resulting activities are carried out by teachers and other classroom staff, such as classroom support workers.

Consultancy and resulting social capital

The questions identified above are applied to give insights into the social capital relationships that pertain in this widely used model.

Do practitioners have the necessary knowledge of others' practice knowledge and skills?

Professionals in consultancy approaches often operate from separate work bases, offering limited opportunity for informal contact, and communicate largely through meetings, phone calls and paper/email exchanges. SLTs usually make planned, rapid, in-and-out visits to schools with limited opportunities for informal contact and shared learning. But, beyond this practical limit there can be more fundamental issues. Health and education services often conceptualise children's individual speech, language and communication needs differently. Health practitioners use a bio-psycho-social model (Goswami 2008) with difficulties seen as developmental health and learning factors, and with improved functional communication and social participation as desired outcomes. Teachers may conceptualise difficulty as a consequence of inadequate or inappropriate learning experiences, with improved access to the curriculum and educational attainments as outcomes to be sought. While both professions would agree on the need to structure classroom experiences to ameliorate and accommodate difficulties, and to offer appropriate support, such underlying differences in understandings are significant.

In the UK SLTs have a broad knowledge of the school curriculum and educational principles from their qualifying studies, but will have limited information about pedagogy. Classroom teachers may have limited knowledge and understanding of speech, language and communication difficulties or language development techniques and little understanding of how to help (Sadler 2005).

Such a lack of underpinning shared knowledge means that consultant and consultee may themselves encounter communication barriers. Teachers may or may not judge information from SLTs to be useful or applicable, and SLTs may or may not be able to mediate information to meet a teacher's specific requirements, which often focus on the literacy difficulties that accompany speech, language and communication problems.

In terms of social capital, professional core subject disciplinary knowledge supplies strong bonding (within profession) capital but weaker, and perhaps inadequate, bridging and linking capital.

Do practitioners have trust and confidence in the practices of practitioners from the other professional group?

Problematic issues around trust and confidence have also been noted. Law et al. (2002) note that SLT 'consultants' are not always particularly experienced practitioners, unlike for example highly proficient managerial, medical or engineering consultants. A teacher might well lack confidence in an inexperienced SLT's decisions and the resulting child plans.

Example 22.1

Why should they believe I know what I'm talking about, when as far as they can see I show up for an hour and write a sheet of recommendations? And I consider I'm not TOO badly off, because I do work in schools so have a good working knowledge of the curriculum and its demands, but I know many of my junior colleagues have no such knowledge and are stared at with disapprobation when they present their decontextualised targets.

Anonymised SLT, web-forum comment.

The relationship between SLTs and class teachers is nominally egalitarian (McCartney 2009) and SLTs have no formal authority within schools. But in seeking to change teachers' behaviour in order to affect a child's classroom experiences, SLTs treat teachers mainly as accountable service delivery agents, rather than as collaborating professionals.

The role thus allocated to teachers is close to that of aide/assistant, where just enough knowledge is transferred to allow specific tasks planned by others to be carried out. This very limited model tends not to recognise or capitalise on teachers' expertise, and may limit a teachers' positive experiences of co-working. Teachers may well resist or contest this role and fail to act on SLT advice.

Example 22.2

Around half of 24 teachers involved in a consultancy approach 'agreed' or 'strongly agreed' with the statement: *'I would have preferred the SLT to work with the child,'* and around two-thirds with the assertion that: *'This method of working expects too much from the class teacher.'*

The 'teacher as assistant' role is exacerbated if, as is likely, the SLT's detailed knowledge of linguistics and assessment practices is privileged above the teacher's knowledge of the child. SLT are (and properly) considered as 'experts', with access to therapies potentially beneficial to children that differ from usual classroom practice. But teachers' equally beneficial insights may not be sought, or offered, and their professional roles and knowledge may remain unrepresented.

Such relationships evidence weak bridging and linking capital connections at co-practice level, and consequent implications for teamwork.

Do practitioners work with others' practice norms at all levels of institutional hierarchies?

The perceived role of an SLT making recommendations within a school is also open to question.

Example 22.3

I worked with an SLT in an ASD [autistic spectrum disorders] unit, and she was very nice and helpful and all that and gave lots of ideas. But I've always just wondered – what was her status?

Teacher on post-graduate model on co-professional working.

As SLTs have no managerial relationship with teachers they cannot ensure compliance with advice or suggestions. This lack of power is a general issue in consultancy approaches (the 'consultant's dilemma'), but usually the consultant has been asked for advice by the consultee who is thus free to 'take it or leave it'. But the teacher or school is not the SLT's client – it is the child. If an SLT considers classroom-based communication development activities to be helpful, they may question a teacher's professional 'right' to avoid complying with advice (Noell and Witt 1999). SLTs in this situation are likely to undervalue the teachers' perspective and teachers to feel they are being coerced.

Example 22.4

[I] *felt like* [a] *go-between from Depute Headteacher to SLT.*

Teacher involved in a consultancy approach.

School managerial practices may also serve to marginalise class teachers' contributions. An individual teacher often does not have contact with an SLT before classroom-based language learning is suggested, or involvement in assessment or decision-making processes. They may be invited to carry out language-learning activities only after a child has been referred to and assessed by an SLT, after their parents and head-teacher have agreed to school-based intervention, and after further discussion and meetings have taken place – all without the teacher's participation. Teachers in such circumstances are routinely excluded from agencies' and professions' linking connections for knowledge exchange and decision-making. It would be unsurprising if this resulted in a lack of any imperative to build strong interprofessional bridges and links or to sustain interventions.

Do practitioners have trust and confidence in other agencies' knowledge and skills, practices, leadership and management at all levels?

SLTs' commitment to evidence-based practice should mean their suggestions are empirically founded, and lead to actions of known effectiveness. In fact, the paucity of evidence means that advice given by an SLT seldom results from exhaustive research and will contain an element of professional opinion. Such advice is therefore open to question by teachers and schools, and a lack of trust and confidence in the SLTs' knowledge base could result.

Consultancy models have also been perceived, rightly or wrongly, as health service managerial attempts to cover up and cope with limited resources, and as 'a pragmatic solution to the problem of coverage' (Law et al. 2002: 154) or 'resource saving strategies' (Gascoigne 2006: 18).

School management and educational agencies may well consider – and resent – a consultancy approach as passing over an SLT's workload to the school.

Example 22.5

Some staff, while reporting that they received information, complained of a lack of consultation on intervention techniques or programmes, which led to a perception of being undervalued, that 'the school was providing a service to the SLTs'.

(Baxter et al. 2009: 225)

The effects of such uncertainties and suspicions concerning another profession's underlying motivation will, it is argued, undermine rather than build and sustain social capital. And where undertaking activities initiated by an SLT, derived from the SLT's knowledge and decisions, is perceived as burdensome, positive social relationships and bridging social capital are unlikely to develop.

The above analysis also suggests that answers to the key bridging and linking questions relating to networks: *Is interprofessional practice, as needed by service users, in place across sites? And do practitioners link at all necessary agency levels?* will at times remain in the negative. This conclusion is further supported by large-scale investigations of co-working in schools (cf. DCSF 2008b: 53–4).

Overly strong bonding, but limited bridging and linking, capital limits practitioners' comfort levels to their central work settings.

Connecting practitioners' social capital and the social capital needed to support service users

Collaborative partnerships require *'a continuous process of nurturing'* (Vangen and Huxham 2003: 6) but, as exemplified, not all practitioners have opportunity to form bridging networks, norms and relations of trust and confidence. There are few examples of child services paying serious attention to fostering sustained, long-term practitioner relationships.

For SLTs and teachers, as for other professional groups, sustaining individual personal links may be an unrealistic goal due to staff turnover, child movement through school, the need to deliver interventions rapidly as needs are identified, the range of possible interventions and expertise, and the very large numbers of children and staff involved. The logistics of nurturing such teams, though potentially most productive, would be daunting.

As evidenced, where policy enjoinders result in coprofessional working with little consideration of practice models, shared perceptions or personal comfort level, good co-working practice is unlikely to develop. Better bridging and linking ties are needed, and would increase the probability of sustaining appropriate actions for children who require joint services. Building better connections could also provide a 'bank' of transprofessional trust and confidence that would transfer to future co-working for children with similar needs. Taking the risk of building bridging and linking social capital would reflect recent understandings of practitioners' roles in co-supporting children, and allow professions and agencies to engage better, more effectively and productively, in working together. Crucially, this would build reciprocal trust and confidence in their ability to connect with the other profession (Field 2009).

To this end, bridging connections must somehow be strengthened, sought within or added to current working contexts – with implications for time and other resources. Further developing linking resources and power, where higher/lower levels of authority support staff at a different level, is also fundamentally important in developing intersector, inter-agency relationships (and in supplying resources to foster bridging social capital). These could, and should, be developed and utilised by education-, social- and health-service managements developing work teams and practitioner networks with known and shared norms and values, and necessary relations of trust, confidence and regard.

Conclusions and Implications

This chapter discusses how professions with different skills, knowledge and sources of legitimacy and authority might work together better for the benefit of children, not the creation of hybrid professions. As such it reflects the present realities of public sector staffing, where it is difficult to envisage the merger, or integration, of all children's sector professions. But the widely used consultancy model discussed here offers few opportunities to form bridging social capital, or relationships likely to support sustained interventions. However challenging to contemplate and implement, establishing the necessary bridging and linking ties at all levels of the institutions and organisations involved appears to necessary for creating partnerships that fully respond to service users' needs.

Social capital theory has been fruitfully taken up and applied by participant education practitioners in Scotland in the activities of the Applied Educational Research Scheme, Schools and Social Capital Network (Catts and Ozga 2005). However, more widely, few children's sector practitioners are likely to have heard of the notion of social capital, let alone realise that its ideas and theory provide a lens to analyse the 'joined-up' knowledge and skills they need in their job and to interpret how social capital functions in their work relations. So, to effectively implement co-practice policy, a useful prerequisite and preparatory step would be for practitioners across children's services to be explicitly introduced to and learn about key ideas in social capital, and for this to occur early in their initial professional education.

Strong statements in policy and governance in the UK are made with the intention of providing and strengthening the bridging and linking capital underpinning those sound collaborative approaches which benefit service users, and to develop the necessary knowledge and skills, authority and legitimacy for interprofessional practice. Such authoritative validation should provide linking forms of social capital, if higher levels of agency authority implement policy by initiating and activating support for co-working practice.

For example, where agencies have developed descriptors of child needs in terms understandable to all staff, with suggested support packages detailing actions to be taken by education, health and other relevant professionals, these provide information that should help bridge, and perhaps link, among services. There are also training models, where teams of cross-agency practitioners demonstrate and discuss good practice with relevant mixes of practitioners. These should provide bridging support for staff in terms of enhanced knowledge, and confidence in specialist interventions. Such approaches also seek to clarify roles and responsibilities and the expectations of staff, and to set up and sustain purposeful relationships of trust and confidence, further enhancing professional bridging social capital.

Cluster and integrated models also exist. Establishing a sustained service network around a key staff team, and providing the necessary time to develop shared norms and values and build relations of trust and regard across the network, should build improved bridging and linking social capital connections among the practitioners concerned, and so enhance the scope and quality of their co-working.

One implication for professionals might be to keep benefits to the child at the centre of decisions concerning models of service. Where staff agree on and schedule actions to be taken, carefully monitor what happens and whether child outcomes are positive, and revise plans accordingly (cf. McCartney et al. 2010), stronger and more effective bridging relationships can result. These emerge from improved confidence derived from the ability to draw on enhanced access to the other's knowledge and skills in equitable social relations. Forbes (2008) similarly suggests that key to making good provision is a model which focuses on individual learners and carefully identifies where different modes of knowledge are needed at different stages in the cycle of co-work.

Co-working is needed at exactly the point where knowledge and skills additional to any single profession are required, and where exclusively valuing and trusting only one set of professional norms, practices and principles is unhelpful. Building practitioners' bridging and linking relations, focused on and driven by resulting benefits for children, would seem a timely imperative in the current moment of changing children's services. The issues uncovered in the SLT/teachers example thus apply to many co-professional partnerships across the children's public sector, as they endeavour to improve environments, provision and outcomes for children through effective, coherent and coordinated planned programmes, and agreed actions.

Exercise

- Consider one example where you experienced or observed co-professional working, or our case example from Baxter et al. (2009).

- Consider which knowledges and skills were needed, and any gaps you can identify.

- Can you suggest any examples of bridging social capital that would help the participants?

- Could (or did) the participants' work contexts support (or hinder?) them in working together, by providing linking social capital opportunities? These usually would come from a higher organisational level.

Recommended reading

http://www.aers.org.uk/aers/index.php?option=com_content&task=view&id=23&Itemid=108

Applied Educational Research Scheme (AERS) Schools and Social Capital Network (SSCN).

http://www.socialcapitalgateway.org

Provides useful resources for all researchers, teachers, students and practitioners interested in social capital, and promotes discussion and ideas-exchange relating to social capital.

www.social-capital.net

The aims of Assist Social Capital, a Scottish company limited by guarantee with charitable status since 2004, are to promote the concept of social capital and its effects in relation to the economy, environment, public services, communities and people's lives.

Chapter 23

Working together for better learning

George Head

Summary points

- Historically, schools have operated in relative isolation from other local authority services.

- Recent initiatives aimed to improve interprofessional working inside and beyond schools, with different models and varying levels of success.

- For schools and other agencies to commit to working together, there has to be some perceived benefit. A commonly recognised gain might be inclusion, which is about children's belonging and achieving. This requires an enhanced form of learning, which can act as the main purpose of working together in schools.

- Such cooperation entails working with parents and pupils, as well as other agencies.

- Structurally, this equates to an open, less bounded type of collaboration based on expansive learning for pupils, families and agencies.

Introduction

Historically, publicly funded schools have operated at a distance from other local authority services and, in some senses, even from the local authority itself. Teachers tend to work in, and therefore 'belong' to, particular schools with long service in one institution being common. Consequently, class teachers' sense of loyalty and obligation belongs to the school in which they work and to local authorities only at a secondary level. Moreover, professional development for teachers tends to be confined to educational issues with incursion into other areas of local authority concern being rare. There are exceptions, however, and policies like *Getting it Right for Every Child* (Scotland) and *Every Child Matters* (England) have provided the stimulus for closer working among children's services (see Chapter 1). Indeed, while in the past local authority staff development tended not to include provision for teachers beyond exclusively educational matters, these policy developments have led to a rethinking of the place and purpose of schools within the wider community.

Since the 1990s one model used by local authorities in the UK to improve cooperation has been through school-based initiatives aimed at bringing children's services closer together. These are the New Community Schools and later Integrated Community Schools initiatives in Scotland, the Extended Schools project in England, extended schools / Full Service Community Network in Northern Ireland, Community Focused Schools in Wales and Full Service Schools in the USA (see Chapter 11).

The policy and practice context of integrated schooling

The innovation of a 'different' kind of school was designed to bring together various children's services in order to provide the appropriate support and care for children and young people throughout their school years and to prepare them for life beyond school. Support and care were to be provided both by bringing other services into these schools (particularly health and social work), and by having an emphasis on the personal and social development of pupils as well as their academic attainment. These measures reflected the complex changes taking place in society generally around this time and in relation to children's rights in particular. Indeed, the Green Paper *Every Child Matters* DfES in England and Scottish legislation (*Standards in Scotland's Schools etc. Act 2000*, *Additional Support for Learning Act 2004*) have their origins in the UN Salamanca Statement on children's right to learn alongside their peers. While the idea of professionals working together to support children is not new, and on the surface appears relatively simple, the reality of practice has proven to be more complex.

At the same time as UNESCO policies on children's rights spawned policies in the UK that could be described as broadly communitarian, the country also underwent a political change in the 1980s and 1990s that saw the emergence of what might be called 'new right' or 'neo-liberal' politics with a focus on the individual. This led to tensions at a philosophical and conceptual level regarding how professionals should work to support and care for children and young people during their school years. For example, O'Brien and Macleod (2010) note that until the late twentieth century, it was widely assumed that the job of schools lay only in teaching the academic curriculum and that pupils' personal and social development took place as a by-product of participating in the learning process. This perspective was reinforced perhaps, by political agendas that emphasised standards and accountability related to a particularly utilitarian view of the purpose of schooling. This is in tension with a parallel development in welfarist approaches to supporting children's development through explicit personal and social education as part of the curriculum, and the provision of learning support and behaviour support for pupils whom schools find difficult to teach (Macleod 2006). A further strand is the growth of pupil support in response to child protection concerns (Todd 2007). These policy initiatives have contributed to the development of additional services in schools but have also created new collaborative challenges.

For example, there may be tensions between *social inclusion* policies, which seek to ensure the provision of increased opportunities and resources to address poverty, and *educational inclusion* practices that are more focused on disability and behaviour, where debates continue on the desirability or not of segregated provision and integration in mainstream schooling. While there might be general agreement that developments in children's services are intended to promote social justice by social and educational inclusion, there does not appear to be a consensus regarding what the practical implications are. Education policy has placed increasing emphasis on inclusion meaning the location of all pupils within mainstream schools. Yet, it seems a significant number of teachers believe that segregated provision is the most appropriate location for young people whose behaviour they find consistently disruptive and difficult (Wilkin et al. 2006). Similarly, while education would be a consideration for social work, psychological, health and other family services, the main focus of support for these agencies might well be the family and the community. Todd (2007: 83) argues that successful inclusion requires schools, other professionals, volunteers, children and families to work together but points out that 'not all multi-agency collaboration results in inclusion'. It is, perhaps, easier to understand why this might be the case than not when policy is examined. *Every Child Matters*, for example, and the *Children Act* (2004) in England are posited on managing children's services to address the five outcomes of:

- being healthy;
- staying safe;
- enjoying life and achieving;
- making a positive contribution;
- economic well-being.   (Todd 2007: 11)

From the different perspectives of education, health and social work alone, it is understandable that there would be different understandings of which of these outcomes and priorities are most important (and their equivalents in other parts of the UK).

Not only are there variations in emphasis as regards shared goals for children's services, but attempts to integrate services within schools have been posited largely on very education-based language, which can signal to other professionals that the majority of the priorities fall outwith their domain. For instance, New Community Schools and Integrated Schools initiatives in Scotland were posited on five national priorities for education of:

- achievement and attainment;
- framework for learning;
- inclusion and equality;
- values and citizenship;
- learning for life.

Again psychological, social work and health professionals are likely to find it harder than teachers to identify with all of these aims and may think that some of their roles are not represented. From the outset, therefore, there may be obstructions to successful inter- and multi-agency working through different understandings of the purposes of these initiatives and the place of the different actors' disciplines within them.

In addition, a considerable degree of flexibility in the organisation of inter-disciplinary collaboration has been allowed so local solutions could be developed to meet the particular needs of each location. In Scotland the initiatives regarding inclusion were seen as a matter of improved access to mainstream schools and services and such aspirations naturally imply a localised approach. While flexibility may have brought advantages in terms of family and community engagement, barriers to effective working together, and hence inclusion, arose from lack of understanding of roles and competing priorities (O'Brien and Macleod 2010).

In both England and Scotland, it has been suggested that adherence to a deficit model of vulnerability is a basic flaw in the structure and operation of the initiatives. Moreover, this view was reinforced through a New Labour concept of social inclusion that admits to society those who are willing to comply with the rules. The overall result of this combination of deficit and restricted membership is that:

> . . . those who choose to remain outside are therefore responsible for their own exclusion and the state/school need no longer hold responsibility for them.
>
> (O'Brien and Macleod 2010: 49)

Furthermore, Todd (2007: 89) argues:

> It is as if the system conspires to see all problems as inherent to the individual rather than as a complex interaction of social practices and institutional, political and cultural influences. It is difficult to see how such a model can support inclusive education.

The dependence of inclusion policies on successful inter- and multi-agency working in collaboration with children, young people and their parents means it is essential to examine the models in operation and indeed the concept of collaboration itself.

Models of working together

Collaboration as a concept is complicated and contested. For example, Laluvein (2010) identified ten variations or types of collaboration. More simply, it is possible to identify a few levels linked to different purposes:

- external collaboration among agencies (including the voluntary sector, parents and pupils) focused on individual children, families or the community as a whole;
- internal collaboration among teachers, other school staff and parents and pupils in order to support pupils in school;
- collaboration between teachers and pupils and among pupils to enrich the learning experience, mainly but not exclusively in the classroom.

Likewise Hargreaves (1994) suggested that there are three kinds of aim or benefits that it is hoped collaboration will achieve:

- *personal* – in terms of increases in moral support and confidence;
- *professional* – by providing opportunities for improved effectiveness, self-reflection, stretching professional boundaries and teacher learning;
- *practical* – through increased efficiency, reduced workload and continuous improvement.

Previously, he had pointed out that there can be limits to the assumed effectiveness of collaboration in what he termed 'bounded collaboration', where participants work within a highly prescriptive context and are allowed little time to question, discuss or develop the materials with which they work (Hargreaves 1992). This concept of 'boundedness' was developed by Stead et al. (2004) in their analysis of inter-agency working which they encountered while researching the varied nature of multiprofessional meetings in three Scottish local authorities. The groups of professionals met to discuss children's personal and behavioural issues. They discussed the support they could provide for young people, at times with the aim of preventing exclusion from school for disciplinary reasons. A comparison of working together in two authorities exemplifies what they termed 'less bounded' and 'more bounded' collaboration (see Example 23.1).

Example 23.1

Wallace City: less bounded
This group comprised a core team who met over a number of years and who invited case-specific staff to contribute as appropriate.

Douglasshire: more bounded
This authority arranged only case-specific meetings attended by only those professionals directly involved with that case. Young people and their parents were also invited.

(Stead et al. 2004)

Stead and colleagues comment that, in the case of Wallace City, the presence of a consistent group of staff meeting regularly as a core team led to increased familiarity, respect for each other as professionals and for the work of the different services, and most important, trust. As a result, this core team took on the features of a cohesive group, sharing responsibility for the decisions they took and developing a shared vision of how they could support the young people referred to the team, thus leading to a 'less-bounded' model of collaboration.

> Shared histories allowed the opportunity for shared reflection and a shared vision of being able to offer support to troubled young people. The combined knowledge of what may be needed and what was available was also a key feature of planning joint work.
>
> (Stead et al. 2004: 46)

In Douglasshire, by contrast, the case-based meetings involved different personnel each time. In this 'more-bounded' model, sharing of information was limited to individual cases and consequently less of a shared vision and understanding developed.

The more-bounded model could be very helpful in handling individual cases, but the focus remained on the particular pupil. The less-bounded model resulted in a wider understanding of how the various agencies could support young people and was more able to consider and perhaps modify more general practice and provision in school. While the trust built through the frequent meetings of the less-bounded group led to innovative solutions for children, young people and their families, there was little evidence of this in the more-bounded authority.

It appears therefore that collaborative processes offer a sense of underlying opportunity, which may benefit from being made explicit and extended to cover the potential for systemic change. Hargreaves (1992: 228) described 'bounded collaboration' as

> . . . collaboration which does not reach deep down to the grounds, the principles or the ethics of practice but which stays with routine advice giving, trick trading and material sharing of a more immediate, specific and technical nature . . .

He has implied here that deeper as well as less-bounded cooperation might well be possible. Similarly, O'Neill (2000: 14) has argued that in limiting collaboration to the routine, there is a danger that we lose out on the chance to explore '. . . the uncertain, the difficult to identify, the less easily understood and the idiosyncratic'. Hence, there is a need to investigate the concept of collaboration as it applies in an educational context and how it may affect learning for both children and professionals.

Collaboration and collective competence

The meaning of collaboration is essentially multidimensional, derived from the range of activities involved in the act of collaboration and from the subsequent effects of such activities. At the simplest level, collaboration comprises a range of closely related acts such as coordinating, consulting, communicating and cooperating and each of these acts were present in the multiprofessional groups examined by Stead et al. (2004).

The value of each of these aspects can be readily understood. Coordination is necessary to ensure that any enterprise runs smoothly and efficiently, and to realise the optimum use of resources, including human resources. Consultation is essential to take account of all relevant viewpoints and information. Communication is necessary to arrange for agreed tasks to be carried out, ensures that everyone knows what they are expected to do and when they have to do it. Finally, participants need to cooperate to execute any agreed and organised activity. Indeed, in the more-bounded example of Douglasshire achieving each of these was the measure of success.

It can further be argued, however, that the elements mentioned above represent the functional aspects of collaboration, but, as the Douglasshire example suggests, participants may not fully realise the effectiveness of their cooperation if they do not participate as fully and regularly in the sharing process as in Wallace. This does not in any way dismiss the importance of the functional aspects of collaboration, but supports the argument that working together presents opportunities that go beyond the procedural.

The commonality of approach in both Douglasshire and Wallace illustrates two further aspects of collaboration that are significant for consideration of the process as having a potential beyond the functional. First, more than one person was involved in each case, with differing roles, expectations and goals. Second, collaboration involved intermediary processes. Something had taken place beforehand to suggest that people needed to work together collaboratively in order to deal with it, resulting in a new context or subsequent set of activities. The concept becomes altogether more fascinating when all aspects are considered together – the multifaceted nature of collaboration, the diversity of people who cooperate in the act, and the antecedent–activity–result process.

Boreham's (2004) discussion of the nature of collaboration and collective activity, developed from his work in the very different context of hospital accident and emergency teams, is enlightening here. He argues that developing a collective knowledge base can lead to 'commonsense-making'. By this he meant not common sense in the everyday usage of taken for granted shared assumptions, but an achievement of the collaborative process to reach a mutual understanding (common sense). This may take thinking beyond the functional and towards looking at what can be accomplished collectively.

Boreham refers to the product of combined knowledge and activities as 'collective competence'. The exact nature of collective competence is dependent on the culture of the group, and its manifestation can be seen as the result of participation within this culture. The argument here is that the surface manifestations are the visible results of a deeper, complex reality involving the cognitive and affective human activities of thinking, feeling and perceiving.

Once individuals acknowledge these factors, they can successfully move away from simply disposing of what has gone before and into the context-enhancing realms of transformation and creativity to achieve a desired outcome. When individuals bring these deeper aspects to the fore, they have the potential, Boreham argues, to develop:

> . . . the group's capacity to overcome the fragmenting tendencies of [its members'] different perceptions . . . by developing a sense of interdependency.   (Boreham 2004: 11)

They create opportunities to do more as a group than they could achieve as a collection of individuals working alongside each other.

Developing a collective understanding through the creation of shared knowledge is central to group effectiveness. At this level of operation – that is at the meta-cognitive rather than functional level – group competencies begin to emerge, and the group becomes more effective as an entity than as a collection of individuals, however highly trained and motivated. This affords individuals the opportunity to move beyond the functional aspects of coordination, cooperation and communication to collective collaboration. Moreover, this reflects what is known about learning, particularly about the creation of meaning essential to the success of groups, both as part of formal education and in other work contexts.

How the different levels of collaboration manifest in practice are perhaps best analysed through an examination of an example from the field of additional support provision (specifically behaviour support), because the need for change in this area is often urgent, requiring educators to undertake self-examination and analysis to develop pedagogy.

Communities of support

Working with children who may be experiencing social, emotional and behavioural difficulties (SEBD) frequently requires teachers to collaborate with a range of interested parties, including children, their parents, other teachers, social workers and educational psychologists. As illustrated in Example 23.2, sometimes the setting for collaboration is formal – e.g. the classroom, referral, planning and review meetings. At other times contact is informal, such as a chat with a parent or other adult, or a telephone conversation with colleagues. Whichever is the case, each individual has the opportunity to make a significant contribution to educating the young person in focus. In this case many of the exchanges began with sharing helpful information, but over time this led to an enhanced understanding of what was being provided and its effectiveness in supporting young people.

Example 23.2 Education support base for secondary students experiencing behavioural difficulties – a community of support

'I used to despair that social work and psychological services either could not attend case reviews or would call off at the last minute. When they did attend, the support they were able to offer the pupils always appeared to me to be minimal and we would end up in fruitless discussions regarding where the young person should be at any one time of the day.

When I considered why, I realised that I was calling these meetings at times that suited me, i.e. within school hours. I also wondered if, from say a social work or psychological services perspective, what we as an educational unit were offering seemed minimal to them.

As a first step, I started calling meetings at times that suited colleagues from other agencies. It was amazing how this simple act led to a more relaxed atmosphere in meetings and eventually to all of us finding that there were supports we could offer that we had not previously imagined'.

[Teacher in charge of support base]

During the meetings referred to in Example 23.2, participants aired problems and considered contradictions in practices and perceptions. They discussed and resolved these to create new understandings and strategies to help young people manage their lives and learning. For example, prior to establishing the more collaborative regime, ongoing discussions about one particular pupil had resulted in agreement that outdoor education would be beneficial. However, limited attention was given to the provision of transport or supervision of the pupil, so nothing came to fruition.

Following the new way of working, time was made available for the pupil to express his opinions and ideas and how he thought he would or would not benefit from particular activities. In response to his input, education arranged appropriate visits and activities, social work organised transport and supervision was shared. As a result of taking part in this series of meetings and similar others, professionals gained new and deeper understandings of their own and each other's roles and practices, and subsequently developed a more cohesive and effective approach. In other words, they created a community of support. Essential to this process was the resolution of the conflicts and contradictions that emerged as professionals interacted.

The difference between the two states – the exchange of information on one hand and shared understanding on the other – highlights the differences between procedural or functional collaboration and deep collaboration. In the first case, people gather together in some context, contribute to the discourse from their own point of view, help to make decisions based on the information generated, and then go off to carry out the actions to which they have agreed. Generally, the various parties approach this context with their own set of priorities and see their contribution as limited to their own area of expertise or knowledge. The kind of material produced at such meetings is generally a list of tasks for some or all of the participants to undertake to support the learning of the young person. All participants have carried out the expected functions of reporting, suggesting and agreeing and view the decisions they make as enhancing provision for the learner. This corresponds with the 'more-bounded' interdisciplinary working illustrated in the Douglasshire example.

In Wallace City, as described by Stead et al. (2004) and Example 23.2, something much more meaningful took place. Individuals no longer simply played their discrete parts, but developed a sense of what the group as a whole was trying to achieve, and directed their efforts and expertise towards reaching this common goal. In Wallace, the shared goal was inclusion in school. Stead et al. cite the example of 'risk-taking' in the case of one pupil who under normal procedures would have been excluded from school. Instead, the inter-agency team 'withdrew' from normal procedures and put in place measures to address the young person's issues. In Example 23.2 a route to full inclusion through the nurturing of learning behaviour and a programme to develop this was devised when the depute head of a mainstream school, support base staff and social work agreed that it was in the best interest of a young person in danger of exclusion (and in keeping with his wishes) that he remain in mainstream schooling with his peers. The support devised required input from all three professional contexts to provide an appropriate range of experiences to reinforce the learning behaviours of planning, decision-making and organising on which the young person was working. The multidisciplinary work became more relevant to the pupil's needs through the generation of shared experiences and trust. In both instances the group evolved into a community with shared understanding of the nature and purpose of the group and a common sense of mutual benefit which helped the individual case but also extended beyond it.

In Example 23.2 the professionals agreed to adopt a solution-focused approach to meetings at which the pupil was first asked to identify 'what had been better' since the last meeting and what he still wanted to address. Thus, the agenda for the meeting became the pupil's priorities rather than those of the professionals. Consequently, the professionals learned from the pupil how they might go about their business in a way that was effective for that pupil. The sense of one party 'doing something to' the other or of having something done to them disappeared, and participants felt more of a sense of group enterprise.

Colleagues in the field of behaviour support suggest that their perceptions and experiences of collaboration are similar. With procedural or functional collaboration, student support is limited to attending meetings, reporting on a student's learning progress, suggesting further programmes of work and thereafter returning to work with the student. With effective collaboration, however, the student leads interaction and each participant contributes in a way that allows the group to generate an understanding of and insight into that student's needs and their own needs, desires and constraints. Once this collective competence has been created within a community of support, it can be recreated more quickly in other cases, leading to more effective support of student learning.

From their study into collaboration among professionals working with children who require learning support, Graham and Wright (1999) identified some of the detailed activities that can help move beyond functional to deeper collaboration, for example:

- giving a knowledge and understanding of my role to others;
- explaining the contribution I make to meeting the needs of pupils;
- talking to other professionals regularly . . . to share knowledge and expertise;
- trying to make sure that a common language is used that can be understood by all professionals and parents;
- acknowledging the importance of the methods used by different professionals;
- getting to know and understand the goals of other professionals.

Graham and Wright distinguished forms of communication with different purposes – planning activities, sharing activities and goal-achieving activities. When learners, teachers, social workers, psychologists and other interested parties work together in this way, they create the opportunity to develop from a supportive group – well-intentioned but constrained – to become a 'community of support' that creates the conditions and strategies necessary to achieve its goals.

Developing a culture of collaboration within schools

Daniels et al. (2000) suggested the concept of teacher support teams (TSTs) as a model for collaboration among teachers. The model indicates that TSTs would be small (perhaps one per school), consisting of perhaps three teachers whom any member of staff may approach about a problem.

The idea of peer support for professionals is not new. Indeed, peer support is an integral part of professions such as counselling. The educational argument is that peer support leads to shared knowledge among teachers and increases the ability of schools to deal with the diverse range of pupils within their catchment areas. Teachers' perceptions of support teams are positive. They claim that team discussion externalises the problem so that it can be considered from a distance, and helps develop strategies. They also claim that the sympathetic ethos of the discussions is cathartic.

Perhaps even more important for creating a culture of collaboration is what happens in the classroom. While the aim of inter- and multi-agency collaboration is to support the inclusion of young people in schools, and the aim of collaboration within schools is to support learning, the underlying principles of sharing, openness and trust are the same. For example, Argyris (1992) emphasised the importance of a secondary phase of learning in which opportunities not available in an initial phase of surface learning are presented. The difference between these levels of learning can be likened to the levels of collaboration described earlier. Similarly,

Bruner's (1996: 20) premise that learning is dependent on the 'ability to understand the minds of others' is applicable to all forms of collaboration. An implication is that teachers may need to problematise their interactions with students and conceptualise them as collaborative episodes in which teaching and learning are coterminous and iterative.

As the majority of teachers in schools, colleges and universities were educated in a behaviourist environment (Pollard and Triggs 1997), this is likely to have had an affect on their own teaching. Educators are therefore liable to continue creating the cultures of individualism and focus on superficial learning. In addition, educational institutions may well constrain learning through prescribing curricula, enforcing necessary timetables and setting exam targets and timing. Consequently, much teacher–student interaction is directed towards control and accountability. Indeed, the very hierarchical structure of such institutions may not only hamper a secondary phase of collaboration and hence learning, but may actually prevent it from taking place (Argyris 1992).

However, organisational barriers to learning can be overcome if what takes place between students and teachers is reconceptualised. Schematically, such rethinking of pedagogy can be represented as follows:

control _____ learning
accountability _____ understanding

This is more likely to be achieved if those in charge enact and support it (Argyris 1992), but it also depends on students and teachers putting it into operation in the everyday learning context. Using a management model based on the assumption that a problem is best solved by those involved in it on a daily basis, the institution ceases to be a hierarchy of command and control and becomes a collegial organisation:

> ...where search is enhanced and deepened, where ideas are tested publicly, where individuals collaborate to enlarge inquiry, and where trust and risk-taking are enhanced.
> (Argyris 1992, p. 153)

Thus, the roles of managers and teachers shift from positions of authority to participants and learners in a culture of investigation, experiment and mutual sense-making. Cranston (2001) has highlighted the need for closer collaboration among school colleagues and for school principals to develop the skills necessary to collaborate in a context of school-based management. In eschewing hierarchical status in favour of academic autonomy and intellectual advancement, school managers, teachers and other relevant professionals work together creating insight and a shared understanding of their function and purpose to become a community of learners.

Communities of learners have their roots within schools and classrooms, and what takes place within them can therefore inhibit or enhance learning. If the interactions between teachers and students operate at the functional level of coordination, cooperation and communication, then the class will likely find itself 'addressing but not necessarily solving problems' (Lloyd et al. 2001: 9). Collaboration at this level may well help to create conditions for learning, but does not guarantee its occurrence. Interactions between pupils and teachers, therefore, should be about generating a shared understanding of why learning in general and the topic being explored at the time are important. The whole school community works to create a vision of where it is heading intellectually and generate appropriate strategies for getting there. Similarly, if this is the dominant culture within the school, there is greater likelihood of collaborating in a deeper, less-bounded way with colleagues from other professions to support inclusion.

Brown et al. (1996) have offered an example of how a community of learners might work. Founded on the theories of Piaget and Vygotsky, the analogy of the relationship between functional and effective collaboration and constructivist and social constructivist approaches to teaching becomes clear. In this model, the teacher and pupils agree on areas and themes for active exploration within an overall context. In acting as researchers on one of these themes or sub-themes, students become the community experts on that theme. They are then in a position to teach others in the classroom and thus contribute to the creation of common knowledge and understanding. To carry out these tasks, learners develop a language that becomes increasingly subject-specific and academic but, crucially, shared as they learn and disseminate their learning.

Conclusions and implications

Schools are examples of learning communities at all levels, so the principles that apply to learning in classrooms apply equally to learning among school staff and between school staff and other professionals. In a community of learners, collaboration takes the form of social support through a variety of expertise. Thus, the approach to learning in classrooms should match that proposed for effective inter-agency working. In a 'more-bounded' context problems are seen as obstacles and barriers to successful collaboration; in 'less-bounded' contexts, problems are features of collaboration that are debated, considered and to which solutions are agreed as a necessary and integral part of the process.

Moreover, the objectives of the learning that takes place in schools are exactly the concerns of all the professionals supporting young people – i.e. learning about healthy living, empathy, how to work with peers, children's and others' rights. In an educational context, therefore, working together for better learning is maybe the most effective approach to supporting young people's inclusion in schools. Similarly, effective collaboration among teachers, pupils and other relevant professionals and lay people in and beyond school is essential to nurture the capacities to cope with life in other contexts.

Exercise

- What would be your priorities to ensure inclusion in education for vulnerable children and young people?
- What do you envisage might be the barriers to effective collaboration put up by pupils, parents, your own and other professionals?
- How might all of the above be addressed in terms of deeper, 'less-bounded' inter-agency working?

Recommended reading

Boreham (2004) explores the concept of collective competence and challenges individual ability and accountability as the sole measure of competence and success within groups.

Daniels (2000) offers an explanation of how effective collaboration might operate using educational theory derived from the work of Vygotsky.

Stead et al. (2004) provides detailed examples of inter-agency working.

Todd (2007) presents a comprehensive critical account of collaboration with pupils, parents and other professionals in school contexts.

Chapter 24

Collaborating to improve the health of looked-after children

Jackie Dougall

Summary points

- Children who are looked after by a local authority, are among the most socially excluded of the child population.
- Looked-after children have greater health needs than their peers, as they are likely to have undetected health concerns and failed to access appropriate services for treatment and follow-up.
- Many of the children will have missed out on routine preventive childhood health screening.
- Provided they have capacity, children have the right to consent to medical assessment and treatment, to agree to sharing of health information (medical confidentiality) and also the right to decline consent.
- A range of professionals and carers have an important role in improving the health of looked-after children.
- Health and well-being is closely connected to other aspects of children's lives, such as education attainment, as well as personal and social support.

Introduction

Children who are unable to be cared for at home for a wide range of reasons, so that the local authority is required to place them away from home, are known as 'looked-after' children. The earlier term 'in care' was officially abandoned as it was stigmatising, but is still in fairly common use. Children who are looked after have greater health needs than their peers, yet are less likely to receive adequate health care and treatment or to be supported in developing their knowledge and skills in making decisions that promote their health and well-being. This chapter will examine health inequalities and the health needs of children placed away from home. It discusses ways health and other services can support the health of looked-after children.

Looked-after children

Parents have the responsibility to safeguard and promote the health and well-being of their children, assisted by support and guidance from health professionals. However, some parents may require additional support from statutory and voluntary organisations to look after their children at home. For others their circumstances may indicate that they can no longer be cared for at home, requiring the local authority to look after them away from home. All such children should have a care plan, which covers all their needs, including health, and is regularly reviewed.

The legal definition of 'looked-after' children and young people varies to some extent across UK jurisdictions, but generally refers to those looked after by the local authority with parental agreement or with a court order (hearings requirement in Scotland). Normally young people leave care before the age of 18, but government guidance covers support for children and young people from birth to age 25, wherever they are looked after (including residential care, foster care, young offender or other secure institutions, boarding school, or those placed with birth parents and other family carers). In Scotland children who are looked after away from home in a care placement provided by the local authority tend to be described as 'looked-after and accommodated', as children supervised at home are also 'looked after'.

Reasons why children are cared away from home

Children may be looked after by the local authority for a range of reasons, which seldom exist in isolation and may be complex. Breakdown in family relationships, inconsistent parenting, parental drug and alcohol misuse, domestic violence, neglect and abuse may result in a child being removed from the family home to be looked after in a care placement (see, e.g. Schofield and Simmonds 2009). Many of these factors are associated with low income, deprivation and social exclusion, resulting in this group of vulnerable children already being disadvantaged prior to being looked after.

The main categories of looked-after children in care placements are:

- those of all ages who enter care and return home quickly;
- children aged under 5 who enter care and are subsequently adopted;
- children raised from an early age in the care system;
- older children who are looked after for some years;
- young people aged 16 and over who have moved on to independent living.

Available health policies on looked-after children

In the UK, local authorities are required to promote the welfare of looked-after children and there is a wide range of policies and guidance relevant to such children. These will be individual to each of the four countries, but they commonly set out how health boards and local authorities have a shared responsibility in helping to support all children to be healthy, stay safe, enjoy and achieve, make a positive contribution and achieve economic well-being.

In addition to setting out key principles and establishing what parents, carers and children in the general population can expect from services, generally the policies and guidance identify the need for:

- robust joint plans agreed between health, education and social-work services, with clarity about overlapping responsibilities for services for looked-after children;
- enabling children who are looked after to live in healthy environments that encourage them to make healthy choices;
- responsive services that provide looked-after children with the right services at the right time to meet their specific health needs and expectations;
- targeted support for looked-after children in view of their generally poor outcomes (discussed below).

Health boards and schools usually designate individuals with special responsibility for looked-after children.

Health of looked-after children

Children are mainly dependent on parents and carers to meet their basic health needs (see Chapter 17). The experience of child abuse and neglect, which are common reasons for becoming looked-after, can adversely affect all aspects of a child's health, growth, intellectual development and mental well-being in the short and long term. The physical health effects of child abuse include injuries such as shaken baby syndrome, non-organic failure to thrive, broken bones, stomach aches and migraines, as well as emotional trauma. Health problems later in life can include heart disease, obesity, liver disease, cancer and chronic lung disease (NSPCC 2010).

The impact of a child moving into a care placement means a change in the adult caring for them and this can result in a loss of knowledge of the child's own and family health history. The number of changes of placement experienced by children can impact on the continuity of their development across all areas of their lives including health (Chambers et al. 2002). Moving between different care placements can result in issues being overlooked, as no one person has a long-term understanding of the child's health needs. Changes in carer may result in lack of an accurate health history, missed or delayed health appointments and the scattering of health records.

Entry into care is usually a traumatic experience and brings with it a huge sense of loss from family and community that can be inadequately recognised within the child care plan. For children who remain in long-term care, creating a sense of belonging and emotional security is vital to their health and well-being. There is a close relationship between educational and health issues, requiring teachers and health professionals to communicate and work together. Looked-after children may experience significant problems at school, due to earlier home problems, having to travel to maintain a stable school placement, loss of friendships and support networks. Rates of truancy and exclusion from school are higher than average, which results in missed opportunities for school-based health promotion sessions on exercise, diet, smoking, alcohol and drugs, sexuality and sex (Polnay and Ward 2000).

For all the above reasons, the physical and mental health of looked-after children is poor in comparison of that of their peers. Evidence suggest that looked-after children experience significantly higher levels of both physical and emotional health problems than their counterparts who are not looked-after (Department of Health 2002; Scottish Executive 2004). This is mainly on account of their family backgrounds, but in addition often their health needs are not detected or attended to. It is more likely that, as children stay in care, pre-existing chronic health conditions will be recognised rather than new health conditions develop.

There has been scant evidence published on the unmet health needs and health care needs of children who live away from home. Two studies give an overview of the health needs gathered from health assessments that children are offered while in care.

In a longitudinal study by Skuse et al. (1999) data was collected from six local authority areas in England who placed children in care, over a one year period 1996–97, across all types of care placements and who were still in care one year and three years later, when follow-up information was gathered. Over half of the children appeared to have an identified physical or health condition of sufficient gravity to require out-patient treatment, suggesting that their health needs were considerably greater than those of the general population. A substantial proportion (26 per cent) had more than one condition and another 26 per cent two or more conditions. Skuse et al. (1999) were unable to identify accurately how many children were substantially disabled, but estimated that 15 per cent required specialist physical care, being either registered disabled, admitted primarily because of a health condition and/or having three or more identified physical/health conditions.

The Edinburgh Residential Care Project (Scottish Executive 2004) gathered information from initial health assessments of 105 children in residential childcare. The average age of the children was 13.9 years. For instance, four-fifths (82 per cent) had physical health problems, most of which had been not recognised prior to assessment. These included minor ailments (warts, acne, menstrual problems), but it should be recognised that these can cause distress and disrupted sleep if advice is not available or accessed. There were also major undiagnosed conditions like asthma, kidney problems and epilepsy. These had more often been identified at some time in the past, but appropriate treatment was disrupted due to early neglected health care when at home and subsequent moves once in the care system. A significant minority had vision problems and all but a few had incomplete childhood screening for visual, hearing and dental issues. Nearly three-quarters had gaps in their childhood immunisations.

One in five of the sample (17 per cent) had learning difficulties. It is essential to be aware of the prevalence of learning disability within the population of children looked after away from home. Large numbers of learning disabled children could, at least partially, explain why local authorities are having difficulty in meeting their education targets for looked-after children. Careful consideration is required on how key health messages are given to the children with learning difficulties and their carers.

There is limited literature concerning the oral health status of vulnerable children, but what evidence there is suggests that vulnerable children have higher levels of untreated dental disease than their peers (Harris et al. 2009). Oral health can have significant impact on the health of children, with the consequences of dental disease including severe pain, loss of sleep, time off school, interference with playing and socialisation. Long-standing disease can result in severe acute and chronic infection and damage to permanent teeth, with the effects of tooth loss in childhood being lifelong. However, dental disease is preventable and treatable.

The mental health of looked-after children

Looked-after children, especially those in residential care, are identified as a group whose mental-health needs are known to be greater than those of their peers. Children in care are much more likely than other children to have experienced risk factors that predispose to the development of mental disorders. A mental or psychiatric disorder is a term used to refer to severe and complex mental-health problems that persist over time and cause a great deal of distress to the child/young person and their families/carers that interferes significantly with every aspect of the children's everyday life and general development. Some of the risk factors are often the reason why they have entered the care system – abuse and neglect, family dysfunction, parental illness, family in acute stress and absent parenting. As well as these factors, many of the children will also have experienced an early life environment, such as socio-economic disadvantage, poverty and homelessness, that also predisposes them to mental-health problems.

McCann et al. (1996) looked at the prevalence and types of psychiatric disorders of all adolescents between the ages of 13 and 17 years in the care of one English local authority. Overall, two-thirds were deemed to have a psychiatric disorder, whereas in a community comparison group the rate was 15 per cent. The figures varied with placement type – 57 per cent of adolescents in foster care and 96 per cent of adolescents in residential care, with the overall prevalence rate across care placement of being 67 per cent. The most common were conduct disorder (28 per cent), anxiety (26 per cent) and major depressive disorder (23 per cent). Children taken into care are greatly at risk of mental illness, but the picture is not bleak. The offer of acceptance and affection by their carers might eventually lead to improved self-esteem and security.

Similarly the Edinburgh Residential Care Project identified that virtually all of their sample had some kind of emotional, behavioural or mental-health problems. These could reflect the reasons for becoming looked after, be a consequence or both. The difficulties were wide-ranging. For instance, two-thirds were assessed as having low self-esteem, while one-quarter self-harmed. One-fifth were currently being seen in child and adolescent mental health services.

Health and well-being is closely connected to other aspects of young people's lives such as education attainment, as well as personal and social support. For example, if a child has toothache, this may result in a disturbed sleeping pattern and impact on the child's ability to concentrate in school, or a child with an unidentified motor impairment may be viewed as clumsy and not be willing to participate in sporting activities.

Impact of risk-taking behaviour on health

Risk-taking behaviours can be viewed as a normal part of adolescent development and in adolescents seeking their own identity. However, it becomes problematic when, for instance, heavy use of alcohol, smoking, drug use and unsafe sexual activity is detrimental to physical and mental health. Such behaviour can result from poor self-esteem and lack of confidence (Dunnet et al. 2006).

A study to examine the health needs of a sample of young people who were looked after by the local authority in Glasgow residential units found that 75 per cent of the young people were smokers, with 27 per cent starting to smoke while in care (The Big Step 2001). This is much higher than that of the peer population. The early commencement of daily smoking indicates that future habitual smoking is likely. This can be the result of various factors – smoking being seen as a way to engage and build friendships, peer pressure, lack of awareness around the damaging effects of smoking, stress, weight management, perceived attractiveness of smoking, and smoking being considered normal and acceptable due to parents and carers smoking. These issues are relevant to all children, but are more significant in care placements due to the vulnerability of the children.

Young people who are looked after have high rates of alcohol and substance misuse. Reasons they give for doing this include to 'forget the bad times', make them relax or boost their confidence (Greisbach and Currie 2001). Many children may have also witnessed parents misusing alcohol and drugs, so may consider it normal (Scott and Hill 2006). In comparison to their peers with regard to misusing alcohol and substances, looked-after young people tend to start at an earlier age and their intake is more frequent. Similarly to smoking, there are concerns that alcohol and substance misuse in a young population may become established and harmful.

Another area where risk-taking behaviour can impact on young people's health is involvement in early sexual relationships, with sexually transmitted infections and high pregnancy rates all too prevalent within looked-after young people. Factors associated are the link to socio-economic deprivation, gaps in knowledge, limited access to the consistent positive adult, having a mother who was pregnant in teenage years, low self-esteem and low educational attainment (Social Care Institute for Excellence 2004).

Perceived long-term effects are not taken into consideration by young people and risk-taking is frequently connected to a high level of self-destructive behaviour, signalling at least a need for an appropriate skilled-based health education, which many do not receive (Griesbach and Currie 2001). Studies have shown young people lacked the opportunity to discuss personal health matters with anyone they could trust, and they often reported they did not feel listened to during health appointments (Bundle 2002; van Beinum, Martin and Bonnett, in Scott and Ward 2005), so are less likely to access support and health services.

Improving the health of looked-after children

Engaging with young people

Looked-after children should have clear expectations to be involved in the discussions and decision-making that affect their lives, including on how to be kept healthy and all aspects of their own health. Care planning entails the ongoing multidisciplinary assessment of the child's needs, and should include careful identification of actions to meet these needs, with reviews at regular intervals to ensure that actions are implemented as agreed. Effective care planning is crucial for improving outcomes for looked-after children and should include aspects that address and improve the child's health.

Medical consent and confidentiality

Local authorities should have guidance in relation to consent to the medical examination and treatment of children who are placed by them and should make these known to the child, health services, the parents, carers and staff. The arrangements for medical consent should be set out in each care plan where a child is placed away from home. These will vary according to the legal status of the child, the age and understanding of the child and whether a local authority does or does not have parental responsibilities for the child. Tensions can arise between respect for young people's privacy or decision-making rights, and their possible needs as vulnerable individuals for support in making complex choices.

In Scotland the starting point for who is entitled to consent to medical treatment for an individual child is Section 2(4) of the Age of Legal Capacity (Scotland) Act 1991. This states that, for any child *under* 16, there is a right to consent to any form of medical treatment and procedure, *if* the doctor, dentist or other medical practitioner takes the view that the child has the capacity to understand *what* the treatment or procedure is *and* its possible consequences. The understanding is in relation to the particular treatment, course of treatment or a certain procedure. When children have the capacity to consent, it can be assumed they are entitled to medical confidentiality and should also be given a choice as to where to get their medicines dispensed. If a doctor, dentist or other medical practitioner takes the view that the child has the capacity to consent, then only the child can consent or refuse consent. The consent or refusal of someone else, such as the parent, is legally irrelevant, although good practice suggests involving the birth family in discussing issues and carrying the treatment forward, if the child is in agreement with that approach. When the medical practitioner considers the child is unable to understand the examination, treatment or procedure and all the possible consequences, the child is not legally capable of agreeing and it is necessary to look elsewhere for consent. Even when children are looked after, this will normally be the child's parents, although sometimes carers can make decisions about day-to-day matters, while in a small minority of cases local authorities obtain full parental responsibilities through a court order.

In England, Wales and Northern Ireland, much of the law affecting consent is not set out in legislation but is common law (i.e. judge-made). The legal right of people to give consent for treatment on behalf of a young person is not wholly extinguished until the young person reaches the age of majority, 18 years, although young people between ages 16 and 18 years are also presumed competent to give consent and should be treated accordingly unless there is evidence to suggest otherwise. No statute governs the rights of young people under 16 to give consent to medical treatment. Ideally, decisions about whether to accept or reject medical treatment should be taken by children together with their parents. Consent for medical treatment of a person under 18 years can come from any one of the following:

- a competent child;
- a person or local authority with parental responsibility;
- a court;
- a person caring for a child but if it is reasonable in the circumstances to safeguard or promote the child's welfare.

Whoever gives consent, the child's wishes are an essential part of assessing what is in their best interest. Competent sustained wishes should not be overridden lightly and all children should be offered the opportunity for their views to be heard and given due consideration.

Across the UK, health professionals have a responsibility to provide emergency treatment, without the necessary consent, if any delay would lead to death or serious harm.

Health information

The loss of personal health information can have significant implications for the immediate and future health and well-being of looked-after children. Birth parents may not recall or may be reluctant to share the child's health or birth family health information with statutory services, particularly when the child is initially placed away from home. Also, due to the frequency with which looked-after children move care placements, there is a risk that health information may be misplaced when the child changes placement, is placed outside their local health area, or when children are admitted to care, discharged and readmitted sometime later.

It is, therefore, crucial that health information of looked-after children is recorded in a detailed and factual manner, as inaccurate record-keeping can lead to wrong decisions by professionals and can adversely affect the child's care. Many areas use a carer-held health book to ensure the person(s) with responsibility for caring for the child has current information on the child's health needs that can be appropriately shared with health professionals.

Health needs should be incorporated into the multi-agency care plan to ensure that actions are followed through irrespective of where the child is placed, and equally important is ensuring that health information is accurate and kept up-to-date and is transferred to the right person, at the right time. Health information, including the birth family's health history, may take on an additional importance when young adults begin to plan their own families.

Services to support the health of looked-after children

All professionals and carers who have contact with looked-after children, including non-health professionals like social workers and teachers, have a role in recognising and promoting the health needs of children, including acting as a good healthy role model. Children have a number of needs – a diet limited in the amount and frequency of sugar, salt and fats, and high in vegetables and fruit; regular tooth-brushing; opportunities and encouragement to participate in physical activity; good sleep pattern; and accessing regular preventive healthcare to enable children to benefit from preventive interventions; and early diagnosis and treatment when necessary. For children to reach optimal health, it is essential that care placements incorporate the key health messages into the child's and placement routine.

Staff and carers have a significant influencing role to educate children to understand the importance of healthcare and to take increasing responsibility for their own health. Staff and carers also have a role in encouraging and supporting children to access health services and to draw the children's attention to their right to give or refuse consent to health examination or treatment and the boundaries of health confidentiality.

The role of primary health care services

It will generally be the responsibility of social workers and carers to ensure that looked-after children are in touch with the appropriate health services. All children should be registered with a General Practitioner (GP). They are personal doctors, primarily responsible for the provision of comprehensive and continuing medical care to patients irrespective of age, sex and illness (Royal College of General Practitioners 2009).

Likewise, all children should be registered with a General Dental Practitioner (GDP) and should access the service regularly for a dental assessment and complete any required treatment. Dentists are healthcare professionals who provide preventive and restorative treatments for problems that affect the mouth and teeth. A GDP typically leads a team made up of dental care professionals such as dental nurse and dental hygienist, and treats a wide range of patients from children to the elderly.

Community pharmacists are expert in medicines and their use, to ensure patients get the maximum benefit from medicines. They are a helpful useful source of information and support to foster carers and residential staff, particularly in relation to the treatment of minor childhood illnesses (e.g. hay fever, threadworms, acne, emergency contraception), and are able to prescribe medicines for specific conditions.

Child and adolescent mental health services (CAMHS) comprise several different mental health professionals – child psychiatrist, clinical nurse specialists, psychologists, occupational therapists; all working together to help young people and their families/carers where there are mental-health problems. The services offered by CAMHS teams can be variable but usually include:

- consultation services to professionals involved with children such as social workers, foster carers, teachers;
- direct work with children, young people, families and carers, including assessment of needs and risks, and provision of therapeutic interventions such as cognitive or family therapy. Most of the work they do is done through an out-patient clinic;
- signposting to other services.

When referring a child to CAMHS it is helpful to provide background information, a description of what is happening, giving examples of specific incidents/events, valid consent and any other relevant information.

Looked-after children (LAC) nurses have a clear role and responsibility to maintain and improve the health and well-being of looked-after children in their care. Working as members of a multidisciplinary team, they have an outstanding opportunity to take a leading role to improve health assessments and develop new and innovative services for children and young people looked after away from home. Most health board and local authority areas across the UK employ LAC nurses. Their precise functions vary, but they are generally involved in activity related to:

- conducting comprehensive health assessments of children, including immunisations, growth, sexual health and mental health;
- providing children and young people with health information and advice;
- supporting young people as they move onto independence;
- provision of training for foster carers and staff;
- guidance and support for foster carers and staff.

(NHS Education Scotland 2008)

Hill et al. (2002) discuss the growing contribution that specialist nurses are making in promoting the health of looked-after children and all the evidence presented points to better outcomes and additional quality through nurse-led health assessments. They can have a valuable role in mediating communication between social workers and teachers, especially where issues of confidentiality arise. LAC nurses have contributed to education initiatives for looked-after children – e.g. to help ensure these include positive health messages.

Health assessments and healthcare planning

A health assessment is an opportunity to assess a child's health needs while taking account of all the background health information available on the child and family health. This will result in a written report on the child health and a health plan to address the child's health needs. The arrangements for looked-after children to be offered a health assessment vary depending on where the child is placed. Many of the policy documents recommend timescales in which a comprehensive health assessment should be undertaken when a child is placed away from home, including the need for a written report and health plan to be available. The requirements for the child to receive a review health assessment again vary according to national and local policy.

Many health board areas have designated health professionals who have a responsibility to assist health boards to fulfil their responsibilities as a commissioner of services to improve the health of looked-after children. The designated doctor role is likely to be undertaken by a senior paediatrician, who has substantial experience of the health needs of vulnerable children and is likely to be a medical advisor to an adoption and fostering service. They will work in close partnership with the LAC nurses.

Partnership working

There is a clear link between health, education attainment, social and future employment prospects of a child, and to address the health needs of looked-after children it is essential for all the key agencies to work in partnership. Using an integrated assessment framework, the needs of the child should be accurately assessed and remain central. There is a requirement for agencies to share information and work in partnership to address the child's needs. This should maximise the opportunity for agencies to provide additional help and support the individual child (e.g. the LAC nurse, social worker and school coordinating efforts to build self-esteem or manage aggression).

Example 24.1

Alison (14 years old) is being placed in a residential unit today, as she is deemed to be out of parental control. She has a history of absconding, drinking alcohol and non-attendance at school. The unit staff are concerned about her general appearance, including her weight. Alison's education attainment is poor. A joint planning meeting took place at school to discuss how carers, teachers, social workers and the LAC nurse could in their separate contacts and roles all work to help Alison improve her self-image and diet, support her to attend school and develop more pro-social friendships.

James (6 years old) is in foster care due to his parents' mental ill-health. He is an insulin-dependent diabetic. He is due to change placement, to reside within another health board area. The new foster carers were given advice by the GP and the diabetic health team about how to manage diabetes, while the LAC nurse ensured that key points in her comprehensive health assessment were conveyed to the child's social worker and new school. The foster carers have a link worker who is providing the carers with guidance and support to help James maintain positive contact with his mother, whose behaviour can be highly variable.

Conclusions and implications

Looked-after children are one of the most vulnerable and socially excluded groups of children within society. The effects of poverty, deprivation, experience of childhood neglect and abuse can have considerable impact on children's current and future health, resulting in this group of vulnerable children already being disadvantaged prior to being looked after. The experience of being looked after can also result in health inequalities due to lack of accurate health information and the ability to access appropriate and consistent health services. Many of the children had undetected health concerns or previously detected health concerns, but had failed to access services due to non-attendance at health appointments or changes in care placements. This can result in a lack of accurate health information being available to health professionals and carers to adequately address the health concern. The mental-health needs of looked-after children are greater than that their peers, with many of the children having experienced some of the risk factors that predispose to mental disorders, prior to being cared for away from home. Some looked-after adolescents engage in the risky problematic use of alcohol and substances, higher incidence of smoking and early sexual relationships and are more likely to lack opportunities to discuss personal health matters with someone they trust.

Most older, looked-after children have the capacity, and hence the entitlement, to consent to medical examination and treatment. This also implies that if they have the capacity they are entitled to withhold consent and have an informed view on whom their health information is shared with. It is crucial for all staff and carers who work directly with looked-after children to recognise they have an important role in ensuring that the children are aware of the issues of consent and act as good role models in relation to health matters. Also, all the key health improvement messages should be incorporated across all aspects of the child's care, as a matter of daily routine.

It is essential for all looked-after children to be registered with a GP and GDP and to access routine health-screening programmes. In addition to mainstream services that all children are entitled to access, many health boards have designated health professionals, usually paediatricians and LAC nurses who will offer and undertake health assessments on looked-after children. The purpose of the health assessments is to assess the child's health needs, while taking account of all the background health information available on the child and their family. This will result in a written report on the child's health and a health plan to address the child's health needs.

Health and well-being is closely connected to other aspects of children's lives such as education attainment, social and future employment prospects of the child, resulting in the need for good partnership working between all agencies, staff and carers who have contact with looked-after children.

Exercise

Discuss with fellow students or colleagues, what you consider your current or future professional role can contribute to improving the health of looked-after children. Consider if there is any local guidance/ policy to support this and where you may access support from.

Recommended reading

NSPCC (2010) 'The impact of abuse and neglect on the health and mental health of children and young people.'

http://www.nspcc.org.uk/Inform/research/briefings/impact_of_abuse_on_health_wda73372.html

Explores long-term effects of abuse and neglect on children's health, growth, intellectual development and mental well-being.

Chapter 25

Issues in interprofessional education

Sally Kuenssberg, Barbara Reid and Raymond Taylor

Summary points

- Interprofessional education is essential to improve mutual knowledge and understanding among the many agencies working with children and families.
- Current confusions about the purposes and definition of interprofessional education need to be clarified.
- A number of barriers to learning must be recognised and allowed for in the planning of effective interprofessional education.
- Interprofessional education should be based on the principles of adult learning and an awareness of group dynamics.
- Increased awareness of ethics, attitudes and values may promote more effective interprofessional practice.

Introduction

This book has explored a wide range of activities included under the umbrella title of 'children's services'. A theme emerging from many of the chapters is the need for more effective collaboration to ensure that the needs of children and their families are being addressed. This chapter considers what kinds of professional education and training can best prepare and support members of different professions and agencies to work in this way.

Challenges of collaborative working

The challenging nature of working in children's services makes significant demands on individual practitioners and agencies. The stresses of dealing with intractable problems against a background of changing rules and procedures, demanding targets, the pressures of audit and inspection, staff shortages and lack of resources can lead to loss of confidence among staff who feel isolated and unsupported

(Parton 2004). Decisions concerning children's lives often require to be taken speedily and in partnership with other professionals in a context that is uncertain, risk-laden and confusing. How individual professionals respond to such challenges will be influenced, at least in part, by their childhood, upbringing and culture, as well as the roles and orientations of their chosen professions.

Intervention in such circumstances requires professionals individually and collectively to draw on not only the knowledge and skills they have acquired during professional formation, but also their own sense of integrity and 'character'. As Lord Laming commented in his first Inquiry Report on the death of Victoria Climbié (Department of Health 2003: p. 3) 'staff doing this work need a combination of professional skills and qualities, not least of which are persistence and courage'. Attempts at collaboration by, for example, childcare practitioners, social workers, community nurses, and police may reveal clashes of views, attitudes and values.

To prevent such clashes becoming barriers to effective working, they need to be confronted in joint training (Example 25.1).

Example 25.1

A child has been smacked. In what circumstances might this be seen as:

- Reasonable punishment?
- The result of momentary loss of control by a parent tested to the limit?
- A child protection matter?
- You may think smacking is necessarily abusive, but if not where does child abuse begin?
- Who should decide? What factors should affect the decision?

This is the kind of issue that can promote constructive discussion of conflicting views in a training session designed for professionals from a range of disciplines.[1]

Professionals working with children will be involved in many different kinds of learning and development throughout their careers – some formal, some less formal:

- initial professional training and qualification;
- integration of initial knowledge and skills in practice under supervision;
- reflective practice with peers;
- expansion of knowledge in specialist areas;
- regular updating of knowledge and expertise;
- 'interprofessional' education and learning with members of other professions to share experiences and develop mutual understanding.

Ensuring that practitioners develop the professional and personal resources to work both as individuals and in teams in the testing environment described above will not

---

[1] For wider examination of issues in relation to smacking readers may wish to review Phillips B. and Alderson P. (2003) 'Beyond "anti-smacking": challenging parental violence', *Child Abuse Review*, 12:282–91.

easily be achieved in a conventional educational setting – library or lecture theatre – nor in the hurly-burly of the working day. This chapter explores ways in which interprofessional education offered at appropriate stages can best help members of different professions and agencies to tackle their demanding work.

Lessons from the past

A series of high-profile inquiry reports over the past 40 years have identified lack of effective interprofessional working as a contributory factor in failures by UK childcare agencies to protect children. Reports on the circumstances surrounding the tragic deaths of children let down by the system echo down the decades – among them Maria Colwell (DHSS 1974), Jasmine Beckford (1985) and Victoria Climbié (Laning 2003). Report recommendations have been taken seriously by governments and have had major influences on the development of child-protection systems. Larger-scale, system-wide failures, for example in Cleveland (1987) and Orkney (1992), have also given rise to changes across the UK.

A number of repeated shortcomings are described in the introduction to the Green Paper *Every Child Matters* (2003) as 'common threads'. These failures included poor record-keeping, inadequate assessment, failure to recognise warning signs and share information, confusion of roles and responsibilities and poor management. Many of the problems relate to inadequacies in basic training and poor communication between agencies (Reder and Duncan 2004). While some of the inquiry reports highlight the training of specific groups, others also recommend training for professionals in working together. Interprofessional education is seen as central to improving practice.

The move towards interprofessional working has come about not only as a reaction to such failures but also from a shift of perspective in UK children's services over the past 20 years. Partly in response to the UN Convention on the Rights of the Child, there has been an increase in child-centred legislation, policies and practice that require all the relevant agencies to cooperate with each other, rather than work in silos. Implementation of 'partnership working' can mean a range of actions from improved communication and better role definition to fully integrated planning and shared budgets (see Chapter 21).

Training for collaboration

It has long been recognised that this kind of collaborative working will not happen by magic but requires sustained efforts to educate and support staff to work in this way.

Concerns emanating from the findings of the Maria Colwell Inquiry (DHSS 1974) led to the formation of Area Child Protection Committees whose remit included a responsibility to promote joint training to 'improve communication and collaboration'. National training programmes were also developed to aid the move towards a more cooperative and collaborative workforce. The Cleveland Inquiry Report (1988: p. 251) made clear that 'training is one of the major needs shown by the Cleveland experience' and argued that while the separate professions should each receive training at student level and continuing in-service training on the subject of child sexual abuse, there was also a need for *joint* training to promote understanding of the roles of other disciplines. For example, the report recommended that police officers and social workers should have joint training for the task of interviewing children. The Munro Review of Child Protection (2011) called for a move from a compliance culture to a learning one and pointed to the need to strengthen multi-agency training.

At a strategic level, *Every Child Matters*, DfSS (2003: SS.17.113 and 114) proposed that within a national framework different agencies should be required to bring staff together for training to promote joint working. This should not be a one-off event, however 'the skills involved in working successfully across organisational boundaries must be given proper recognition in both the initial and continuing training of staff'. The Green Paper emphasised the degree of change necessary, including the introduction of common occupational standards across children's services and a 'common core' of training both for professionals working mainly with children and families and for those with a wider remit such as GPs and the police. Similarly, in her book on child neglect, Horwath (2007: p. 231) argues strongly that effective multidisciplinary working depends on training to support collaborative practice.

The wide-ranging review of children's services *For Scotland's Children* (Scottish Executive 2001) recognised joint training as 'the most effective local mechanism to improve collaborative working' (p. 82) and commended a number of organisations such as Child Protection Committees and New Community Schools where this was already happening.

Barriers

The aspirational titles of policy documents, such as *Every Child Matters* (2003) and *Getting it Right for Every Child* (2005a), express strong determination to bring about change, but it has proved difficult to convert these good intentions into action. It is important to recognise a number of difficulties involved in providing interprofessional education for the wide range of different professionals who deliver services to children. Particularly where problems have arisen, it is not surprising that individuals may feel inhibited and defensive about coming together with colleagues from other agencies to reflect on their practice and analyse problems.

Mindsets

One barrier to effective interprofessional education originates in the earliest stages. Typically initial education and training is 'uniprofessional' and contacts with other professions during academic teaching are nil or minimal. This creates from the beginning a worldview that is difficult to break down in later years. Such mindsets arising from separate disciplinary education and training are likely to become embedded in practice and are very difficult to alter. Fundamental differences in attitude to, for example, the interests of children and adults, the importance of children's views or the balance between sharing information and respecting confidentiality tend to inhibit constructive dialogue and shared understanding. Practice placements or work shadowing arrangements may offer opportunities to work alongside other professions, but often in an unplanned and unanalysed way. Failure to address the need for collaboration at an early stage in professional education may lead different staff groups to develop dependence on their own rules and procedures and defensive working practices.

Complexity

Another issue is the complexity of children's services and the number of agencies involved. As Parton (2004: p. 88) points out, the Jasmine Beckford Inquiry (1985) focused on problems of communication between *two* caseworkers, whereas nearly twenty years later the Victoria Climbié Report (Laning 2003) revealed the difficulties within *a labyrinth of relationships* between caseworkers and several layers of management in different organisations involved in this single case. The professionals in the main disciplines – social work, education, health, police, law – differ in their initial training, roles and responsibilities, priorities, professional accountabilities and often values and ethical standpoints. In a literature review exploring interdisciplinary practice, McCallin (2001) demonstrates that in health service settings alone many tensions arise among professionals at different levels in multiple specialties responsible for varying aspects of patient care. Besides such professional and positional differences, Huxham (2003) identifies further obstacles to collaboration between people working in different organisations, including lack of common aims, absence of shared targets, different cultures, value bases and professional 'languages' and concerns about power often linked to control over funding. All these factors 'create areas of potential confusion and misunderstanding' and bringing these diverse groups together in an environment conducive to learning presents a considerable challenge (Humes 2006: p. 1).

Professional identity

In their study of professionalism in integrated children's services Anning et al. (2006) refer to the definition of professionalism by Sims et al. (1993), which includes the following characteristics:

- a systematic body of knowledge;
- a self-regulating code of ethics;
- control over entry to the profession;
- extended education leading to specific qualifications.

These are central to the development of a sense of professional identity, which may be challenged when individual professionals are required to work collaboratively with colleagues from other disciplines and are expected 'to confront, articulate and lay to one side the distinctiveness of their long established 'tribal' beliefs and behaviours,' (Anning et al. 2006: p. 71). Other differences affect communication at learning events, for example status differences.

Institutional factors

There are also significant institutional factors that present obstacles to improving the current position in relation to interprofessional education. A review undertaken by the Integrated Children's Services in Higher Education Project concluded that the complexity of higher education structures, including the divisions between subject disciplines, lack of coordination among professional regulatory frameworks and inconsistency of funding streams, can all present barriers to learning. While the project was cautious about the statistical significance of its findings, it noted that those Higher Education Institutions in which interprofessional education in children's issues was being actively addressed tended to be the newer institutions with a close connection to local communities, institutions involved in the development of foundation degrees, or older institutions with a tradition of providing teacher education (Higher Education Academy 2008). Three other factors found to be important for the promotion of interprofessional working and learning were:

- leadership from senior academics who could influence their counterparts in external agencies;
- the employment of specialist academics who were not linked to particular faculties and thus could work across boundaries to support interprofessional learning;
- 'brokers' i.e. individuals often with community development expertise, who helped make connections between different disciplines (Wenger 1998).

Other studies have noted the important role that faculty teachers, practical placements and practice teachers play in fostering awareness of the importance of interprofessional collaborative practice (Department of Health 2003). The emerging picture suggests that those professions and academic institutions that actively promote interprofessional practice have a cadre of individuals who are not only able to face the everyday challenge of understanding and adopting the established culture, but also have the capacity to formulate and articulate a desirable future culture (Engeström 1999).

Image

In addition, childcare work is undervalued in the UK. Very low levels of competence and qualification have traditionally been tolerated within some areas of children's services and staff working in low status, part-time jobs with poor career progression have, until recently, had limited access to ongoing training and development (Brannen et al. 2007). This image is now improving and changing. Numbers of qualified staff and levels of qualification have increased, in part through regulation and inspection. Other problems, such as shortage of funding and the related reluctance of agencies to release workers to participate in joint training events, unfortunately reduce the opportunities to participate in interprofessional education.

The rest of this chapter will consider the kind of strategies, processes and teaching methods needed to overcome these barriers and support effective interprofessional education for practitioners working in children's services.

Interprofessional education

Background

Interprofessional education in the United Kingdom had its roots in the 1960s and is characterised by the emergence of initiatives between different professionals in what Barr (2001) refers to as 'parallel interprofessional movements'. The World Health Organisation was proactive in encouraging developments in interprofessional education as early as 1973 with an Expert Committee review, which promoted the strategy of 'Health for All by the Year 2000'. The importance of interprofessional education also ran through the White Paper *Working Together: Learning Together* (Department of Health, 2001b). The Laming Report on the death of Victoria Climbié (Laning, 2003) suggested that in order to protect and safeguard children, policy support for interprofessional working must include resourcing of interprofessional learning. A major policy driver promoting interprofessional education was the NHS Plan of 2000, which recommended that all health professionals should have common learning with other professions at each stage of their professional development (Carpenter and Dickinson 2008). The Quality Assurance Agency has also sought to ensure that common elements are included in the curricula of, for instance, nursing and social work. Safeguarding boards have expanded training where a range of professions attend together.

Shared training has slowly grown over the decades and has been particularly strong in relation to early years services for which many qualifying child studies programmes exist. Otherwise it remains largely limited to short courses as part of continuing professional development, particularly in relation to child abuse and neglect.

Definitions

Like cooperation itself, interprofessional education may occur in varied ways and to different degrees. This is reflected in the different terms used to define it, whose meanings may be interpreted variously or overlap. For instance Bruner (1991) defines collaboration as 'a process that cannot be achieved by one single agent'. Others define collaboration in terms of a continuum and emphasise the importance of shared knowledge and common understanding. Yet others emphasise the importance of developing consensus in relation to values.

The Royal College of Nursing literature review (Clifton et al. 2006) notes that the range of descriptions of 'interprofessional education' includes a variety of confusing prefixes with 'inter', 'multi' and 'trans' used almost at random, which parallel the confusion of 'inter' terminology in relation to practice (see Chapter 21). The review accepted the following definition from the UK Centre for the Advancement of Interprofessional Education:

> The application of principles of adult learning to interactive, group-based learning, which relates collaborative learning to collaborative practice within a coherent rationale which is informed by understanding of interpersonal, group, organisational and inter-organisational relations and processes of professionalisation. (Clifton et al. 2006: p. 3)

Emphasising the idea of progression in a professional career, Carpenter and Dickinson (2008) distinguish four levels of professional training and education:

1. *uniprofessional* – involves only members of a single profession;
2. *multiprofessional* – two or more professions learn in parallel;
3. *interprofessional* – two or more professions learn with and from each other;
4. *transprofessional* – boundaries are crossed or merged.

Similarly a progression is described from *common learning* (following a similar curriculum) via *shared learning* (alongside each other) to *interactive learning*.

Purposes

The basic purposes of interprofessional education are to enable participants to know about and work with the roles of other professionals. In some cases, there can be additional expectations of preparedness to take on part of the role of another profession or follow a career route involving more than one profession (Carpenter and Dickinson 2008). There are dangers of a mismatch between the aspirations of course providers and those attending, so it is important to be clear especially whether aims are about mutual understanding or role blurring. The concept of interprofessional education can include an additional expectation of improvement, i.e. learning 'from and about each other to improve collaboration and consequently the quality of care' (Clifton et al. 2006: p. 3).

Learning strategies

Timing

As previously pointed out, the lack of interprofessional education in pre-qualification training may impede collaboration among different professional groups later on as young professionals enter practice. If, however, in the early years of study there was a core module that promoted a 'common' understanding by all those working with children of some of the basic issues relating to children, some of the misconceptions and distrust which develop early in the careers of professionals might be reduced. Ideally, therefore, shared interprofessional learning to promote team working should start in the initial stages of professional education (McCallin 2001). One major initiative designed to achieve this objective is the Common Core, which has been developed by the Children's Workforce Development Council (http://www.cwdcouncil. org.uk/common-core). First published in 2005, the Common Core sets out the skills and knowledge that all those working with children and young people should have:

- effective communication and engagement with children, young people and families;
- child and young person development;

- safeguarding and promoting the welfare of the child;
- supporting transitions;
- multi-agency working;
- sharing information.

These six areas of expertise offer a single framework to support integrated working, professional standards and training and qualifications across the children's workforce. Similar standards are being developed in other countries of the UK (Scottish Government 2011). These are being used to create simpler and more accessible careers paths (Northern Ireland Care Council 2011).

At later stages, this should be followed up by high-quality induction and carefully structured programmes of early professional development, which covers the first five years of a professional's career and is an important stage in continuing professional development, before professionals begin to develop more specialist knowledge and expertise (Taylor et al. 2011).

In-service training to provide updates on the implementation of legal and policy changes can be greatly enriched by the participation of staff from different professional standpoints. Similarly, cross-disciplinary groups can benefit from the opportunity to develop joint approaches to difficult social issues such as child offending, sexual abuse of children or the effects of drug and alcohol misuse.

Working in groups

Because working together involves people with different group allegiances (to their agency and/or profession) coming together in a mixed team, network or meeting, it is valuable to have an understanding of how groups function and how tensions and conflicts within and between groups can be ameliorated. Positive and negative stereotypes are likely to be present even before students begin training. Group experiments have shown that contact between groups with distinct separate identities is insufficient by itself to overcome suspicions and differences. It is important to build a new identification with the multidisciplinary enterprise and to increase interpersonal empathy in order to help break down stereotypes and misunderstandings about others (Crisp and Beck 2005; Christian et al. 2006).

Principles of adult learning

Interprofessional education is grounded in adult learning theory and has a task-centred or problem-based orientation. Both Knowles et al. (1984) and Kolb (1995) emphasise the demands that are placed on the learner – self-direction, reflection, teamwork, effective communication and adaptability. The key principles of adult learning include using real experiences of the learners, setting tasks and allowing the learners to solve scenarios in a discursive, team-based learning situation. Use is made of learning from direct practice or simulations. Reflective learning is encouraged by such means as a personal journal, regular feedback and peer debriefing, and discussions to promote the exchange of views. Such learning relies on the creation of a non-threatening learning environment that can support the exchange of real experience. It must also demonstrate relevance between work, learning and experience.

The learner has to believe that the organisation will embrace the results of such learning. Interprofessional education is most effective when there is strong organisational support for those taking part. By using this process of learning, collaboration is encouraged and the workforce is more likely to be responsive to required changes in practice such as improved communication.

Active learning with real problems

The Integrated Children's Services in Higher Education Project found that among effective 'tools' being used to promote interprofessional learning were Problem-based Learning and Action Learning Sets (Higher Education Academy 2008).

Problem-based Learning (PBL) is essentially about learning through tackling live issues. Participants work on a case or situation in small groups. They investigate and generate the information necessary to respond to the problems involved (see Recommended reading). When PBL is used as part of interprofessional education, a non-threatening training environment is particularly important. The structure of sessions should enable those taking part to reflect on and discuss their different professional roles and responsibilities. It can also be helpful to facilitate open exchange about the emotive and, at times, distressing nature of work with children who are in need.

Action Learning is based on the relationship between reflection and action, usually with the structured attention and support of a group. Put simply, it is about solving problems and getting things done (Fry et al. 2000). An Action Learning Set comprises a group of around eight people who meet on a regular basis to discuss issues of current concern and mutual importance. Sets are convened by a facilitator who agrees ground rules on important matters such as confidentiality and timekeeping. The focus is on the issues and problems that individuals bring and planning future action (Example 25.2).

Example 25.2

The work of Burgess (1999) provides illustrations of how sessions can be structured in stages (see Recommended reading). For instance:

- Group members make bids to discuss challenges they are facing in their work, such as how to deal with an aggressive parent or new manager.
- The group chooses two or three issues to focus on.
- Members seek clarification of the problems in the first case.
- Ideas are shared about how to deal with the problems.
- An action plan is agreed.
- Stages 3–5 are repeated for the other issues.

Developing a shared language

Training sessions that bring together a range of professionals form the ideal context within which to develop an understanding of what different professionals mean when they use terms such as 'risk', 'harm' or 'abuse'. Similarly, the training environment is the ideal setting to explore different professional perspectives on significant matters. For example, reflection on the term 'threshold of concern' (judgements about the extent to which a child is in need) is useful in so far as it requires professionals to articulate when and why to intervene in the life of a family (Beckett 2008). This will stimulate an exchange of views between different professionals on what is and is not acceptable.

The ethical dimension

As noted by Turnell and Edwards (1999; p. 197)

> Workers pursuing collaborative strategies often operate at the periphery of the protocols and conventions of normal agency practice and make decisions which are in the best interests of a range of stakeholders rather than blindly following the procedure of any one particular agency (see also Chapter 4).

Staff involved in many aspects of childcare work, particularly the most demanding situations where children are thought to be at risk, are required to apply particular virtues, like respect and fairness (Lonne et al. 2009). They have to think clearly and wisely in situations where emotions are fraught, information is lacking and yet urgent action may be required. Interprofessional education is one way of heightening shared awareness of the values that professionals apply when handling dilemmas. This includes deciding whether intervention is necessary to protect a child or prioritising the needs of one child over another in the allocation of a limited resource such as an early years place.

Learning with the 'new' technologies

Some of the practical challenges of providing interprofessional education for staff of many agencies can be overcome through the use of technology. Increasingly, distance learning makes use of a variety of forms of technology from the written word to the computer, including handheld electronic equipment such as smart phones. The advantages of these new methods for the learner are that they are flexible, convenient and can be fitted in with other commitments – work, family and other activities. They also offer the opportunity to interact with a greater number of people.

An increasing number of educational establishments are integrating distance learning/eLearning with on-campus courses. Blended learning and new pedagogies have been developed, most notably at the Open University (Salmon 2001; 2002). eLearning has the potential to strengthen and enliven distance learning and can be used in conjunction with more traditional face-to-face learning. Many methods of virtual learning encourage meaningful exchanges between participants – web communities, discussion boards, blogs, chatrooms and electronic voting systems.

Web-based models allow for the development of a central resource library, which can be available online at any time and to all members. This also allows for immediate updating/uploading and for the addition of links to extra materials for those who wish to learn in greater depth. However, this needs a webmaster who can control content, is aware of the issues being discussed and who can ensure that resources are up to date.

A shared set of competences

With the demands for closer working and closer learning among different groups of professionals there has been a move by policy-makers towards national standards and outcomes. There has also been consideration of the development of competence models for interprofessional education and a variety of approaches have been considered. A competence is a description of an action, behaviour or outcome, which can be demonstrated, and for each competence there are performance indicators, which can provide the evidence that the competence has been achieved.

Barr (2001) distinguishes between the various competence models used by different professions and has summarised them as:

- *common* – those held by most or all professional groups;
- *complementary* – those that distinguish between one profession and another;
- *collaborative* – those necessary for effective joint working.

The advantages of a competence model are that it provides clear guidelines about the desired outcome, agreed standards and a framework to assess personal development. This approach also identifies areas that may require additional learning and or support. It should also be noted that the issue of competency-based education is contested and some have argued that it enables the *status quo* to be maintained while creating an 'illusion' of change (Heron and Chakrabarti 2002).

As Barr suggests, the competences for interprofessional education need to promote effective and collaborative working practices. Professionals are enabled to articulate their own role and understand the role of others, as well as share ideas about ways to develop collaborative working within complex areas of work. Training can help professionals to develop more specific competences, such as how to chair case conferences and interdisciplinary meetings or handle conflicting perspectives on care and treatment.

Impact of interprofessional education

The evidence about the impact of interprofessional education is mixed. Huxham (2003) acknowledges that collaborative practice is not a panacea and can lead to disappointment and inertia due to the failure to achieve any shared meaningful purpose. However, she also says that many practitioners find simply it helpful to understand that the problems they are experiencing are inevitable. Given the right circumstances, there can be positive outcomes from collaborative engagement, which can result in advantage and synergy for all parties. These themes closely parallel Wenger's theory of 'communities of practice,' which are characterised by mutual engagement (co-participation), a joint enterprise (shared accountability), and shared repertoire (common discourses and concepts) (Anning et al. 2006). Such groups can derive much insight and support from opportunities to share experience and reflect on practice in a safe environment.

Lockyer and Stone (1998: p. 267) commend the value of the regular in-service training events, which offer volunteer children's panel members in Scotland 'the opportunity to share experience, debate issues with other agencies and renew and reinforce the commitment to service.' Anning et al. (2006) observed that over time, through experience of working together, barriers between professionals were eroded and new forms of shared professional identity emerged. Bringing people together in supported common objectives over a period of time can help them to 'break down stereotypes, build mutual knowledge and understanding and consider how to work with differences across organisational and professional boundaries' (Charles and Horwath 2009). For instance, an interprofessional education programme for doctors, nurses and social workers in Bristol led to fewer negative perceptions of the others. Certain conditions appear to foster positive learning about each other, including equal status in the programme, clear common goals and active efforts by teaching staff to examine typifications. The immediate effects of interprofessional education may differ from longer-term consequences (Carpenter and Dickinson 2008).

Conclusions and implications

Interprofessional education seeks to promote a common understanding of children's needs and circumstances that will contribute to the delivery of better integrated and more holistic services to children and their families. Increasingly the importance of a common core of skills, knowledge and competences is being promoted by UK governments, particularly through the *Every Child Matters* agenda and its equivalents elsewhere in the UK. However, as this chapter has demonstrated, opportunities for this kind of training are still patchy and a much more strategic approach is required. Pre-qualification training for all childcare professions should include a common core of knowledge to lay the foundations for genuine partnership working. This should be followed up by career-long opportunities for joint professional development and sharing of experience to increase confidence in fellow practitioners, address interprofessional misunderstandings and learn about the processes that can undermine or underpin positive collaboration. All this will promote joint accountability for ensuring that children's needs are met. To implement such a programme will require cooperation between governments, providers of education and training, local authorities and individual professional groups. The provision of adequate and consistent funding is crucial, particularly in times of increasing financial stringency. Only in this way can childcare professionals be prepared and be supported to carry out their essential and challenging work in the best interests of children.

Exercise

Read the scenario below. Find out about the knowledge and roles of the professionals with whom you are less familiar. Using role-play or discussion, consider how they might work in a more integrated way.

We are the parents of an eight-year-old boy with autism. We have contact with a range of professionals: a speech and language therapist, a nurse, child psychologist, child psychiatrist, special needs teacher, social worker and audiologist. They often ask us much the same questions or make appointments on the same date. Sometimes we wonder if they speak to each other. It can be very frustrating.

Recommended reading

Barr, H. (2011) Developing Interprofessional Education in Health and Social Care Courses, Occasional Paper 12, London, Health Science and Practice Project Centre.

http://www.cwdcouncil.org.uk/common-core
  Higher Education Academy (2008)
  For guidance on harmonising higher education structures and professional curricula.

http://www.gla.ac.uk/departments/thescottishforumforprofessionalethics/events/events0708/

www.heacademy.ac.uk/resources/detail/resource_database/id362_Imaginative_Curriculum_Guide_Problem_Based_Learning

http://www.robinburgessolpd.co.uk/downloads/actionoutline.doc/view
  All give details on problem-based and action learning methods

Chapter 26

Working together in children's services: constants and changes

Malcolm Hill, George Head, Andrew Lockyer, Barbara Reid and Raymond Taylor

The policy context

This book has been produced at a time of major change in the UK and international context, particularly related to the onset of recession from 2008 and the replacement of a new Labour government in Westminster after ten years by a Conservative – Liberal Democrat coalition government. The former has increased pressures on family income and resources. The latter introduced major reductions in funding to the public sector. The UK government has sought to promote what it hopes will be a compensating development in voluntary sector and volunteer effort (not the same) as part of the 'Big Society'. A number of more specific radical policy initiatives have included a shift to health service commissioning by GP and other health professionals, alterations in teacher education and training, greater autonomy for school heads, devolution to localities and a 'bonfire' of quangos, like the National CAMHS Support Service. The government is committed to reducing centralised recording and accountability procedures, which virtually all professional groups have complained about.

It is neither our role nor intention to comment from a party political perspective on this changed environment, but we are aware that throughout the history of the welfare state there has always been a plurality of providers of children's services, including private schools, medical care, leisure facilities and residential care. Similarly, recurrent tensions have been present about the respective parts to be played by public, charitable and private organisations, as well as self-help and mutual aid initiatives. Voluntary organisations have long made major, if fluctuating, contributions to child welfare provision, though in recent decades many have relied more on income from public sources than from fund-raising, bequests and so on. Periods of expansion of public expenditure, some of it passed on to non-governmental agencies and often crucial for them, have alternated with times of retrenchment. Similarly, governments have repeatedly espoused the value of local communities, while finding it hard to relinquish opportunities to insist on what they think is desirable. The boundaries and internal structures of the NHS and local authorities have been subject to periodic alteration.

We suspect, therefore, that the current changes will not be the last and that commitment to public services, alongside others, will be reaffirmed, as it was in the late

1940s and late 1990s, albeit doubtless in a different form. As ever, professionals working with children need to be able to adjust to policy shifts and reorganisations. The legal duties remain and, are likely to remain, to keep children's welfare at the forefront of thinking and action. The UN Committee on the Rights of the Child in 2002 and again in 2008 made clear their expectation that the best interests of children be 'adequately integrated' as a 'primary consideration' in all policy and legislation affecting children (2008: p. 7). The eminent judge, Dame Elizabeth Butler-Sloss (2010), argued that in times of austerity it is particularly vital for government measures to take account of the welfare of children. Naturally, opinion will vary about precisely what is best for children and how to achieve that, though various chapters in this book have pointed to the importance of reducing poverty, support for responsive parenting and access to quality education and healthcare from a young age.

We do not wish to suggest that everything changes, nor that change is inevitably cyclical. There have been continuities over the past 60 years, among which have been a strong commitment to children's welfare and a desire to increase opportunities for all children, even if the means of doing so have been oft disputed. Moreover, significant positive developments have occurred, for example greater emphasis on children's rights including, but not confined to, their participatory rights to comment on and influence decisions affecting them. The creation of four Children's Commissioner Offices has symbolised this increased recognition of children's rights and also provided formal mechanisms for furthering children's interests and representing their views in the public domain (Chapter 2). Early intervention is receiving renewed attention. It is a well-founded and long-standing policy aim, since at least the US intensive Head Start programme of the 1960s and similar initiatives like High/Scope Perry, which led not only to gains in education for the children, but in the long run reduced offending and improved employment prospects (Zigler and Styfco 1994).

The first decade of the twenty-first century witnessed a number of distinct trends in children's services in the UK. One of these was a substantial increase in overall resources and the numbers of most key professionals – doctors, nurses, teachers, police, social workers and so on. With the onset of economic problems after 2008 and the advent of the Coalition government committed to substantial reduction of expenditure, that the 'time of plenty' is over, at least for some years to come. Another key development has been the extension of devolution, which has led to greater diversification in policy in the four main jurisdictions and some differences in targets of expenditure. As all the main parties are now committed to devolution, this trend is not likely to be reversed. The question is whether it will now stabilise or further divergence will occur.

Children's professionals and agencies working collaboratively

A key feature of the past 10 years has been the emphasis of both central and devolved governments on cooperation between services in the children's fields, with aspirations that they become more joined-up, joint or integrated. Some elements of policy have been persuasive about collaboration, but certain measures have legally required it (as in the form of Children's Trusts in England and Wales) or made financial grants contingent on joint planning or action. In years to come, policy may put less emphasis on service integration and the terminology may change, but sadly recurrent child abuse enquiries over 40 years have indicated that, at the very least, effective communication and information sharing is a persistent requirement for safeguarding children at risk. At times of financial constraint, agencies may be tempted to look to others to help make up shortfalls, but limited resources also tend to engender a focus on one's core professional task so there may be less time and energy to look outwards.

A major theme of this book has been the ways in which different kinds of professional working with children relate to each other. In a number of circumstances close working together is not needed or desirable. However, overlap and contact is often unavoidable, just as children's lives do not divide up neatly into silos. It is not possible for any single profession or service to meet all the needs and fulfil the rights of children and their families, while many issues such as safeguarding children's welfare, health education and tackling youth crime require the input of several agencies. Hence cooperation is necessary and has taken place to a greater or lesser extent, for better or for worse, ever since the evolution of formal services. The police, for example, have increasingly recognised that their role in protecting children as citizens and addressing crime by young people is dependent on working collaboratively with other professions, especially to try to prevent family and neighbourhood difficulties leading young children to set out on criminal or antisocial pathways (Chapter 10). Several chapters have pointed to the need to take account of the full range of services beyond education, health and social work. For instance, recreational and sports facilities, libraries and various forms of youth and outreach work can provide vital opportunities for children to learn, develop social skills and make valuable supportive connections.

Yet research and experience reviewed in this book has shown that there are many barriers to collaboration and that efforts to work more closely tend to have varied and usually mixed results (Chapter 21). Hence it is vital to understand the complex processes involved in cooperation and the different factors at work when collaborating between different organisations (perhaps in different sectors – public, private or NGO), across professional boundaries or both. Equally, there are times for specialist work to be carried on in parallel and other times when coordination or joint work is desirable. Integration across whole service areas requires careful preparation and a multiple strategy including organisational restructuring, information sharing, mentoring and shifts in professional cultures (Chapter 5). Even then, the history of integrated services in the early years shows how hard it can be to reconcile multiple objectives, such as tackling poverty, ensuring a healthy start to life, providing high-quality education and offering good social care (Chapter 8). Several chapters in this book have reviewed research evidence and different kinds of theory that should help ensure that managers and practitioners are better able to decide when and how close working is necessary and how it can work well (Chapters 4 and 22). It is important that awareness of such a knowledge base is made accessible in professional training and to people in the field as well as to policy makers.

For many years efforts have been made to enable students on different kinds of professional education programmes to meet and share learning, stimulated particularly by findings of poor communication and misunderstandings when children have been ill treated (Chapter 25). Success in inter-disciplinary training has been limited in scope and scale, owing in part to different patterns of mixing academic and 'on the job' learning, in teacher, medical, nursing and social work education for instance. Other inhibiting factors have been differing specific requirements from professional education regulatory bodies and the large and growing extent of essential knowledge and skills necessary for any particular occupation. Continued efforts are needed and should be accompanied by wisdom gained about how people with contrasting remits, goals, specialist language and so on can interact productively and not reinforce negative stereotypes. There may be scope for new professional configurations, as has been witnessed in the development of early years workers drawing on a mix of previously separate expertise. The role of social pedagogue, widespread on the continent and introduced tentatively in a few parts of the UK, has the potential to enhance working across interfaces to help the whole child develop in varied areas of his/her life (Chapter 6).

Cooperation involving children services is not only a matter of relations between different children's organisations in the same area. Collaboration across agency geographical boundaries is also important because families move, while differences in entitlement can lead to a 'geographical lottery' where, for instance, sports and music or subsidised transport for children are much more readily available in one area than in an adjacent one. In general separate agencies cherish their autonomy, but efficiency considerations and cutbacks have prompted some local authorities to work closely together or even merge responsibility for services as in inner London. A common view at the time of writing is that fewer police forces are needed, so that mergers are desirable. No easy answer exists about the ideal size of local, health or police authorities. Large size facilitates economies of scale, cross-subsidisation for the benefit of poorer sub-districts and consistency of policies across a substantial area. On the other hand, small can be beautiful with regard to responsiveness to local opinion and needs, as well as avoidance of what may be experienced as excessive bureaucracy and large political fiefdoms.

Coordination problems also arise at the interface between children's and adult services. Young people with mental-health problems or who offend often encounter gaps and difficult adjustments as they pass from the responsibility of child and adolescent mental health services and youth justice agencies to adult systems, sometimes with an abrupt change at a specific age threshold. Many young people in foster and residential care continue to find it difficult to manage when the time comes to leave, often prematurely, despite the development of through-care and after-care programmes intended to support their practical and social coping as young adults. Likewise, policies exhorting joint working by agencies at the transition to adulthood and personalisation practices have only partially overcome the deficiencies in support and confusion often experienced by young people with learning disabilities and their families (Chapters 20).

Similarly, problems can arise when adult services seeking to help individuals who are parents do not recognise or respond to the effects of the adults on their children. Cleaver et al. (2007) found that housing, substance misuse and domestic violence issues were frequently present in child abuse cases, but the relevant adult-focused agencies were not routinely involved at any stage of the child protection process.

The legal, theoretical and research bases for work with children

In this book we have not attempted the anyway impossible task of covering all the knowledge areas that are important for professionals, since that is the remit of more specialist texts. However, we have outlined the legal basis for children's services, which embodies key principles that all should seek to put into practice. British legislation and policy has been influenced by and must take account of international treaties, most notably the UNCRC and European law embodied in the Human Rights Act 1998. It is also important that internationally agreed standards are followed, such as those of the Council of Europe that emphasise decriminalisation of young people and diversion from formal processes, wherever possible (Chapter 7).

Within the different jurisdictions of the UK the policy frameworks vary in detail, as is the intention of devolved government, but a great deal of consistency exists in policy documents (and academic thinking) about the key dimensions of children's lives that should be at the heart of professional activities alongside the specific tasks of each particular role. These include ensuring that children are safe and well, assisting them to learn, listening to them, treating their views with respect and supporting them to be responsible for themselves and towards others. Attending to the views of children not only reflects their entitlement to participate, but is one vital key to ensuring services are relevant and effective. The location and layout of services, signage, responses by both receptionists and professional staff, as well as young people's prior experience of informal help and guidance, all affect the likelihood of service uptake and influence the extent to which individual young people will respond to professional efforts (Chapter 2). Likewise, careful balancing of children's wishes and adults' perceptions of what is best for them is required when lawyers and others are involved in representing children (Chapter 13). Mechanisms for taking account of children's views more collectively have proliferated in recent years, for instance in school councils. It is important to avoid tokenism and be clear about the purposes of such developments, which can be multiple and do not always fit with children's and young people's own expectations (Chapter 12).

For some time now, many policy-makers and practitioners have espoused a commitment to 'evidence-based' work. The precise terminology and meanings may change in future, but it seems highly probable that research evidence will continue to play a vital part in informing policy and practice. Most of our chapters have incorporated relevant empirical findings, though naturally these have required summarising and interpreting. In the health field, research has provided valuable findings at widely different levels. It has identified simple measures that can help parents, recognised the value of lay expertise and shown what kinds of early intervention programmes are helpful (Chapters 16 and 17). Research has also made clear that good and poor health outcomes are inextricably linked to wider inequalities and risks. Furthermore, careful analysis of international comparative data by Wilkinson and Pickett (2009)[1] has indicated that in countries with lower levels of inequality than the UK not only do 'poor' children do better, but the whole of society benefits.

The book has included a number of concepts (with their associated research bases), which can help form a common currency for those of different disciplinary backgrounds working with children. Ideas about attachment, resilience and desistance, for instance, help professionals understand the factors and processes that enable children to lead happy or troubled lives, or that can aid in overcoming difficulties (Chapters 18 and 19). They also illuminate the close interaction between family relationships and children's care, emotions, learning and behaviour. When problems arise in one of these areas, it is common for them to be connected to difficulties in others. These overlaps are particularly evident when children's upbringing is seriously problematic on account of abuse, neglect and/or being looked after in public care (Chapter 24). That interconnectedness of problems and the reasons for them is part of the reason why professionals with expertise in one aspect of children's lives need to cooperate with others who specialise in another aspect.

It is clearly important for professionals to understand how individual children develop and the kinds of needs and rights they have. However, the ways in which these play out is crucially affected by their family, neighbourhood and societal environments. Hence much professional activity will be affected by influences and resources in the local and wider community. Access to safe, suitable informal spaces and to organised activities are crucially affected by household income and quality of the local neighbourhood (Wager et al. 2009). Schools can play a major role in providing a base for free or low-cost additional services and linking children to other resources. However, attempts to create a more inclusive role for early years provision and schools as a community hub have been only partially successful and require more imaginative ways of locating formal learning and teaching within a broader set of children's needs and services (Chapters 11 and 23).

Looking beyond the child to the local and wider environment also means that those working with children can benefit from exposure to a range of academic disciplines as well as professional disciplines. Psychology, including its ecological, social and community variants, has a major part to play but the past two decades have seen a burgeoning contribution from sociology and anthropology, sometimes linked to historical and philosophical analyses about the position of children *vis à vis* adulthood and wider society. Within geography, unprecedented attention to how children make sense of and make use of formal and informal spaces and routes has been sufficient to warrant a journal dedicated to the topic. Examples of key socially oriented conceptual frameworks have been given in the book. Chapter 15 highlighted the importance of understanding changes in family practices alongside

---

[1] There have, however, been criticisms of the selection and interpretation of evidence.

demographic and household changes. Professionals can gain from understanding the opportunities and constraints of social networks, including such notions as reciprocity and peer support, and also help children and young people to make better use of or revive existing relationships (close and distant) or develop new positive ones (Chapter 9). Network theory links to the notions of social capital that help inform understanding of relationships between professionals and organisations as well as within communities. It has been pointed out, though, that social capital thinking may underplay children's perspectives and some of the negative consequences of trusting social groupings (e.g. exclusion of outsiders) (Portes 1998; Morrow 1999).

At the same time as the academic underpinnings of ecological approaches and social contexts have been strengthening, significant developments have occurred in the opposite direction with regard to what goes on inside a child's body and brain. New insights from studies in neuroscience have valuable implications for understanding the complex relationships between parenting, stress, events in the brain and outcomes for children. Leckman and March (2011) conclude that the processes discovered do not suggest crude genetic or molecular determinism, but that very early experiences including abuse affect brain functioning, which in turn contributes to later responses to stress and ability to learn. Similarly, as a sociologist, Prout (2005) pointed to the need to avoid oversimple dualisms and eschew both biological and social determinism by focusing on the interactions between human biology and cultural constructions. Examples of such an interactive approach have involved analysis of the ways in which conceptions of children's bodies impact on their experiences (Horschelmann and Colls 2009).

Ideas about childhood, adulthood and citizenship

Underpinning all policies with respect to children are ideas about childhood, which we view as 'socially constructed' in that they are shaped by prevailing ideas and values, often different from those adhered to in the past or in other cultures. Implicitly or explicitly, a number of chapters have shown how academic thinking, policy and practice have been affected by competing conceptions of children – along spectra of deficiency to competence, passivity to agency, innocence to innate 'badness', vulnerability to threat, among others. Thus, it is vital to constantly question and debate presuppositions in order to avoid the dangers of idealisation and negative stereotyping. Professionals have a duty here not only to be vigilant about their own patterns of thinking but also to contribute to public debates, where oversimplification is a ready resort.

A frequent assertion is that, for all their differences, everyone working with children can unite in a common goal of furthering children's best interests. Certainly it is vital in talk of working together not to forget what it is all about and to recognise a shared purpose. At the same time, we must recognise that both professionals and lay people hold divergent aspirations for children, so that promoting children's welfare may entail very different and sometimes conflicting aims – or means to reach those aims. This is illustrated by views about faith schools or the best way to enhance social mobility, for instance. Thus, it is valuable for regular debate to occur in various media about what is best for children, as far as possible based on fair representation of viewpoint, mutually respectful processes and genuine efforts to set preconceptions and self-interest to one side.

Notions about childhood are linked to ideas about adulthood. This is illustrated by the age-old concept of citizenship, which has featured in different guises in several recent policy initiatives (Chapter 14). Some have held citizenship to be a characteristic acquired only once adulthood has been achieved, so that in this view children are future citizens, but not current holders of that status. This has been one of the main emphases in citizenship education – namely, that children need adequate preparation for later adult responsibilities. An opposite view is that children are citizens now, with the same entitlements and responsibilities as adults. This is qualified by competence requirements but the main point is that children should not be prevented from doing things like voting or choosing not to go to school on the basis of age alone. A middle viewpoint is that children are citizens in the making, so they gradually acquire participatory rights and responsibilities as they gain in competence (Lockyer 2010). Studies have shown that most children have a sense of duty towards others and their local community. They are predisposed to an active concept of citizenship and many do engage in volunteering (IVR 2008).

Some children's services have long welcomed the contributions of adult volunteers as active citizens in providing support to or mentoring children, parents or families as a whole. More specialist roles may be undertaken, as by volunteer (as opposed to paid) teaching assistants and volunteer special constables. In some contexts, the use of volunteers has evoked concerns about insufficient training or that they undermine properly funded work. It is important to clarify when and how professionals and volunteers can engage in productive collaboration.

Approaches to the role of professionals working with children and their families

A range of views exist about the appropriate relationship between a practitioner and a member of the public, symbolised in part by various terms used to depict the latter – e.g. patient, client, service user, consumer, customer, partner. Any particular individual's stance will reflect many different influences, including the profession to which they belong, personal values, evidence of service effectiveness, feedback about satisfaction and so on. This book has included chapters with different emphases and orientations in order to reflect that diversity. Here we briefly consider some of the critical considerations.

At the risk of oversimplification, two places on the spectrum may be described as 'expert' and 'empowerment' based. Certain individuals and types of professional tend to espouse a more expert approach, whereby the main role of professionals is to understand the need, issue or problem and provide or suggest an answer or solution, drawing on their theoretical, empirical and practical knowledge and experience. For instance, certain textbooks on child and adolescent mental health sometimes begin with understanding the 'presenting problem' from the child and family's viewpoint, but thereafter the thrust of assessment involves the professional gathering evidence to identify symptoms and categorise the problem through a diagnosis that fits with standard 'disorders' or 'conditions'. Key elements in assessment are formal mental state examinations and psychometric assessment, alongside personal, medical and family history. Likewise, professional actions are framed in terms of treatment or management by the practitioner or service, though some interventions do involve a degree of working together on the issue (e.g. solution focused therapy) (Goodman and Scott 2005; Dogra et al. 2008).

Even if done sensitively, this can be criticised for being top-down, giving insufficient attention to people's own perspectives, not building on or up capacities, or even of creating power-based relationships. Also, diagnostic and other labels may lead professionals to think about children as having a single primary identity that is relatively fixed and can lead to self-fulfilling prophecies. For instance, research has shown how teacher expectancies can significantly affect pupil performance (Johnston-Wilder and Collins 2008). Problems that are at least in part influenced by the social context in which they occur may be individualised and pathologised (Davis 2011). Of course, there can be situations, especially in an emergency, when someone else taking control is to be welcomed. Furthermore, while children and parents want their wishes and lay understandings respected, they often look to professionals to deploy their knowledge and practice wisdom, whether about quadratic equations or concerning the nature and causes of problems and about what may be good ways to deal with them.

The empowerment approach aims to work from the perspective of the person(s) to be taught or helped. As noted in the Introduction, this orientation has become influential in a range of settings (Rixon 2008a). As far as possible, the capacities of users, students, patients or clients to deal with the matters under consideration are to be tapped into and enhanced. This position is seen as more equal and democratic than the traditional expert role. Arguably, additional expertise is required to adopt the empowerment mode, since it relies on communication skills to engage more fully with service users and convey specialist knowledge in a less direct way. When it works well, people can be strengthened not only to handle present problems better but also future challenges. Similarly, actively engaged learners develop longer-term motivations and strategies for knowledge acquisition. The focus of empowerment may be a child, parents or the family as a whole. Pinkerton and Katz (2003) suggest that family support needs to be based on partnership with parents and children, which involves respect for both. A key role is to reach out to vulnerable families and help strengthen their social resources.

Yet it can be argued that empowerment models may deny actual power differences, give a false sense of equality and divest professionals of responsibility. In some circumstances it may be necessary to deploy professional authority or a legal sanction to override the autonomy of the individual because otherwise serious harm will occur, as in some circumstances of abuse, bullying or violence. Moreover, tensions occur when seeking to reconcile 'partnership' relationships with parents and children, if their (perceived) interests or views do not coincide. It is often possible to take account of the views of both adults and children and seek resolution or compromise, but at times it is necessary to act against one or both in the interests of a child's health or safety.

A slightly different but related model is that of 'inclusion'. This has been applied quite generally in the notion of social inclusion with the aim of ensuring that children are not 'excluded' from the usual benefits or acceptance in society because of poverty, disability, ethnicity or other factors. Within education an inclusive approach seeks to emphasise the positives in individuals and to cater for the 'needs of a wide range of children within diverse classrooms' (Forlin 2010: p. 247). Alongside values about respect and variety, it requires a certain kind of expertise based on understanding children's many differences in background and orientation to learning, as much as inculcation of curriculum specific knowledge.

Davis (2011) illustrates the contrast between 'expert' and 'empowerment/inclusive' approaches by the examples of circle time (where children share experiences and views in class) and cognitive behavioural therapy (which involves professionals seeking to motivate children or parents to change their ways of thinking and acting). He states that the first envisages the adult role as facilitating learning and dialogue, while in the latter the adult's role is to ensure that children (or adults) 'know the correct way to behave' (p. 68).

Within a range of service areas, traditional expert models have been criticised for using 'deficit' and 'risk' models, which stress deficiencies that need correcting or overcoming. The problems may be seen as residing largely in the person concerned, though it is also recognised that there are environmental health and social risks or external barriers to learning. Alternative models put more emphasis on the strengths and capacities of individuals, families and communities.

Naturally, those who lean to the more expert or empowerment, deficit or strength perspectives are often aware of the complexities. Many health professionals do not espouse fully so-called 'medical models' of mental health and disability (Connors and Stalker 2003; Davis 2011). They take a holistic, inclusive view of children and give them opportunities to discuss their feelings, wishes and opinions. Many health-promotion activities are founded on consultation and evidence about young people's views, as in relation to sex education, mental health or alcohol use (e.g. Day 2008; Ingram and Salmon 2010). As stated at the outset, we believe it is most helpful to seek to work with the positives in situations and as far as possible in constant dialogue taking account of service users' viewpoints, but it is also important not to ignore weaknesses and hazards.

Much of the foregoing applies equally to children and adults. A similar spectrum can be recognised when considering orientations specifically towards children. In the past the predominant mode has been for professionals to regard their primary duty as optimising children's development, health, learning etc. based on practitioners' own judgements or diagnoses about needs and problems. The growth of children's participatory rights in law and society, as well as of academic perspectives stressing children's agency, have supported a more participatory approach. Even so, the UNCRC and legislation within the UK require professionals and decision-makers to make children's welfare and interests the primary consideration or, on some issues, the paramount influence (O'Halloran 1999). This is why judicial systems dealing with disputes concerning children usually have mechanisms to ensure that a child's wishes are effectively represented, while decisions ultimately centre on the child's interests.

Prout (2011), a leading critic of developmental approaches to children, has recently argued that it is necessary to move beyond dualisms, such as structure and agency, nature and culture, discourse and materiality. He believes it is vital to recognise the plurality of childhoods and interrelationships not only between the various actors involved in a child's life but also between the biological and social. This requires professionals to be able to manage ambiguity and complexity. A child's experience is not the product of genetics, a natural unfolding of development, family environment, exercise of individual choices etc., but a complicated amalgam of all of these. Prout advocates the use of actor–network theory, which attends to the web of relationships in which individuals are embedded. Crucially, this theory includes connections and disconnections with artefacts and technologies as well as human relationships, which echoes the consideration of varied tools, material and interpersonal, in Vygotskian education (see Chapter 4). Davis (2011) has also argued that a 'post-modern' perspective is desirable, which recognises the complexity and diversity of both children and the service nexus.

Working beyond the individual

Many professionals work primarily or exclusively with individual children and families, or with groups of children, notably in schools. However, many of the chapters in this book have highlighted how children's well-being and prospects are greatly affected by wider processes in society, including central, devolved and local government policies. This raises the question of when and how professionals – acting alone or together – should attempt to tackle problems on a community, population or even national level. In some instances (e.g. health promotion, youth work, community policing) there is a specific remit to work in that way.

Cooper (2008) argues that both Conservative and New Labour administrations have focused too much on individuals in their strategies to tackle youth crime and antisocial behaviour. He argued that it is necessary to understand the problematic impact on young people's lives of income poverty and neighbourhood decline. Similar points have been made in relation to tackling health inequalities and educational disadvantage.

Dominelli (2011) indicates that practitioners should consider the interaction between individual and collective needs, taking account of convergences and divergences. She argues that practitioners should assist people to challenge attitudes and processes that isolate, marginalise or oppress them (e.g. on the basis of race, ability, class or age), while promoting commonalities that cross social divisions. Similarly Moss (2008) highlights the importance of reflecting on how social divisions based on such characteristics as race, gender and sexuality may affect children's access to and experience of services. This can involve:

- awareness raising – e.g. about the needs of disabled children;
- advocating on behalf of individuals or groups who are marginalised or discriminated against;
- helping local groups organise to help each other, handle social problems or campaign (Holman 2001; Ferguson and Woodward 2009).

For instance, many public health nurses in Canada see poverty as having a major influence on the problems they are dealing with and believe it is part of the role of regional health authorities to raise awareness about child and family poverty and to seek to change public policies in the interests of child health (Cohen and McKay 2010).

While professional bodies can and do aim to influence national policies at UK and devolved levels (as illustrated by intense debates about health and education service reform), the main scope for many practitioners to affect environments beyond the individual or family lie at the local or neighbourhood level. A wide range of activities are possible from the highly specific, like developing play facilities, to broad-based economic regeneration and supporting or creating social networks and organisations. The police and youth workers have established outreach and activity-based projects aiming to increase pro-social connections and skills in disadvantaged community with a view to reducing stress, conflict and violence within the home and on the street.

Craig (2007), though, cautions about the danger that seeking to build up the social, political and economic capacities of communities has often not had much benefit for local people but served more the interests of the powerful, the state or even of large charitable organisations.

Furthermore, many community development activities have been largely conducted by adults even when children have been potential beneficiaries. Some areas have developed children's fora, youth councils and other organisations to represent children's views, but despite this the great majority of children have no contact with councillors, police or decision-makers and have little idea how to influence their local community and environment (Matthews 2001; Christensen and O'Brien 2003). Two main kinds of impeding factors can be recognised:

1. The tendency of adults to regard children and young people as irrelevant or threats to community well-being.

2. The alienation of many young people and their lack of power and confidence (Kettle 2008).

Increasingly, though, it has come to be expected that children can and should be involved in crucial decisions about policies and services affecting them.

Final remarks

Working effectively and respectfully with children and their families will always involve a complex mix of legal, policy and/or agency imperatives, theoretical and empirical knowledge, accumulated professional or clinical wisdom, personal and shared values and critical awareness and reflection. Working well with others for the sake of children requires careful thought and empathy to ensure that differences in expertise, aims, approach and organisational context complement and enhance each other, rather than obscure or obstruct the shared wish to optimise children's lives. We hope this book makes a contribution to that vitally important enterprise.

Recommended reading

There is a growing body of general purpose journals about children and many are now available electronically through libraries. *Children & Society* contains articles on a wide range of policies and services related to children, mainly but not exclusively in the UK. The *Journal of Children's Services* has a focus on research evidence about child development and service evaluations, but also covers relevant legal and policy matters. *Childhood* and *Children's Geographies* attend to children's everyday lives and include papers relating to different parts of the world. *The International Journal of Children's Rights*, as its name suggests, has a focus on rights and legal matters, but covers a wide range of issues. *Youth Policy* concentrates on policy and practice related to young people. Articles on policies relevant to children and families are to be found at times in journals such as *Social Policy* and *Society* and *Critical Social Policy*.

Many journals are targeted at particular professional audiences, but often publish items of interest to a wider audience – e.g. *Journal of Educational Enquiry; Journal of Child Psychology and Psychiatry; Child: care, health and development; Child and Family Social Work; Journal of Social Welfare and Family Law.* Some deal with specialist topics – e.g. *Child Abuse Review, Youth Justice, Adoption & Fostering, Journal of Family Therapy.*

Valuable sources of information about children's lives and use of services are to be found in cohort studies that follow up representative samples of children from birth or an early age. The Millennium study has a wealth of data on children in the UK born in 2000 (Hansen et al. 2010a). The samples in Scotland, Wales and Ireland were 'boosted' in number so that they were adequate for analysis and separate reports have been published for these countries in addition to UK overviews. The Growing Up in Scotland study is gathering information on somewhat younger children. (http://www.crfr.ac.uk/gus/).

For information on children at a later age, the Avon Longitudinal Study of Parents and Children (ALSPAC) includes many details about the health and development of children born in the early 1990s. http://www.bristol.ac.uk/alspac/ The organisation Young People in Focus (formerly the Trust for the Study of Adolescence) provides access to research findings on young people aged 10–25. http://www.studyofAdolescence.org.uk/

Bibliography

11 Million (2009a) *Business Plan of 11 Million* (Children's Commissioner for England), London, July.

11 Million (2009b) *Child Rights Impact Assessment of the Equality Bill*, 11 Million (Children's Commissioner for England), London, May.

Ainsworth, M. D. S. (1979) 'Infant–mother attachment', *American Psychologist*, Vol. 34, No. 10, pp. 932–37.

Alderson, P. (2000) '*School students*' views on school councils and daily life at School', *Children and Society* 12(2), pp. 121–34.

Aldgate, J. (2002) 'Evolution not revolution: family support services and the Children Act 1989', in *Approaches to Needs Assessment in Children's Services*, Ward, H. and Rose, W. (eds), London: Jessica Kingsley Publishers.

Aldgate, J. (2011) 'Ensuring that every child really does matter', in R. Taylor, M. Hill and F. McNeill (eds) *21st Century Social Workers: A resource for early professional development*, London: Venture Press.

Aldgate, J., Jones, D., Rose, W. and Jeffery, C. (2006) *The Developing World of the Child*, London: Jessica Kingsley.

Alexander, C. (2008) *(Re)thinking 'Gangs'*, London: Runnymede Trust.

Allan, J., Ozga, J. and Smith, G. (eds) (2009) *Social Capital, Professionalism and Diversity*. Rotterdam: Sense.

Allan, J. and Smyth, G. (2009) 'Connections: children's social capital and diversity', in J. Allan, J. Ozga and G. Smith (eds) *Social Capital, Professionalism and Diversity*, Rotterdam: Sense, pp. 193–205.

Allen, G. (2011) *Early Intervention: the next steps*: an independent report to HM Government, London, http://media.education.gov.uk/assets/files/pdf/g/graham%20 allens%20review%20of%20early%20intervention.pdf.

Andrews, D. and Bonta, J. (2003) *The Psychology of Criminal Conduct* (3rd edition), Cincinnati, OH: Anderson Publishing.

Andrews, D., Zinger, I., Hoge, R., Bonta, J., Gendreau, P. and Cullen, F. (1990) 'Does correctional treatment work? A clinically relevant and psychologically informed meta-analysis', *Criminology*, 28, pp. 369–404.

Anglin, J. (2002) *Pain, Normality and the Struggle for Congruence*, New York: Haworth Press.

Anisfield, E., Casper, V., Nozyce, M. and Cunningham, N. (1990) 'Does infant carrying promote attachment? An experimental study of the effects of increased physical contact on the development of attachment', *Child Development*, 61, pp. 1617–27.

Annette, J. (2010) 'Democratic citizenship and lifelong learning' in Crick and Lockyer *op. cit.*

Anning, A., Cottrell, D., Frost, N., Green, J. and Robinson, M. (2006) *Developing Multi-professional Teamwork for Integrated Children's Services*, Buckingham: Open University Press.

Anning, A., Cottrell, D., Frost, N., Green, J. and Robinson, M. (2010) *Developing Multi-professional Teamwork for Integrated Children's Services*, Buckingham: Open University Press.

Antonovsky, A. (1987) *Unravelling the Mystery of Health*, San Francisco: Jossey-Bass.

Argyris, C. (1992) *On organizational learning*, Oxford: Blackwell.

Arshad, R., Forbes, J. and Catts, R. (2007) 'The role of social capital in Scottish educational policy', *Scottish Educational Review*, 39(2), pp. 127–37.

Association of Chief Police Officers (2010) *Children and Young People Strategy 2010–2013*, www.acpo.police.uk.

Audit Commission (2008) *Are we there yet?* London: Audit Commission.

Axford, N. (2010) 'What's in a service?', *Child and Family Social Work*, 15(4), pp. 473–82.

Axford, N. and Whear, R. (2008) 'Measuring and meeting the needs of children and families in the community: Survey of parents on a housing estate in Dublin, Ireland', *Child Care in Practice*, 14(4), pp. 331–53.

Bachman, M., O'Brien, M., Husbands, C., Shreeve, A., Jones, N., Watson, J., Reading, R., Thoburn, J. and Mugford, M. (2009) 'Integrating children's services in England: national evaluation of children's trusts', *Child: Care, Health and Development*, 35(2), pp. 257–65.

Backett-Milburn, K., Wilson, S., Bancroft, A. and Cunningham-Burley, S. (2008) 'Challenging childhoods: young people's accounts of "getting by" in families with substance use problems', *Childhood*, 15, pp. 461–79.

Baer, J. C. and Martinez, C. D. (2006) 'Child maltreatment and insecure attachment: a meta-analysis', *Journal of Reproductive and Infant Psychology*, Vol. 24, No. 3, pp. 187–97.

Baker, K. and Sutherland, A. (2009) *Multi-agency Public Protection Arrangements and Youth Justice*, Bristol: Policy Press.

Bakermans-Kranenburg, M. J., van IJzendoorn, M. H. and Juffer, F. (2003) 'Less is more: meta-analyses of sensitivity and attachment interventions in early childhood', *Psychological Bulletin*, 129, pp. 195–215.

Bancroft, A., Carty, A., Cunningham-Burley, S. and Backett-Miburn, K. (2002) *Support for the Families of Drug Users*, Edinburgh: Scottish Executive.

Bannister, J., Pickering, J., Batchelor, S., Burman, M., Kintrea, K. and McVie, S. (2010) *Troublesome Youth Groups, Gangs and Knife Carrying in Scotland*, Edinburgh: Scottish Government.

Barber, J. (2003) *Social Work with Addictions*, Basingstoke: Macmillan.

Barnard, M. and McKeganey, N. (2004) 'The impact of parental problem drug use on children: what is the problem and what can be done to help?', *Addiction*, Vol. 99, pp. 552–59.

Barnes, M., Newman, J. and Sullivan, H. (2007) *Power, Participation and Political Renewal*, Bristol: Policy Press.

Barnsley Metropolitan Borough Council (2005) *Remaking Learning: Leading Change for Success*, Barnsley: Barnsley MBC.

Barr, H. (2001) *Inter-professional Education Today, Yesterday and Tomorrow*, London: Higher Educational Academy.

Barry, M. (2006) *Youth Offending in Transition*, Abingdon: Routledge.

Batchelor, S. (2009) 'Girls, gangs and violence: assessing the evidence', *The Probation Journal*, 56(4), pp. 399–414.

Baxter, S., Brookes, C., Bianchi, K., Rashid, K. and Hay, F. (2009) 'Speech and language therapists and teachers working together: exploring the issues', *Child Language Teaching and Therapy*, 25(2), pp. 215–34.

Bayat, M. (2007) 'Evidence of resilience in families of children with autism', *Journal of Intellectual Disability Research*, 51(9), pp. 702–14.

Becher, H. (2008) *Family Practices in South Asian Muslim Families: Parenting in a Multi-Faith Britain*, Basingstoke: Palgrave.

Beck, U. (1992) *Risk Society*, London: Sage.

Beckford Report. (1985) *A Child in Trust*, Wembley, London: Borough of Brent.

Beckett, C. (2007) *Child Protection*, London: Sage.

Beckett, C. (2008) 'Risk, uncertainty and thresholds in contemporary risk assessment', in M. Calder (ed.) *Safeguarding Children*, London: Routledge.

Belsky, J., Barnes, J. and Melhuish, E. (eds) (2007) *The National Evaluation of Sure Start – Does Area-based Early Intervention Work?*, Bristol: The Policy Press.

Benzies, K. and Mychasiuk, R. (2009) 'Fostering family resiliency', *Child and Family Social Work*, 14(1), pp. 103–14.

Beresford, B. (2004) 'On the road to nowhere? Young disabled people and transition', *Child: Care, Health and Development*, 30(6), pp. 581–87.

Bertram, T., Pascal, C., Bokari, S., Casper, M. and Holterman, S. (2002) *Early Excellence Centre Pilot Programme: Second Evaluation Report 2000–2001*, DfES Research Report RR361, London: HMSO.

Berzins, S. C. (2010) 'Vulnerability in the transition to adulthood: defining risk based on youth profiles', *Children and Youth Services Review*, 32, pp. 487–95.

Beyer, S. (2008) *Transition from School to Employment. What Works?* Llias, 2008.

Bignall, T., Butt, J. and Pagarani, D. (2002) *'Something to do': The development of peer support groups for young black and minority ethnic disabled and deaf people*, York: The Policy Press.

Bilson, A. and White, S. (2005) 'Representing children's views and best interests in court: an international comparison', *Child Abuse Review*, 14(4), pp. 220–39.

Birch, J., Curtis, P. and James, A. (2007) 'Sense and sensibilities: in search of the child-friendly hospital', *Built Environment*, 33(4), pp. 405–16.

Bisson, J., Jenkins, P. L., Alexander, J. and Bannister, C. (1997) 'Randomised controlled trial of psychological debriefing for victims of acute burn trauma', *British Journal of Psychiatry*, Vol. 171, pp. 78–81.

Black, C., Homes, A., Diffley, Sewel, K. and Chamberlain, C. (2010) *Evaluation of Campus Police Officers in Scottish Schools*, Edinburgh: Scottish Government.

Black, D. (1998) 'The limitations of evidence', *Journal of the Royal College of Physicians of London*, 32(1), pp. 23–6.

Blaffer-Hrdy, S. (1999) *Mother Nature*, New York: Chatto and Windus.

Blomquist, K. (2007) 'Health and independence of young adults with disabilities. Two years later', *Orthopaedic Nursing*, 26(5), pp. 296–309.

Bochel, C., Bochel, H., Someville and Worley, C. (2008) 'Marginalised or enabled voices? "User Participation" in policy and practice', *Social Policy and Society*, 7(2).

Boreham, N. (2004) 'A theory of collective competence: challenging the neo-liberal individualisation of performance at work', *British Journal of Educational Studies*, 52(1), pp. 5–17.

Borgonovi, F. (2010) 'A life-cycle approach to the analysis of the relationship between social capital and health in Britain', *Social Science and Medicine*, 71(11), 1927–34.

Borland, M., Laybourn, A., Hill, M. and Brown, J. (1998) *Middle Childhood*, London: Jessica Kingsley.

Bottoms, A. and Dignan, J. (2004) 'Youth justice in Great Britain', *Crime and Justice*, 31, pp. 21–183.

Bottoms, A. and Kemp, V. (2007) 'The relationship between youth justice and child welfare in England and Wales', in M. Hill, A. Lockyer and F. Stone (eds) *Youth Justice and Child Protection*, London: Jessica Kingsley.

Bourdieu, P. (1986) 'The forms of capital', in J. G. Richardson (ed.) *Handbook of Theory and Research for the Sociology of Education*, New York: Greenwood, pp. 241–58.

Bourdieu, P. and Wacquant, L. J. D. (1992) *An Invitation to Reflexive Sociology*, Chicago: University of Chicago Press.

Bowlby, J. (1973) *Separation: Anxiety and Anger*. Vol. 2 of *Attachment and Loss*, London: Hogarth Press.

Bowlby, J. (1982) *Attachment*. Vol. 1 of *Attachment and Loss*, 2nd edition, London: Hogarth Press.

Bowlby, J. (1980) *Loss: Sadness and Depression*. Vol. 3 of *Attachment and Loss*, London: Hogarth Press.

Bradshaw, J. and Mayhew, E. (eds) (2005) *The Well-being of Children in the UK*, London: Save the Children.

Braithwaite, J. (1999) 'Restorative justice: assessing optimistic and pessimistic accounts', in Tonry, M. (ed.) *Crime and Justice: A Review of Research*, Chicago, IL: University of Chicago Press.

Brannen, J., Mooney, A., Brockmann, M. and Statham, J. (2007) *Coming to Care: The work-family lives of those working with vulnerable children*. Policy Press: Bristol.

Brannen, J., Moss, P. and Mooney, A. (2004) *Working and Caring in the Twentieth Century: Change and Continuity in Four-generation Families*, Basingstoke: Palgrave.

Brannen, J. and Nilsen, A. (2002) 'Young people's time perspectives: from youth to adulthood', *Sociology*, 36(3), pp. 513–37.

Brannen, J. and Nilsen, A. (2006) 'From Fatherhood to Fathering: Transmission and Change among British Fathers in Four-generation Families', *Sociology*, 40, pp. 335–52.

Brendan Nagle, D. (2006) *The Household as the Foundation of Aristotle's Polis*, Cambridge: Cambridge University Press.

Broadhurst, K., Duffin, M., Taylor, E. and Burrell, A. (2009) *Gangs and Schools*, Birmingham, NASUWT.

Bronfenbrenner, U. (1979) *The Ecology of Human Development*, Cambridge, Mass: Harvard UP.

Brown, A. L., Metz, K. E. and Campione, J. C. (1996) 'Social interaction and individual understanding in a community of learners: the influence of Piaget and Vygotsky', in A. Typhon and J. Vonèche (eds) *Piaget – Vygotsky: the social genesis of thought*, Hove: Psychology Press.

Brown, K. and White, K. (2006) *Exploring the Evidence Base for Integrated Children's Services*, Edinburgh: The Scottish Government.

Brownrigg, A., Soulsby, A. and Place, M. (2004) 'Helping vulnerable children to become more resilient', *International Journal of Child and Family Welfare*, 7(1), pp. 14–25.

Bruner, C. (1991) *Thinking Collaboratively: Ten Questions and Answers to Help Policy-makers Improve Children's Services*, Washington, DC: Education and Human Services Consortium.

Bruner, J. (1996) *The culture of education*, Boston: Harvard University Press.

Brunnberg, E. and Pećnik, N. (2007) 'Assessment process in social work with children at risk in Sweden and Croatia', *International Journal of Social Welfare*, 16(3), pp. 231–41.

Buckley, H. (2000) 'Beyond the rhetoric: a "working" version of child protection practices', *European Journal of Social Work*, 3(1), pp. 13–24.

Bui, Hoan N. and Morash, Merry (2007) 'Social capital, human capital, and reaching out for help with domestic violence: a case study of women in a Vietnamese-American community', *Criminal Justice Studies*, 20(4), pp. 375–90.

Bukowski, W. M. (2003) 'Peer relationships', in M. Bornstein, D. Lucy, C. L. M. Keyes and K. A. Moore, *Well-being*, London: Lawrence Erlbaum.

Bundle, A. (2002) 'Health information and teenagers in residential care: a qualitative study to identify young people's views', *Adoption and Fostering*, 26(4), pp. 19–25.

Burgess, R. (1999) 'Reflective practice: action learning sets for managers in social work', *Social Work Education*, 18(3), Sept. 1999, pp. 257–270.

Burnett, R. (2005) 'Youth offending teams', in T. Bateman and J. Pitts (eds) *Youth Justice*, London: Russell House Publishing.

Burns, J. and Rapee, R. (2006) 'Adolescent mental health literacy: Young people's knowledge of depression and help seeking', *Journal of Adolescence*, 29, pp. 225–39.

Buston, K. (2003) 'Adolescents with mental health problems: what do they say about health services', *Journal of Adolescence*, 25, pp. 231–42.

Butland, B., Jebb, S., Kopelman, P., McPherson, K., Thomas, S., Mardell, J. et al. (2007) 'Foresight', *Tackling obesities: future choices – project report*. London: Department of Innovation Universities and Skills.

Butler, I. and Drakeford, M. (2010) 'Children and young people's policy in Wales', in P. Ayre and M. Preston-Shoot (eds) (2010) *Children's Services at the Crossroads*, Lymne Regis: Russell House Publishing.

Butler-Sloss, E. (2010) 'A child's place in the Big Society', *Family Law*, 40, pp. 938–43.

Butt, J. and Box, L. (1998) *Family Centred – a Study of the Use of Family Centres by Black Families*, London: Race Equality Unit.

Bynner, J. (2001) 'Childhood risks and protective factors in social exclusion', *Children and Society*, 15(5), pp. 285–301.

Byrne, J., Conway, M. and Ostermeyer, M. (2005) *Young People's Attitudes and Experiences of Policing, Violence and Community Safety in North Belfast*, Belfast: Northern Ireland Policing Board.

CAFCASS (2008) *Annual Report and Accounts*, London: CAFCASS.

Cabinet Office, *Modernising Government*, Cm 4310, (1999) accessed http://www.archive.official-documents.co.uk/document/cm43/4310/4310.htm (21.2.05).

Cairns, B. (2004) *Fostering Attachments: Long-term Outcomes in Family Group Care: A Study of Long-term Outcomes in Family*, London, British Association of Adoption and Foster Care.

Cairns, K. (2003) *Attachment, Trauma and Resilience: Therapeutic Caring for Children*, London: BAAF.

Cairns, L. (2006) 'Participation with purpose', in K. Tisdall, J. Davies, M. Hill and A. Prout (eds) *Children, Young People and Social Inclusion*, Bristol: Policy Press.

Cairns, L. (2009) 'Investing in children: support young people as researchers', in *Researching with Children and Young People*, E. K. M. Tisdall, J. D. Davis and M. Gallagher (eds), London: Sage.

Cameron, A. and Lart, R. (2003) 'Factors promoting and obstacles hindering joint working: a systematic review of the research evidence', *Journal of Integrated Care*, 11(2).

Canavan, J., Coen, L., Dolan, P. and Whyte, L. (2009) 'Privileging practice: facing the challenge of integrated working for outcomes for children', *Children and Society*, 23(5), pp. 377–88.

Carnochan, J. and McCluskey, K. (2010) 'Violence, culture and policing in Scotland', in *Policing Scotland*, 2nd edition, D. Donnelly and K. Scott (eds), Devon: Willan Publishing.

Carpenter, J. and Dickinson, H. (2008) *Interprofessional Education and Training*, Bristol: Policy Press.

Carpenter, J., Griffin, M. and Brown, S. (2005) *The Impact of Sure Start on Social Services*, Research Report SSU/2005/FR/015, Nottingham: DfES.

Cassidy, J., Yair, Z., Brandi, S., Sherman, L. J., Butler, H., Karfgin, A., Cooper, G., Hoffman, K. T. and Powell, B. (2010) 'Enhancing attachment security in the infants of women in a jail-diversion program', *Attachment and Human Development*, 12(4), pp. 333–53.

Catan, L., Coleman, J. and Dennison, C. (1997) *Getting Through*, Brighton: Trust for the Study of Adolescence.

Catchpole, R. (2008) 'Working together for children's mental health', in *Child and Adolescent Mental Health Today*, C. Jackson, K. Hill and P. Lavis (eds), Brighton: Pavilion.

Caton, S. and Kagan, S. (2007) 'Comparing transition expectations of young people with moderate learning disabilities with other vulnerable youth and their non-disabled counterparts', *Disability and Society*, 22(5), pp. 473–88.

Catts, R. and Ozga, J. (2005) *Centre for Educational Sociology Briefing Paper 36 – What is social capital and how might it be used in Scottish Schools?* Edinburgh: CES, The University of Edinburgh.

CCfE (2010) *Annual Business Plan of the Children's Commissioner for England*, London, 2010.

CCfW (2009) *Annual Report and Accounts of the Children's Commissioner for Wales*, Swansea, 2009.

Chamberlain, T., Golden, S. and Walker, F. (2010) *Implementing Outcome Based Accountability in Children's Services*, Slough: NFER.

Chambers, H., Howell, S., Madge, N. and Olle, H. (2002) *Healthy Care: Building An Evidence Base for Promoting the Health and Well-Being of Looked after Children and Young People*, London: National Children's Bureau.

Chandler, T. (2006) 'Working in multi-disciplinary teams', in *Contemporary Issues in the Early Years*, Pugh, G. and Duffy, B. (eds), London: Sage.

Chapman, B. and Hough, M. (1998) *Evidence Based Practice: A Guide to Effective Practice*, London: Home Office.

Chapman, S. (2007) *Public Health Advocacy and Tobacco Control: Making Smoking History*, Oxford: Blackwell.

Chapman, T. and O'Mahony, D. (2007) *Youth and criminal justice in Northern Ireland*, in G. McIvor and P. Raynor (eds) 'Developments in social work with offenders', *Research Highlights 22*, London: Jessica Kingsley.

Charles, M. and Horwath, J. (2009) 'Investing in inter-agency training to safeguard children', *Children and Society*, 23(5), pp. 364–76.

Charles, N. and James, E. (2005) 'He earns the bread and butter and I earn the cream: job insecurity and the male breadwinner family', *Work, Employment and Society*, 19, pp. 481–502.

Charsley, K. (2005) 'Unhappy husbands: masculinity and migration in transnational Pakistani marriages', *Journal of the Royal Anthropological Institute*, 11, pp. 85–105.

Chase, E. (2010) 'Agency and silence: young people seeking asylum alone in the UK', *British Journal of Social Work*, 40(7), pp. 2050–68.

Chaskin, R. J. (2008) 'Resilience, community and resilient communities', *Child Care in Practice*, 14(1), pp. 65–74.

Chattoo, S., Atkin, K. and McNeish, D. (2004) *Young People of Pakistani Origin and Their Families: Implications for Providing Support to Young People and Their Families*, Centre for Research in Primary Care University of Leeds in collaboration with Barnardo's funded by the Community Fund.

Chess, S. and Thomas, A. (1991) 'The New York longitudinal study (NYLS): the young adult periods', *Canadian Journal of Psychiatry*, Vol. 35, No. 6, pp. 557–61.

Children's and Young People's Unit (2000) *Tomorrow's Future: Building a Strategy for Children and Young People*, London: Children and Young People's Unit.

Children in Scotland and University of Edinburgh (2010a) *Having a Say at Schools: Research briefing paper 1, Local Authorities and Pupil Councils*, http://www.havingasayatschool.org.uk/promoting.html (27.5.10)

Children in Scotland and University of Edinburgh (2010b) *Having a Say at Schools: Research briefing paper 2, Characteristics of Pupil Councils*, http://www.havingasayatschool.orh.uk/promoting.html (27.5.10)

Children in Scotland and University of Edinburgh (2010c) *Having a Say at Schools: Research briefing paper 3, The Adult Adviser to Pupil Councils*, http://www.havingasayatschool.org.uk/promoting.html (27.5.10)

Children in Scotland and University of Edinburgh (2010d) *Having a Say at Schools: Research briefing paper 4, Pupil Council 'Effectiveness' Processes*, http://www.havingasayatschool.org.uk/promoting.html (27.5.10)

Children in Scotland and University of Edinburgh (2010e) *Having a Say at Schools: Research briefing paper 5, Pupil Council Effectiveness Outcomes*, http://www.havingasayatschool.org.uk/promoting.html (27.5.10)

Children's Parliament (2007) *A consultation with young people about the recommendations of the Cool With Change project*, Edinburgh: CRFR.

Children's Parliament (2010a) *Hearing the Views of Children: Lothian and Borders Police youth strategy*, Edinburgh: Children's Parliament. http://www.childrensparliament.org.uk/assets/new/pdfs/cp_police_report.pdf

Children's Parliament (2010b) *Children's Hearings Reform: the views of children*, Edinburgh: Children's Parliament. http://www.childrensparliament.org.uk/assets/new/pdfs/cp_childrens_hearings_report.pdf

Christensen, P. (2002) 'Why more "quality time" is not on the top of children's lists: the "qualities of time" for children'. *Children and Society*, 16, pp. 77–88.

Christensen, P. and O'Brien, M. (eds) (2003) *Children in the City*, London: Routledge Falmer.

Christian, J., Poerter, L. W. and Moffitt, G. (2006) 'Workplace diversity and group relations: an overview', *Group Processes and Intergroup Relations*, 9(4), pp. 459–66.

Chugg, R. (2009) 'Managed networks and integrated children's services – case study of Devon', *Journal of Integrated Care*, 17(6), pp. 37–45.

Churchill, H. (2007) 'Children's services in 2006', in K. Clarke, T. Maltby and P. Kennett (eds) *Analysis and Debate in Social Policy*, 2007, Bristol: Policy Press.

Clark, A. and Moss, P. (2001) *Listening to Young Children: The Mosaic Approach*, London: Joseph Rowntree Foundation and National Children's Bureau.

Clark, C. and Hawkins, L. (2010) *Young People's Reading: The Importance of the Home Environment and Family Support. More Findings from our National Survey*, London, National Literacy Trust.

Clarke, K. (2006) 'Childhood, parenting and early intervention: a critical examination of the Sure Start programme', *Critical Social Policy*, 26(4), pp. 699–721.

Cleaver, H., Nicholson, D., Tarr, S. and Cleaver, D. (2007) *Child Protection, Domestic Violence and Parental Substance Misuse*, London: Jessica Kingsley.

Cleaver, H., Walker, S., Scott, J., Cleaver, D., Rose, W., Ward, H. and Pithouse, A. (2008) *The Integrated Children's System*, London: Jessica Kingsley.

Cleland, A. and Sutherland, E. (2009) *Children's Rights in Scotland*, Edinburgh: W. Green.

Cleveland Report 1988: The report of Lord Justice Butler-Sloss on her inquiry into child abuse in Cleveland, HMSO London, Cm 412.

Clifton et al. (2006) *The Impact and Effectiveness of Inter-professional Education in Primary Care – an RCN literature review*, London: Royal College of Nursing.

CoE (Council of Europe) (2005) *Report by MR Alvarao Gil-Robles Commissioner for Human Rights on his visit to the United Kingdom*, Geneva: European Commission.

Coalition for Community Schools (no date) *Community schools: partnerships for excellence*. Available online at http://76.227.216.38/assets/1/Page/partnershipsforexcellence.pdf (accessed 9 November 2010).

Cockburn, T. (2009) 'Children and deliberative democracy in England', in *A Handbook of Children and Young People's Participation*, B. Percy-Smith and N. Thomas (eds) Abingdon: Routledge.

Coghlan, D. and Brannick, T. (2005) *Doing Action Research in your own Organisation*, London: Sage.

Cohen, B. E. and McKay, M. (2010) 'The role of public health agencies in addressing child and family poverty', *The Open Nursing Journal*, 4, pp. 6–71.

Cohen, B., Moss, P., Petrie, P. and Wallace, J. (2004) *A New Deal for Children? Re-forming Education and Care in England, Scotland and Sweden*, Bristol: The Policy Press.

Cohen, S. (2004) 'Social relationships and health', *American Psychologist*, Vol. 59(8), pp. 676–84.

Coleman, J. (1988) 'Social capital in the creation of human capital', *American Journal of Sociology*, 94 (suppl.), S95–S120.

Coleman, J., Catan, L. and Dennison, C. (2004) 'You're the last person I'd talk to', in J. Roche and S. Tucker (eds) *Youth in Society*, London: Sage.

Colley, H. (2003) *Mentoring for Social Inclusion*, London: Routledge/Falmer.

Commission for Social Care Inspection (CSCI) (2007) *Growing up Matters: Better Transition Planning for Young People with Complex Needs*, London: CSCI.

Connell, J. and Klem, A. M. (2000) 'You can get there from here: using a theory of change approach to plan urban education reform', *Journal of Educational and Psychological Consulting*, 11(1), pp. 93–120.

Connors, C. and Stalker, K. (2002) *Children's Experiences of Disability: A Positive Outlook*, Edinburgh: Scottish Executive.

Connors, C. and Stalker, K. (2003) *The Views and Experiences of Disabled Children and Their Siblings*, London: Jessica Kingsley.

Cook, M., Crowley, A. and Thomas, N. (2008) *Evaluating the Children's Commissioner for Wales*, Swansea: Children's Commissioner for Wales.

Cooper, B. (2011) 'Criticality and reflexivity; best practice in uncertain environments', in J. Seden, S. Matthews, M. McCormick and A. Morgan (eds) *Professional Development in Social Work*, London: Routledge.

Cooper, C. (2008) 'Rethinking the "problem of youth"', *Youth and Policy*, 103, pp. 81–92.

Cooperrider, D. L., Whitney, D. and Stavros, J. M. (2008) *Appreciative Inquiry Handbook: for Leaders of Change*, Brunswick: OH Crown.

Corby, B. (2006) *Child Abuse*, Maidenhead: Open University Press.

Coussee, F., Bradt, L., Roose and Bouverne-de-Bie, M. (2010) 'The emerging social pedagogical paradigm in UK child and youth care', *British Journal of Social Work*, 40, pp. 789–805.

Cox, J. L., Holden, J. M. and Sagovsky, R. (1986) 'Detection of postnatal depression. Development of the 10-item Edinburgh postnatal depression scale', *British Journal of Psychiatry*, 150, pp. 782–86.

Cradock, G. (2004) 'Risk, morality, and child protection: risk calculation as guides to practice', *Science, Technology, and Human Values*, 29(3), pp. 314–31.

Craig, G. (2007) 'Community capacity building', *Critical Social Policy*, 27(3), pp. 335–59.

Craig, G., Adamson, S., Ali, N., Ali, S., Atkins, Dadze-Arthur, A., Elliott, C., McNamee, S. and Murtuja, B. (2007) *Sure Start and Black and Minority Ethnic Populations*, Research Report NESS/2007/FR/020, London: HMSO.

Craig, P., Macintyre, S., Michie, S., Nazareth, I. and Pettigrew, M. (2010) *Developing and Evaluating Complex Interventions*, London: Medical Research Council.

Craig, W., Pepler, D. and Blais, J. (2007) 'Responding to bullying: what works?' *School Psychology International*, 28(4), pp. 465–77.

Cranston, N. C. (2001) 'Collaborative decision-making and school-based management: challenges, rhetoric and reality', *Journal of Educational Enquiry*, 2(2), pp. 1–24.

Creekmore, M. (2007) 'Child welfare and juvenile justice in the USA: a practice perspective', in M. Hill, A. Lockyer and F. Stone (eds) *Youth Justice and Child Protection*, London: Jessica Kingsley.

Crick, B. (2010) 'Civic republicanism and citizenship: the challenge for today' in Crick and Lockyer, *op. cit.*

Crick, B. (2000) *Essays on Citizenship*, London: Continuum.

Crick B. (1962) *In Defence of Politics*, 5th edition (2000), London and New York: Continuum.

Crick B. (2003) 'The English Citizenship Order 1999: context, content and presuppositions', in A. Lockyer, B. Crick and J. Annette (eds) *Education for Democratic Citizenship*, Aldershot: Ashgate.

Crick, B. and Lockyer, A. (eds) (2010) *Active Citizenship*, Edinburgh: Edinburgh University Press.

Crick, B. and Porter A. (eds) (1978) *Political Education and Political Literacy*, London: Longman.

Crisp, R. J. and Beck, S. R. (2005) 'Reducing intergroup bias: the moderating role of ingroup identification', *Group Processes and Intergroup Relations*, 8(2), pp. 173–85.

Crompton, R. (2006) *Employment and the Family: the Reconfiguring of Work and Family Life in Contemporary Societies*, Cambridge University Press.

Cummings, C., Dyson, A. and Todd, L. (2004) *Evaluation of Extended Schools Pathfinder Projects. Research Report 530*, London: DfES.

Cummings, C., Dyson, A. and Todd, L. (2011) *Beyond the School Gates: Can Full Service and Extended Schools Overcome Disadvantage?* London: Routledge.

Cummings, C., Dyson, A., Muijs, D., Papps, I., Pearson, D., Raffo, C., Tiplady, L., Todd, L., with Crowther, D. (2007) *Evaluation of the Full Service Extended Schools Initiative: Final Report. Research report RR852*. Report for DfES (London).

Cunningham, S. and Lavalette, M. (2004) 'Active citizens or irresponsible truants? School student strikes against the war', *Critical Social Policy*, 24(2), pp. 255–69.

CYPS (2003) http://www.communities.gov.uk/publications/communities/2003citizenship surveychildren.

D'Cruz, H. (2004) 'The social construction of child maltreatment. The role of medical practitioners', *Journal of Social Work*, 4(1), pp. 99–123.

Dahl, R. (1956) *A Preface to Democratic Theory*, Chicago, University of Chicago Press.

Daily Mail (2010) 'Now Britain is the fattest country in Europe', September 25, http://www.dailymail.co.uk/news/article-1314807/How-Britain-fattest-country-Europe-fifth-overweight-world.html?ito=feeds-newsxml

Daily Telegraph (2010) '20 mph limit has not made roads safer', October 2, http://www.telegraph.co.uk/news/uknews/road-and-rail-transport/8038821/20mph-limit-has-not-made-roads-safer.html

Daly, K. (2003) 'Restorative justice: the real story', in G. Johnstone (ed.) *A Restorative Justice Reader*, Cullompton: Willan Publishing.

Daniel, B., Vincent, S., Farrall, E. and Arney, F. (2009) 'How is the concept of resilience operationalised in practice with vulnerable children?' *International Journal of Child and Family Welfare*, 12(1), pp. 2–21.

Daniel, B. and Wassell, S. (2002) *Assessing and Promoting Resilience in Vulnerable Children*, London: Jessica Kingsley.

Daniels, H. (2001) *Vygotsky and Pedagogy*, London: Routledge.

Daniels, H. (2008) *Vygotsky and Research*, London: Routledge.

Daniels, H. (2010) 'The mutual shaping of human action and institutional settings: a study of the transformation of children's services and professional work', *The British Journal of Sociology of Education*, Vol. 31, No. 4.

Daniels, H., Creese, A. and Norwich, B. (2000) 'Supporting collaborative problem-solving in schools', in H. Daniels (ed.) *Special education reformed*, London: Falmer Press.

Daniels, H., Leadbetter, J., and Warmington P., with Edwards, A., Brown, S., Middleton, D., Popova, A. and Apostolov, A. (2007) 'Learning in and for multi-agency working', *Oxford Review of Education*, Vol. 33, No. 4, pp. 521–38.

Davies, J. M. (2011) *Integrated Children's Services*, London: Sage.

Davies, J. and Wright, J. (2008) 'Children's voices', *Child and Adolescent Mental Health*, 13(1), pp. 26–31.

Davies, L., Krane, J., Collings, S. and Wexler, S. (2007) 'Developing mothering narratives in child protection practice', *Journal of Social Work Practice*, 21(1), pp. 23–34.

Davies, L., Williams, C. and Yamashita, H. with Man-Hing, K. (2006) *Impact and Outcomes: taking up the challenge of pupil participation*, London: Carnegie Foundation, http://www.participationforschools.org.uk (31.5.10).

Davis, J. (2006) 'Disability, childhood studies and the construction of medical discourses', in Lloyd et al.

Davis, J. M. (2011) *Integrated Children's Services*, London: Sage.

Davren, M. (2007) 'Child and adolescent mental health services and the strategic context', *Child Care in Practice*, 13(4).

Day, C. (2008) 'Children's and young people's involvement and participation in mental health care', *Child and Adolescent Mental Health*, 13(1), pp. 2–8.

Department for Children, Schools and Families (DCSF) (2007) *The Children's Plan: Building Brighter Futures*. Cm 7280. (London, The Stationery Office.)

Department for Children, Schools and Families (DCSF) (2008a) *21st century schools: a world class education for every child.* (London, DCSF Publications.)

Department for Children, Schools and Families (DCSF) (2008b) *The Bercow report: a review of services for children and young people (0–19) with speech, language and communication needs.* www.dcsf.gov.uk/bercowreview Accessed 09/07/08.

Department for Children, Schools and Families (DCSF) (2008c) *2020 Children and Young People's Workforce Strategy*, Nottingham: DCSF.

Department for Education and Skills (2002) *Classification of Special Educational Needs. Consultation Document*, Http://www.dfes.gov.uk/sen.

Department for Education and Skills (2003) *Every Child Matters*, London: DfES.

Department for Education and Skills (DfES) (2004) *The Children Act*, London: HMSO.

Department of Health (2001a) *Valuing people: a new strategy for learning disability for the 21st Century*, London: HMSO.

Department of Health (2001b) *Working together, learning together: a framework for lifelong learning for the NHS*, London: DH.

Department of Health (2002) *Promoting the Health of Looked-After Children*, London: Department of Health.

Department of Health (2004) *National Service Framework for Children, Young People and Maternity Services*, London: HMSO.

Department of Health (2007) *Valuing People now: from Progress to Transformation*, London: Department of Health.

Department of Health (2008) *Transition: Moving on Well*, London: Department of Health.

Department of Health and the Home Office (2003) *The Victoria Climbié Inquiry (The Laming Report)*, Cm. 5730, London: The Stationery Office.

Detrick, S. (ed.) (1991) *The United Nations Convention on the Rights of the Child: A Guide to the Travaux Preparatoires*, Dordrecht: Martinus Nijhoff.

Deuchar, R. (2009) *Gangs: Marginalised Youth and Social Capital*, Stoke-on-Trent: Trentham Books.

DH 11. (1974) Report of the Committee of Inquiry into the Care and Supervision Provided in Relation to Maria Colwell, London.

Dickens, J. (2010) *Social Work and Social Policy*, London: Routledge.

Dobbie, W. and Roland G. Fryer, J. (2009) *Are high-quality schools enough to close the achievement gap? Evidence from a bold social experiment in Harlem*, NBER working paper No. 15473. Report for National Bureau of Economic Research (Cambridge MA).

Doek (2008) 'Foreword' in Invernizzi and Williams *op. cit.*

Dogra, N., Parkin, A., Gale, F. and Frake, C. (2008) *A Multi-disciplinary Handbook of Child and Adolescent Mental Health*, London: Jessica Kingsley.

Dominelli, L. (2011) 'Anti-oppressive practice', in R. Taylor, N. Hill and F. McNeill (eds) *Early Professional Development for Social Workers*, Birmingham: Venture Press.

Donaldson, T. and Harbison, J. (2006) 'The Children (N.I.) Order 1995 10 Years on', *Child Care in Practice*, 12(3), pp. 299–308.

Donnelly, D. (2008) *Municipal Policing in Scotland*, Dundee: Dundee University Press.

Donnison, D. (2010) 'Power and public services: for customers or citizens?' in Crick and Lockyer *op. cit.*

Dozier, M. (2003) 'Attachment-based treatment for vulnerable children', *Attachment and Human Development*, Vol. 5, No. 3, pp. 253–57.

Dozier, M., Lindhiem, O., Lewis, E., Bick, J., Bernard, K. and Peloso, E. (2009) 'Effects of a foster parent training program on young children's attachment behaviours: preliminary evidence from a randomized clinical trial', *Child and Adolescent Social Work Journal*, 26(4), pp. 321–32.

Dozier, M., Peloso, E., Lewis, E., Laurenceau, J. and Levine, S. (2008) 'Effects of an attachment-based intervention of the cortisol production of infants and toddlers in foster care', *Development and Psychopathology*, 20(3), pp. 845–59.

Dozier, M., Stovall, K. C., Albus, K. E. and Bates, B. (2001) 'Attachment for infants in foster care: the role of caregivers' state of mind', *Child Development*, Vol. 72, No. 5, pp. 1467–77.

Drury, J. (2003) 'Adolescent communication with adults in authority', *Journal of Language and Social Psychology*, 22(1), pp. 66–73.

Drury, J. and Dennison, C. (1999) 'Representations of teenagers among police officers', *Youth and Policy*, 66, pp. 62–87.

Dryfoos, J. G., Quinn, J. and Barkin, C. (eds) (2005) *Community Schools in Action: Lessons from a Decade of Practice*, Oxford: Oxford University Press.

Dumbrill, G. C. (2006) 'Parental experience of child protection intervention: a qualitative study', *Child Abuse and Neglect*, 30(1), pp. 27–37.

Dunn, J. (2004) *Children's Friendships: the Beginnings of Intimacy*, Oxford: Blackwell.

Dunnett, K., White, S., Butterfield, J. and Callowhill, I. (eds) (2006) *Health of Looked-after Children and Young People*, Dorset: Russell House Publishing.

Duquette, D. (1992) 'Child Protection Legal Processes: Comparing the United States and Great Britain', *University of Pittsburgh Law Review*, 54(1), pp. 240–94.

Duquette, D. (1994) 'Scottish children's hearings and representation of the child', in S. Asquith and M. Hill (eds) *Justice for Children*, Dordrecht: Martinus Nijhoff.

Duquette, D. (2007) 'Children's justice: a view from America', in M. Hill, A. Lockyer and F. Stone (eds) *Youth Justice and Child Protection*, London: Jessica Kingsley.

Dyson, A. and Todd, L. (2010) 'Dealing with complexity: theory of change evaluation and the full service extended schools initiative', *International Journal of Research and Method in Education*, 33(2), pp. 119–34.

Easton, C., Morris, M. and Gee, G. (2010) *LARC2: Integrated Children's Services and the Common Assessment Framework Process*, Slough: NFER.

Ecclestone, K. (2001) *Learning in a comfort zone: cultural and social capital in outcome-based assessment regimes*, Paper presented at the British Educational Research Association Conference, University of Leeds. 13–15 September.

Edwards, A. (2004) 'The new multi-agency working: collaborating to prevent social exclusion of children and families', *Journal of Integrated Care*, 12(5).

Edwards, A. (2010) *Being an Expert Professional Practitioner: the Relational Turn in Expertise*, Dordrecht, Springer.

Edwards, A., Barnes, M., Plewis, I. and Morris, K. et al. (2006) *Working to Prevent the Social Exclusion of Children and Young People: Final Lessons from the National Evaluation of the Children's Fund: RR 734*, London: DfES.

Edwards, A., Daniels, H., Gallagher, T., Leadbetter, J. and Warmington, P. (2009) *Improving Inter-professional Collaborations: Multi-agency Working for Children's Wellbeing*, London: Routledge.

Edwards, A. and Kinti, I. (2010) 'Working relationally at organisational boundaries: negotiating expertise and identity', in *Activity Theory in Practice: promoting learning across boundaries and agencies*, H. Daniels, A. Edwards, Y. Engeström and S. Ludvigsen (eds) London: Routledge, pp. 126–39.

Edwards, A., Lunt, I. and Stamou, E. (2010) 'Inter-professional work and expertise: new roles at the boundaries of schools', *British Educational Research Journal*, 36(1), pp. 27–45.

Edwards, P., Green, J., Roberts, I. and Lutchmun, S. (2006) 'Deaths from injury in children and employment status in family: analysis of trends in class specific death rates', *BMJ*, 333: 119 doi:10.1136/bmj.38875.757488.4F (published 7 July 2006).

Ehrenreich, B. and Hochschild, A. (2003) *Global Woman: Nannies, Maids and Sex Workers in the New Economy*, London: Granta.

Emond, R. (2002) 'Understanding the resident group', *Scottish Journal of Residential Child Care*, 1, pp. 30–40.

Engeström, Y. (1995) 'Innovative learning in work teams: analysing cycles of knowledge creation in practice', in Y. Engeström, R. Miettinen and R. L. Punamaki (eds) *Perspectives on Activity Theory*, Cambridge: Cambridge University Press.

Engeström, Y. (1999) *Perspectives on Activity Theory*, New York: Cambridge University Press.

Engeström, Y. (2007) 'Putting activity theory to work: the change laboratory as an application of double stimulation', in *The Cambridge Companion to Vygotsky*, H. Daniels, M. Cole and J. V. Wertsch (eds) Cambridge: Cambridge University Press.

Engeström, Y., Engeström, R. and Kerosuo, H. (2003) 'The discursive construction of collaborative care', *Applied Linguistics*, 24(3), pp. 286–315.

Ennew, J. and Hastadewi, Y. (2002) *Seen and Heard*, http://sca.savethechildren.se/South_East_Asia/Publications/Child-participation/ (31.5.10)

Erickson, L. D., McDonald, S. and Elder, G. (2009) 'Informal mentors and education', *Sociology of Education*, 82, pp. 344–67.

Exworthy, M. and Halford, S. (eds) (1999) *Professionals and the New Mangerialism in the Public Sector*, Buckingham, Open University Press.

Fagg, J., Curtis, S., Stansfeld, S., Cattell, V., Tupuola, A. and Arephin, M. (2008) 'Area social fragmentation, social support for individuals and psychosocial health in young adults: evidence from a national survey in England', *Social Science and Medicine*, 66(2), pp. 242–54.

Fahmy, E. (2006) *Young Citizens*, Aldershot: Ashgate.

Fallon, B. J. and Bowles, T. (2001) 'Family functioning and adolescent help-seeking behaviour', *Family Relations*, 50(3), pp. 239–45.

Farmer, E. (2010) 'What factors relate to good placement outcomes in kinship care?', *British Journal of Social Work*, 40(2), pp. 426–44.

Farrall, S., Bottoms, A. and Shapland, J. (2010) 'Social structures and desistance from crime', *European Journal of Criminology*, 7(6), pp. 546–70.

Farrall, S. and Maruna, S. (2004) 'Desistance-focused criminal justice policy research', *The Howard Journal*, 43(4), pp. 358–67.

Farrington, D. (2007) 'Childhood risk factors and risk focused prevention', in M. Magure, R. Morgan and R. Reiner (eds) *The Oxford Handbook of Criminology*, Oxford: OUP.

Feinberg, J. (1980) 'The child's right to an open future', in W. Aiken and H. LaFollette (eds) *Whose Child? Parental Rights, Parental Authority and State Power*, Totowa, NJ: Rowman and Littlefield.

Ferguson, I. and Woodward, S. (2009) *Radical Social Work in Practice*, Bristol: Policy Press.

Ferguson, L., Follan, M., Macinnes, M., Furnivall, J. and Minnis, H. (2010) 'Residential childcare workers' knowledge of reactive attachment disorder', *Child and Adolescent Mental Health*, Vol. 16, No. 2, 2011, pp. 1011–109.

Ferguson, N., Douglas, G., Lowe, N., Murch, M. and Robertson, M. (2004) *Grandparenting in Divorced Families*, Bristol: Policy Press.

Ferri, E. and Saunders, A. (1991) *Parents, Professionals and Pre-school Centres: a Study of Barnardo's Provision*, London: National Children's Bureau with Barnardo's.

Field, F. (2010) *The Foundation Years: Preventing Poor Children Becoming Poor Adults*, London: HM Government.

Field, J. (2003) *Social Capital*, Abingdon: Routledge.

Field, J. (2009) 'A social capital toolkit for schools? Organisational perspectives on current social capital research', in J. Allan, J. Ozga and G. Smith (eds) *Social Capital, Professionalism and Diversity*, Rotterdam: Sense, pp. 21–35.

Fine, B. (2001) *Social Capital Versus Social Theory. Political Economy and Social Science at the Turn of the Millennium*, London: Routledge.

Fisher, P. A., Gunnar, M. R., Dozier, M., Bruce, J. and Pears, K. C. (2006) 'Effects of therapeutic interventions for foster children on behavioural problems, caregiver attachment, and stress regulatory neural systems', *Annals of the New York Academy of Sciences*, 1094: 215–25.

Fitzgerald, R. (2010) 'Active Citizenship: Gender Equality and Democracy', in Gick and Lockyer (2010) *op. cit.*

Fitzpatrick, C. (2009) 'Looked-after children and the criminal justice system', in *Critical Perspectives on Safeguarding Children*, K. Broadhurst, C. Grover and J. Jamieson (eds) Chichester: Wiley.

Flaquer, L. (2000) 'Is there a southern European model of family policy?' in A. Pfenning and T. Bahle *Families and Family Policies in Europe. Comparative Perspectives*, Peter Lang: Frankfurt am Main.

Flouri, E., Buchanan, A., Tan, J-P., Griggs, J. and Attar-Schwartz, S. (2010) 'Adverse life events are a socio-economic disadvantage, and adolescent psychopathology: The role of closeness to grandparents in moderating the effect of contextual stress', *Stress*, 13(5), pp. 402–12.

Foley, P. and Rixon, A. (2008) *Changing Children's Services*. Bristol: Policy Press.

Fonagy, P., Steele, M., Higgit, A. and Target, M. (1994) 'The theory and practice of resilience', *Journal of Child Psychology and Psychiatry*, 35(2), pp. 231–57.

Fonagy, P., Steele, H. and Steele, M. (1991) 'Maternal representations of attachment during pregnancy predict the organization of infant–mother attachment at one year of age', *Child Development*, Vol. 62, pp. 891–905.

Foot, J. and Hopkins, T. (2010) *A Glass Half-full: How an Asset Approach can Improve Community Health and Well-being*, Report for IDeA (London).

Forbes, J. (2006) 'Types of social capital: tools to explore service integration?' *International Journal of Inclusive Education*, 10(6), pp. 565–80.

Forbes, J. (2008) 'Knowledge transformations: examining the knowledge needed in teacher and speech and language therapist co-work', *Educational Review*, 60(2), pp. 141–54.

Forbes, J. and McCartney, E. (2010) 'Social capital theory: a cross-cutting analytic for teacher/therapist work in integrating children's services?' *Child Language Teaching and Therapy*, 26(3), 321–34.

Forbes, J. and Watson, C. (2009) *Service Integration in Schools: Research and Policy Discourses, Practices and Future Prospects*, Rotterdam: Sense.

Forlin, C. (2010) 'Future directions for teacher education for inclusion', in C. Forlin (ed.) *Teacher Inclusion for Education*, London: Routledge.

Foster, J., Newburn, T. and Souhami, A. (2005) *Assessing the Impact of the Stephen Lawrence Inquiry*, Home Office Research Study 294, London: Home Office.

France, A., Hine, J., Armstrong, D. and Camina, M. (2004) *The OnTrack Early Intervention and Prevention Programme: from theory to action. Home office Online Report 10/04*, London: Home Office.

France, A., Munro, E. R., Meredith, J., Manful, E. and Beckhelling, J. (2009) *Effectiveness of the New Local Safeguarding Boards in England*, Loughborough: Loughborough University.

France, A. and Utting, D. (2005) 'The paradigm of "risk and protection-focused prevention" and its impact on services for children and families', *Children and Society*, 19, pp. 77–90.

Fraser, M. W. (ed.) (2004) *Risk and Resilience in Childhood*, Washington: NASW.

Freake, H., Barley, V. and Kent, G. (2007) 'Adolescents' views of helping professionals', *Journal of Adolescence*, 30, pp. 639–53.

Freeman, I. (2009) 'Electronic sharing of information on children: the Scottish and English experiences', *Journal of Integrated Care*, 17(2), pp. 22–25.

Frejka, T., Sobotka, T., Hoem, J. M. and Toulemon, L. (2008) 'Summary and general conclusions: childbearing trends and policies in Europe', *Demographic Research*, 19(2), pp. 5–14.

Friesen, B. (2007) 'Recovery and resilience in children's mental health', *Psychiatric Rehabilitation Journal*, 31(1), pp. 38–48.

Frost, N. and Stein, M. (2009a) *Understanding Children's Social Care*, London: Sage.

Frost, N. and Stein, M. (2009b) 'Outcomes of integrated working with children and young people', *Children and Society*, 23(5), pp. 315–19.

Fry, H., Ketteridge, S. and Marshall, S. (2000) *A Handbook for Teaching and Learning in Higher Education*, London: Kogan Page.

Fukkink, R. and Hermans, J. (2009) 'Children's experiences with chat support and telephone support', *Journal of Child Psychology and Psychiatry*, 50(6), pp. 759–766.

Fukuyama, F. (2001) 'Social capital, civil society and development', *Third World Quarterly*, 22(1), 7–20.

Fulcher, G. (1989) *Disabling Policies? A Comparative Approach to Education Policy and Disability*, London: The Falmer Press.

Furlong, A., Cartmel, F., Biggart, A., Sweeting, H. and West, P. (2003) *Youth transitions: Patterns of Vulnerability and Processes of Social Inclusion*, Edinburgh: The Stationery Office.

Garrett, P. M. (2003) *Remaking Social Work with Children and Families*, London: Routledge.

Gascoigne, M. (2006) *Supporting Children with Speech, Language and Communication Needs Within Integrated Children's Services*, Royal College of Speech and Language Therapists Position Paper, London: RCSLT.

Gass, K., Jenkins, J. M. and Dunn, J. (2006) 'The sibling relationship as protective for children experiencing life events: a longitudinal study', *Journal of Child Psychology and Psychiatry*, 48, pp. 167–75.

Geldard, K. and Geldard, D. (2009) *Relationship Counselling for Children, Families and Young People*, London: Sage.

Gelsthorpe, T. (2006) 'Extended schools – the story so far', in J. Piper (ed.) *Schools Plus to Extended Schools*, Coventry: ContinYou.

Ghaziani, R. (2010) 'School design: researching children's views', *Childhoods Today*, 4(1), pp. 1–27.

Gibbons, J. (1991) 'Children in need and their families: outcome of referral to social services', *British Journal of Social Work*, 21(3), pp. 221–27.

Gibbs, I. and Sinclair, I. (2000) 'Bullying, sexual harassment and happiness in residential children's homes', *Child Abuse Review*, 9(4), pp. 247–56.

Gillies, V. (2007) *Marginalised Mothers: Exploring Working-Class Experiences of Parenting*, London: Routledge.

Gillies, V. and Edwards, R. (2006) 'A qualitative analysis of parenting and social capital: comparing the work of Coleman and Bourdieu', *Qualitative Sociological Review*, 11, pp. 42–60.

Gilligan, R. (1999) 'Working with social networks', in Hill, M. (ed.) *Effective Ways of Working with Children and Their Families*, London: Jessica Kingsley.

Gilligan, R. (2001) *Promoting Resilience: A Resource Guide on Working with Children in the Care System*, London: BAAF.

Gilling, D. (2000) 'Policing, crime prevention and partnerships', in *Core Issues in Policing*, F. Leishman, B. Loveday and S. P. Savage (eds) Harlow: Pearson.

Giordano, P. C., Cernkovich, S. A. and J. L. Rudolp (2002) 'Gender, crime and desistance: toward a theory of cognitive transformation', *American Journal of Sociology*, 107(4), pp. 990–1064.

Glaister, A. and Glaister, B. (eds) (2005) *Inter-agency Collaboration in Providing for Children*, Edinburgh: Dunedin.

Glass, N. (1999) 'Sure Start: the development of an early intervention programme for young children in the UK', *Children and Society*, 13(4), pp. 257–65.

Glisson, C. and Hemmelgarn, A. (1998) 'The effects of organisational climate and interorganisational coordination on the quality and outcomes of children's service system', *Child Abuse and Neglect*, 22(5), pp. 401–21.

Glover, V. and O'Connor, T. G. (2002) 'Effects of antenatal stress and anxiety: implications for development and psychiatry', *British Journal of Psychiatry*, 180, pp. 389–91.

Goldthorpe, L. (2004) 'Every Child Matters: a legal perspective', *Child Abuse Review*, 13, pp. 115–36.

Goodman, R. and Scott, S. (2005) *Child Psychiatry*, Oxford: Blackwell.

Gordon, G. and Grant, J. (1997) *How We Feel*, London: Jessica Kingsley.

Goswami, U. (2008) 'Foresight Mental Capital and Wellbeing Project', *Learning Difficulties: future challenges*, The Government Office for Science, London. http://www.foresight.gov.uk/Mental%20Capital/Wellbeing_and_work.pdf Accessed 9 September 2010.

Goulbourne, H., Reynolds, T., Solomos, J. and Zontini, E. (2010) *Transnational Families: Ethnicities, Identities and Social Capital*, London: Routledge.

Graetz, J. (2010) 'Autism grows up: opportunities for adults with autism', *Disability and Society*, 25(1), pp. 33–47.

Graham, J. and Wright, J. A. (1999) 'What does "inter-professional" collaboration mean to professionals working with pupils with physical difficulties?', *British Journal of Special Education*, 26(1), pp. 37–41.

Granovetter, M. (1973) 'The strength of weak ties', *American Journal of Sociology*, 78(6), pp. 1360–80.

Grayling, T., Glaister, S., Hallam, K., Graham, D. and Anderson, R. (2002) *Streets Ahead: Safe and Liveable Streets for Children*, London: IPPR.

Greeff, A. (2005) *Resilience*, London: Crown House.

Green, J., Stanley, C., Smith, V. and Goldwyn, R. (2000) 'A new method of evaluating attachment representations in young school age children: The Manchester Child Attachment Story Task', *Attachment and Human Development*, Vol. 2, No. 1, pp. 48–70.

Greishbach, D. and Currie, C. (2001) *Health Behaviours of Scottish Schoolchildren, Report 7: Control of Adolescent Smoking in Scotland*, Edinburgh: University of Edinburgh.

Growing up in Scotland (2007) 'Sources of formal and informal support for parents of young children' GUS *Growing Up in Scotland Research Findings No 4*, http://www.scotland.gov.uk/Publications/2007/01/08145545/1 accessed 14 November 2010.

Guggenheim, M. (2005) *What's Wrong with Children's Rights?* Cambridge, MA: Harvard University Press.

Hallam, A. (2008) *The Effectiveness of Interventions to Address Health Inequalities in the Early Years*, Edinburgh: The Scottish Government.

Hallett, C., Murray, C. and Punch, S. (2003) 'Young people and welfare: negotiating pathways', in C. Hallett and A. Prout (eds) *Hearing the Voices of Children: Social Policy for a New Century*, London: Falmer Routledge.

Halpern, D. (2005) *Social Capital*, Cambridge: Polity Press.

Hamilton, D. (2011) 'Child poverty in the uk: issues and answers', in R. Taylor, M. Hill and F. McNeill (eds) *21st Century Social Workers: A Resource for Early Professional Development*, London: Venture Press.

Hansen, K. (2005) *Not So Nuclear Families: Class Gender and Networks of Care*, London: Rutgers University.

Hansen, K., Jones, E., Joshi, H. and Budge, D. (2010a) *Millenium Cohort Study Fourth Survey*, London: Institute of Education.

Hansen, K., Joshi, H. and Dex, S. (eds) (2010b) *Children of the 21st Century: The First Five Years*, Bristol: Policy Press.

Hardiker, P. (2002) 'A framework for conceptualizing need and its application to planning and providing services', in *Approaches to Needs Assessment in Children's Services*, H. Ward and W. Rose (eds) London: Jessica Kingsley Publishers.

Harding, L. F. (1996) *Family, State and Social Policy*, Basingstoke, Macmillan.

Hargreaves, A. (1992) 'Cultures of teaching: a focus for change', in A. Hargreaves and M. G. Fullan (eds) *Understanding Teacher Development*, London: Cassell.

Hargreaves, A. (1994) *Changing Teachers, Changing Times: Teachers' Work and Culture in the Postmodern Age*, London: Cassell.

Harris, F. R. (2006) *The Baby Bust: Who will do the work? Who will pay the taxes?* Maryland: Rowman and Littlefield.

Harris, J., Balmer, R. and Sidebottom, P. (2009) 'British Society of Paediatric Dentistry: a policy document on dental neglect on children', *International Journal of Paediatric Dentistry*.

Hart, R. (1992) *Children's Participation: The Theory and Practice of Involving Young Citizens in Community Development and Environmental Care*, London: Earthscan.

Harvey, R. (2002) 'The UK before the UN Committee on the rights of the child', *ChildRIGHT*, October, issue no 190, pp. 9–11.

Hawkins, R. and Maurer, K. (2010) 'Bonding, bridging and linking: how social capital operated in New Orleans following hurricane Katrina', *British Journal of Social Work*, 40(6), pp. 1777–93.

Hawkins-Rodgers, Y. (2007) 'Adolescents adjusting to a group home environment: a residential care model of reorganising attachment behaviour and building resiliency', *Children and Youth Services Review*, 29, pp. 1131–41.

Hawthorne, J., Jessop, J., Pryor, J. and Richards, M. (2003) *Supporting Children Through Family Change: A Review of Interventions and Services for Children of Divorcing and Separating Parents*, York: JRF.

Hawton, K. and Williams, K. (2002) 'Influences of the media on suicide', *BMJ*, 325, pp. 1375–6.

Hay, D. F., Asten, P., Mills, A., Kumar, R., Pawlby, S. and Sharp, D. (2001) 'Intellectual problems shown by 11-year-old children whose mothers had postnatal depression', *The Journal of Child Psychology and Psychiatry*, 42, pp. 871–89.

Hayden, C. (2007) *Children in Trouble*, Basingstoke: Palgrave Macmillan.

Head, G. (2007) *Better Learning, Better Behaviour*, Edinburgh: Dunedin Academic Press.

Healy, K. (2010) 'Recognising and enabling social workers to promote child wellbeing', *Australian Social Work*, 63(2), pp. 141 4.

Hearn, J., Pöso, T., Smith, C., White, S. and Korpinen, J. (2004) 'What is child protection? Historical and methodological issues in comparative research on *Lastensuojelu*/child protection', *International Journal of Social Welfare*, 13(1), pp. 28–41.

Heatherington, R. (2002) *Learning from Difference. Comparing Child Welfare Systems, Partnership for Families and Children Project*, Ontario: Wilfred Laurier University.

Henderson, P. (2010) *Creative Methodologies*, paper at Children and Young People's Participation Seminar, Rio di Janeiro, Brazil 13.5.10.

Henderson, P. and Glen, A. (2005) 'From recognition to support: community development workers in the United Kingdom', *Community Development Journal*, 41(3), pp. 277–92.

Henderson, P. and Thomas, N. (2002) *Skills in Neighbourhood Work*, London: Routledge.

Henderson, S., Holland, J., McGrellis, S., Sharpe, S. and Thomson, R. (2007) *Inventing Adulthoods: A biographical approach to youth transitions*, London: Sage.

Heron, G. and Chakrabarti, M. (2002) 'Impact of Scottish vocational qualifications on residential child care: Have they fulfilled the promise?', *Social Work Education*, 21(2), pp. 83–197.

Hibel, L. C., Granger, D. A., Blair, C. and Cox, M. J. (2009) 'Intimate partner violence moderates the association between mother–infant adrenocortical activity across an emotional challenge.', *Journal of Family Psychology*, Vol. 23, No. 5, pp. 615–25.

Higher Education Academy (2008) *Integrated Children's Services in Higher Education Project Summary*, The Higher Education Subject Centre for Social Policy and Social Work (SWAP): University of Southampton.

Highet, G. and Jamieson, L. (2007) *Cool with Change: young people and family change*, Final Report http://www.crfr.ac.uk/reports/CWC%20final%20report%202007.pdf

Hill, C., Wright, V., Sampeys, C., Dunnett, K., Daniel, S., O'Dell, L. and Watkins, J. (2002) 'The emerging role of the specialist nurse: promoting the health of looked-after children', *Adoption and Fostering*, 26(4), pp. 35–43.

Hill, M. (1999) 'What's the problem? Who can help?' *Journal of Social Work Practice*, 13(2), pp. 135–45.

Hill, M. (2002) 'Network assessments and diagrams: a flexible friend for social work practice and education', *Journal of Social Work*, 2(2), pp. 233–54.

Hill, M. (2006) 'Children's voices on ways of having a voice', *Childhood*, 13(1), pp. 69–89.

Hill, M. (2009a) 'Change and continuity, contradiction and compatibility: children and their families in the United Kingdom', in T. Maundeni, L. L. Levers and G. Jaques (eds) *Changing Family Systems: A Global Perspective*, Gabarone: Bay Publishing.

Hill, M. (2009b) 'The place of child placement research in policy and practice', in G. Schofield and J. Simmonds (eds) *The Child Placement Handbook*, London: BAAF.

Hill, M., Lockyer, A., Morton, P., Batchelor, S. and Scott, S. (2002) 'Safeguarding children in Scotland: the perspectives of children, parents and safeguarders', *Representing Children*, 15(3), pp. 169–83.

Hill, M., Lockyer, A., Morton, P., Batchelor, S. and Scott, S. (2003) 'Safeguarding children's interests in welfare proceedings: the Scottish experience', *Journal of Social Welfare and Family Law*, 25(1), pp. 1–25.

Hill, M., Lockyer, A. and Stone, F. (eds) (2007a) *Youth Justice and Child Protection*, London: Jessica Kingsley.

Hill, M., Stafford, A., Seaman, P., Ross, N. and Daniel, B. (2007b) *Parenting and Resilience*, York: Joseph Rowntree Foundation.

Hill, M. and Tisdall, K. (1997) *Children and Society*, Harlow: Longman.

Hill, M., Turner, K., Walker, M., Stafford, A. and Seaman, P. (2006) 'Children's perspectives on social exclusion and resilience in disadvantaged communities', in E. K. M. Tisdall, J. M. Davis, M. Hill and A. Prout (eds) *Children, Young People and Social Inclusion*, Bristol: Policy Press.

Hillman, M. (2006) 'Children's rights and adult wrongs', *Children's Geographies*, Vol. 4, No. 1, pp. 61–7.

Hillman, M., Adams, J. and Whitelegg, J. (1991) *One False Move: a Study of Children's Independent Mobility*, London: Policy Studies Institute.

Hitching, J. (2008) *Maintaining Your Licence to Practise*, Exeter: Learning Matters.

Hoare, J., Parfrement-Hopkins, J., Britton, A., Hall, P., Scribbins, M. and Flatley, J. (eds) (2010) *Children's experience and attitudes towards the police, personal safety and public spaces: findings from the 2009/10 British Crime Survey interviews with children aged 10 to 15*, Supplementary Volume 3 to Crime in England and Wales 2009/10, London: Home Office.

Hobcraft, J. (2009) 'Circumstances of young adults; results from the Generations and Gender Programme', *How Generations and Gender Shape Demographic Change: Towards Policies Based on Better Knowledge*, Geneva: United Nations Economic Commission for Europe.

Hodges, J., Steele, M., Hillman, S., Henderson, K. and Kaniuk, J. (2003) 'Changes in attachment representations over the first year of adoptive placement: narratives of maltreated children', *Clinical Child Psychology and Psychiatry*, Vol. 8, No. 3, pp. 351–87.

Hoffman, K. T., Marvin, R. S., Cooper, G. and Powell, B. (2006) 'Changing Toddlers' and Preschoolers' Attachment Classifications: The Circle of Security intervention', *Journal of Consulting and Clinical Psychology*, 74(6), pp. 1017–26.

Holland, J. (2009) 'Young people and social capital', *Young*, 17, pp. 331–50.

Holland, J., Reynolds, T. and Weller, S. (2007) 'Transitions, networks and communities: the significance of social capital in the lives of children and young people', *Journal of Youth Studies*, 10(1), pp. 97–116.

Holloway, S. L. and Valentine, S. L. (eds) (2000) *Children's Geographies*, London: Routledge.

Holman, B. (1988) *Putting Families First – Prevention and Childcare*, Basingstoke: Macmillan.

Holman, B. (2001) 'Neighbourhood projects and preventing delinquency', *Youth Welfare*, 1(1), pp. 45–52.

Home Office (2000) *Report of Policy Action Team 12: Young People*, London: Home Office.

Horschelmann, K. and Colls, R. (eds) (2009) *Contested Bodies of Children and Youth*, Chichester: Wiley.

Horwath, J. (2007) *Child Neglect: Identification and Assessment*, Basingstoke: Palgrave MacMillan.

Houston, S. (2010) 'Building resilience in a children's home', *Child and Family Social Work*, 15(3), pp. 357–68.

Howard, S. and B. Johnson (2000) 'What makes the difference? Children and teachers talk about resilient outcomes for children "at risk"', *Educational Studies*, 26(3), pp. 321–37.

Howe, D. (2011) *Attachment Across the Life Course*, Basingstoke: Palgrave Macmillan.

Howison, C. (2003) *Destination of early leavers: evidence from the Scottish school leaver's survey*, Special Centre for Educational Research Briefing Number 28, Edinburgh: Centre for Educational Research.

Hoyle, C. (2008) 'Restorative justice, victims and the police', in *Handbook of Policing*, T. Newborn (ed.), Cullompton: Willan.

Hudson, B. (2003) 'From adolescence to young adulthood: the partnership challenge for learning disability services in England', *Disability and Society*, 18(3), pp. 259–76.

Hudson, B. (2006) 'Making and missing connections: learning disability services and the transition from adolescence to adulthood', *Disability and Society*, 21(1), pp. 47–60.

Hughes, D. (2007) *Attachment Focused Family Therapy*, New York: Norton and Company.

Hughes, D. (1997) 'The importance of the family of origin to the child in care', MSc in *Child Protection and Welfare* dissertation, Trinity College, Dublin.

Humes, W. (2006) '*Research Perspectives On Service Integration*', Children's services in Scottish Schools: Research Seminar Proceedings, Aberdeen: University of Aberdeen.

Hutchby, I. and Moran-Ellis, J. (2001) *Children, Technology and Culture*, London: Routledge.

Hutchison, E. D. and Charlesworth, L. W. (2000) 'Securing the welfare of children: policies past, present and future', *Families in Society*, 81(6), pp. 576–85.

Huth, E. J. and Murray, T. J. (2006) *Medicine in Quotations*, Philadelphia: American College of Physicians.

Huxham, C. (2003) 'Theorizing collaborative practice', *Public Management Review*, Vol. 5, Issue 3, Routledge.

Iles, N. and Lowton, K. (2010) 'What is the perceived nature of parental care and support for young people with cystic fibrosis as they enter adult health services', *Health and Social Care in The Community*, 18(1), pp. 21–9.

Ingram, J. and Salmon, D. (2010) 'Young people's use and views of school-based health drop-in service in areas of high deprivation', *Health Education Journal*, 69(3), pp. 227–35.

Institute for Volunteering Research (2008) *Young People Help Out*, London: IVR.

Invernizzi, A. and Williams, J. (2008) *Children and Citizenship*, London: Sage.

Ipsos Mori (2009) *Children's and young people's access to online content on mobile devices, games consoles and portable media players*, http://www.ofcom.org.uk/advice/media_literacy/medlitpub/medlitpubrss/online_access.pdf (27.5.10).

Irwin, S. (2009) 'Family contexts, norms and young people's orientations: researching diversity', *Journal of Youth Studies*, 12, 337–54.

Jack, G. (1997) 'Discourses of child protection and child welfare', *British Journal of Social Work*, 27(5), pp. 659–78.

Jackson, C., Hill, K. and Lavis, P. (eds) (2008) *Child and Adolescent Mental Health Today*, Brighton: Pavilion.

Jackson, P. (2004) 'Rights and representation in the Scottish Children's Hearings system', in J. McGhee, M. Mellon and B. Whyte, *Meeting Needs Addressing Deeds – Working with Young People who Offend*, Glasgow: NCH.

Jahnukainen, M. and Järvinen, T. (2005) 'Risk factors and survival routes – social exclusion as a life-historical phenomenon', *Disability and Society*, 20(6), 667–80.

James, A. (2008) 'Children, the UNCRC, and family law in England and Wales', *Family Court Review*, 46(1), pp. 53–64.

James, A., Curtis, P. and Birch, J. (2008) 'Care and control in the construction of children's citizenship' in Invernizzi and Williams *op.cit.*

James, A. and Prout, A. (eds) (1998) *Constructing and Reconstructing Childhood*, 2nd edition, London: Falmer Press.

Jamieson, L. (1987) 'Theories of family development and the experience of being brought up', *Sociology 21*, pp. 591–607.

Jamieson, L. (2005) 'Boundaries of intimacy', in S. Cunningham-Burley and L. McKie (eds), *Families in Society: Boundaries and Relationships*, Bristol: Policy Press, pp. 189–206.

Jamieson, L., Anderson, M., McCrone, D., Bechhofer, F., Stewart, R. and Li, Y. (2002) 'Cohabitation and commitment: partnership plans of young men and women', *Sociological Review*, 50, pp. 354–75.

Jamieson, L., Morgan, D., Crow, G., Allan, G. (2006) 'Friends, neighbours and distant partners: extending or decentring family relationships?', *Sociological Research Online*, 11.

Janze, N. (1999) 'A comparative approach to public childcare for children living away from home in Germany and England', *European Journal of Social Work*, 2(2), pp. 151–163.

Jelphs, K. and Dickinson, H. (2008) *Working in Teams*, Bristol: Policy Press.

Johnston, L., MacDonald, R., Mason, P., Riddell, L. and Webster, C. (2000) *Snakes and Ladders: Young People, Transition and Social Exclusion*, Bristol: The Policy Press.

Johnston-Wilder, S. and Collins, J. (2008) 'Children negotiating identities', in J. Collins and P. Foley (eds) *Promoting Children's Well-being*, Bristol: Policy Press.

Jones, G. (2002) *The Youth Divide: Diverging Paths to Adulthood*, York: Joseph Rowntree Foundation.

Jones, G. (2009) *Youth*, Cambridge: Polity Press.

Jones, P., Moss, D., Tomlinson, P. and Welsh, S. (eds) (2008) *Childhood: Services and Provision for Children*, Harlow: Pearson Education.

Jordan, A., Carlile, O. and Stack, A. (2009) *Approaches to Learning*, Maidenhead, Open University Press.

Juffer, F., Bakermans-Kranenburg, M. J. and van IJzendoorn, M. H. (2008) *Promoting Positive Parenting: An Attachment-based Intervention*, New York, Taylor and Francis Group/Lawrence Erlbaum Associates.

Kaga, J., Bennett, J. and Moss, P. (2010) *Caring and Learning Together – A Cross-national Study on the Integration of Early Childhood Education within Education*, Paris: UNESCO.

Kearney, B. (2000) *Children's Hearings and the Sheriff Court*, Edinburgh: Butterworths.

Kearney, H. F. (2006) *The British Isles: a History of Four Nations*, Cambridge: Cambridge University Press.

Kellett, M. (2010) *Rethinking Children and Research*, London: Continuum.

Kellogg Foundation (2004) *Logic Model Development Guide*, (Battle Creek, MI, W. K. Kellogg Foundation).

Kelly, G. and Pinkerton, J. (1996) 'The Children (Northern Ireland) Order 1995: prospects for progress', in M. Hill and J. Aldgate (eds) *Child Welfare Services*, London: Jessica Kingsley.

Kettle, J. (2008) 'Children's experiences of community regeneration', in P. Jones, D. Moss, P. Tomlinson and S. Welch (eds) *Childhood: Services and Provision for Children*, Harlow: Pearson Education.

Keys, S. (2006) 'Student choices and values in England', *European Journal of Education*, 41(1), pp. 85–96.

Khoo, E. G., Hyvonen, U., Nygren, L. (2002) 'Child welfare or child protection: uncovering Swedish and Canadian orientation to social intervention in child maltreatment', *Qualitative Social Work*, 1(4), pp. 451–71.

Kilbrandon, C. S. (1964) *Report of the Committee on Children and Young Persons, Scotland*, (Kilbrandon Report), Cmnd 2306.

Kim, L., Corlett, L., Thompson, L., Law, J., Wilson, P., Gillberg, C. and Minnis, H. (2010) 'Measuring attachment in large populations: a systematic review', *Education and Child Psychology*, Vol. 27, No. 3, pp. 22–32.

Kina, V. J. (2010) 'Participant or protagonist? The impact of the personal on the development of children and young people's participation', Ph.D. thesis, Durham: Durham University.

Kingdon, D., Hansen, L., Finn, M. and Turkington, D. (2007) 'When standard cognitive-behavioural therapy is not enough' *Psychiatric Bulletin*, 31, pp. 121–23.

Kirk, S. (2008) 'Transitions in the lives of young people with complex health needs', *Child: Care, Health and Development*, 34(5), pp. 567–75.

Kirkpatrick, I., Ackrody, S. and Walker, R. (2005) *The New Managerialism and Public Service Professions*, Basingstoke: Palgrave Macmillan.

Kirton, D. (2009) *Child Social Work: Policy and Practice*, London: Sage.

Kiwan, D. (2010) 'Active citizenship multiculturalism and mutual understanding', in Crick and Lockyer, *op. cit.*

Kjørholt, A. and Bjerke, H. (2008) Paper presented at ESF seminar Children's Participation in Decision-Making, Berlin June 2008. Further information about this project can be found at http://www.ntnu.no/noseb/english/research/projects/childrenascitizens (27.5.10).

Knowles, M. S. et al. (1984) *Andragogy in Action. Applying Modern Principles of Adult Education*, San Francisco: Jossey Bass.

Knowsley Council (2008) *Future Schooling in Knowsley – a Strategy for Change 2008–2010*, Knowsley: Knowsley Council.

Kohli, R. K. S. (2007) *Social Work with Unaccompanied Asylum Seeking Children*, Basingstoke: Palgrave.

Kohli, R. and Mitchell, F. (eds) (2007) *Working with Unaccompanied Asylum Seeking Children*, Basingstoke: Palgrave.

Kolb, D. A. (with J. Osland and I. Rubin) (1995) *The Organizational Behaviour Reader*, Englewood Cliffs, NJ: Prentice Hall.

Koslowski, A. (2010) 'Working fathers in Europe: earning and caring', *European Sociological Review*, Advance Access published online on 11 February 2010, doi:10.1093/esr/jcq004.

Laluvein, J. (2010) 'School inclusion and the "community of practice"', *International Journal of Inclusive Education*, 14(1), pp. 35–48.

Laning, Lord. (2003) *The Victoria Climbie Inquiry*, London: Stationery Office.

Lansdown, G. (2002) 'The participation of children', reprinted in *Changing Childhoods*, H. Montgomery, R. Burr and M. Woodhead (eds) Milton Keynes: Open University Press.

Lansdown, G. (2005) *The Evolving Capacities of the Child*, Florence: UNICEF Innocenti Research Centre.

Lavis, P. (2008) 'Child and adolescent mental health service structures and policy', in *Child and Adolescent Mental Health Today*, C. Jackson, K. Hill and P. Lavis (eds) Brighton: Pavilion.

Law, J., Lindsay, G., Peacey, N., Gascoigne, M., Soloff, N., Radford, J. and Band, S. (2002) 'Consultation as a model for providing speech and language therapy in schools – a panacea or one step too far?', *Child Language, Teaching and Therapy*, 18, pp. 145–163.

Leadbetter, J., Daniels, H., Edwards, A., Martin, D., Middleton, D., Popova, A., Warmington, P., Apostolov, A. and Brown S. (2007) 'Professional learning within multi-agency children's services: researching into practice', *Educational Research*, 49(1), pp. 83–98.

Leckman, J. F. and March, J. S. (2011) 'Developmental neuroscience comes of age', *Journal of Child Psychology and Psychiatry*, 52(4), pp. 1–5.

Lee, M., Chan, A., Bradby, H. and Green, G. (2002) 'Chinese migrant women and families in Britain', *Women's Studies International Forum*, 25, pp. 607–18.

Leigh, S. and Miller, C. (2004) 'Social work and the third way: social work with children and families', *Journal of Social Work*, 4(3), pp. 245–67.

Lerpiniere, P. (1999) 'Counselling for drug misuse' in *Illegal Drug Use in the United Kingdom*, C. Stark, B. A. Kidd and R. A. D. Sykes (eds).

Lewis, A. (2010) 'Silence in the context of "child voice"', *Children and Society*, 24(1), pp. 14–23.

Liebmann, M. (2008) *Restorative Justice*, London: Jessica Kingsley Publishers.

Lindon, J. (2005) *Understanding Child Development: Linking Theory and Practice*, London: Hodder.

Lindsay, D. (2007) 'Prioritisation: an educationalist's perspective', in (2007) *Prioritising Child Health*, S. Roulstone (ed.), London: Routledge.

Ling, R. and Yttri, B. (2006) 'Control, emancipation, and status: the mobile telephone in teens'; parental and peer relationships', in R. Kraut, M. Brynin and S. Kiesler (eds) *Computers, Phones, and the Internet: Domesticating Information Technology*, Oxford: Oxford University Press, pp. 219–34.

Lister, R. (2007) 'Why citizenship: where, when and how children?', *Theoretical Inquiries in Law*, 8(2), pp. 693–718.

Lister, R. (2008) 'Unpacking children's citizenship' in Invernizzi and Williams *op.cit.*

Lister, R., Smith, N., Miton, S. and Cox, L. (2003) 'Young people talk about citizenship', *Citizenship Studies*, 7(2), pp. 235–53.

Little, A. (2002) *The Politics of Community: Theory and Practice*, Edinburgh: Edinburgh University Press.

Littlechild, B. (2008) 'Child protection social work: risks of fears and fears of risks – impossible tasks from impossible goals?', *Social Policy and Administration*, 42(6), pp. 662–75.

Liveability (2008) *Freedom to Live: Transition for Disabled Young People*: Liveability's report on disabled young people moving towards adulthood, Bedford: New North Print.

Livingstone, S. (2009) *Children and the Internet: Great Expectations Challenging Realities*, Cambridge: Polity.

Lloyd, E. (1997) 'The role of the centre in family support', in *Social Action with Children and Families – A Community Development Approach to Child and Family Welfare*, C. Cannan and C. Warren (eds), London: Routledge.

Lloyd, E. (2008) 'The interface between childcare, family support and child poverty strategies under New Labour: tensions and contradictions', *Social Policy and Society*, 7(4), pp. 479–94.

Lloyd, G., Stead, J. and Cohen, D. (2006) *Critical New Perspectives on ADHD*, London: Routledge.

Lloyd, G., Stead, J. and Kendrick, A. (2001) *Hanging in There*, London: National Children's Bureau.

Locke, J. [1689] *Two Treatises on Government*, ed. P. Laslett 1963, Cambridge: Cambridge University Press.

Lockyer, A. (2010) 'Young people as active political citizens', in Crick and Lockyer *op.cit.*

Lockyer, A. and Stone, F. (1998) *Juvenile Justice in Scotland*, Edinburgh: T. and T. Clark.

Loewenstein, K. (2011) 'Going beyond traditional educational models', *Journal of Continuing Education in Nursing*, 42(3), pp. 103–104.

Longelly, P., Bachman, M., Shreeve, A., Reding, R., Thoburn, J., Mugford, M., O'Brien, M. and Husbands, C. (2009) 'Is it feasible to pool funds for local children's services in England?' *Journal of Health Services Research and Policy*, 14(1), pp. 27–34.

Lonne, B., Parton, N., Thomson, J. and Harries, M. (2009) *Reforming Child Protection*, London, Routledge.

Lorenz, W. (1991) The new German Children and Young People Act, *British Journal of Social Work*, 21(3), pp. 329–39.

Lorenz, W. (1994) *Social Work in a Changing Europe*, London: Routledge.

Lorenz, W. (2006) *Perspectives on European Social Work: From the Birth of the Nation State to the Impact of Globalization*, Budrich: Opladen.

Lorenz, W. (2008) 'Paradigms and politics: understanding methods paradigms in an historical context: the case of social pedagogy', *British Journal of Social Work*, 38(4), pp. 625–44.

Lowe, N. and Douglas, G. (2007) *Bromley's Family Law*, Oxford: University Press.

Loxley, A. (2007) *Collaboration in Health and Welfare*, London: Jessica Kingsley.

Lundy, L. (2007) 'Voice is not enough: conceptualising Article 12 of the UN Convention on the Rights of the Child', *British Educational Research*, 33(6), pp. 927–42.

Lupton, R. (2010) 'Area-based initiatives in English education: What place for place and space?', in C. Raffo, A. Dyson, H. Gunter, D. Hall, L. Jones and A. Kalambouka (eds) *Education and Poverty in Affluent Countries*, London: Routledge.

Luthar, S. S. (2003) *Resilience and Vulnerability: Adaptation in the Context of Childhood Adversities*, Cambridge: Cambridge University Press.

McAra, L. and McVie, S. (2005) 'The usual suspects: street life, young people and the police', *Criminal Justice*, 5(5), pp. 5–36.

McAra, L. and McVie, S. (2010) 'Youth crime and justice: key messages from the Edinburgh Study of Youth Transitions and Crime', *Criminology and Criminal Justice*, 10(2), pp. 179–209.

McCallin, A. (2001) 'Interdisciplinary practice – a matter of teamwork: an integrated literature review', *Journal of Clinical Nursing*, 10, 419–28.

McCann, J., James, A. and Wilson, S. et al. (1996) 'Prevalence of psychiatric disorders of young people in the care system', *BMJ*, 313, pp. 1529–30.

McCarthy, M. (1957) *Memoirs of a Catholic Girlhood*, San Diego: Harcourt Press.

McCartney, E. (2009) 'Joining up working: terms, types and tensions', in J. Forbes and C. Watson (eds) *Service Integration in Schools: Research and Policy Discourses, Practices and Future Prospects*, Rotterdam: Sense, pp. 23–36.

McCartney, E., Ellis, S., Boyle, J., Turnbull, M. and Kerr, J. (2010) 'Developing a language support model for mainstream primary school teachers', *Child Language Teaching and Therapy*, 26(3), pp. 359–74.

McCubbin, H. I., Thompson, A. I. and McCubbin, M. A. (1996) *Family Assessment: Resiliency, Coping and Adaptation*, Madison: University of Wisconsin Publishers.

McDonald, R. and Marsh, J. (2005) *Disconnected Youth?*, Basingstoke: Palgrave Macmillan.

McIntosh, J. and N. McKeganey (2001) 'Identity and recovery from dependent drug use: the addicts' perspective', *Drug: Education, Prevention and Policy*, 8(1), pp. 47–59.

McIvor, G. (2010) 'What works with women who offend?', in *21st Century Social Workers*, R. Taylor, M. Hill and F. McNeill (eds), London: Venture Press.

McLeod, A. (2008) *Listening to Children*, London: Jessica Kingsley.

McLeod, A. (2010) 'A friend and an equal', *British Journal of Social Work*, 40, pp. 722–88.

McMahon, E., Reulbach, U., Keeley, H., Perry, I. and Arensman, E. (2010) 'Bullying victimisation, self harm and associated factors in Irish adolescent boys', *Social Science and Medicine*, 71(7), pp. 1300–1307.

McNeill, F. (2004) 'Desistance, rehabilitation and correctionalism', *The Howard Journal*, 43(4), pp. 420–36.

McNeill, F. (2009a) 'Supervising young offenders: what works and what's right?', in *Youth Offending and Youth Justice*, M. Barry and F. McNeill (eds), London: Jessica Kingsley.

McNeill, F. (2009b) 'What works and what's just?', *European Journal of Probation*, 1(1), pp. 21–40.

McNeill, F. (2010) 'Youth justice: policy, research and evidence', in J. Johnstone and M. Burman (eds) *Youth Justice*, Edinburgh: Dunedin.

McNeill, F. and S. Maruna (2007) 'Giving up and giving back: desistance, generativity and social work with offenders', in *Developments in Social Work with Offenders*, G. McIvor and P. Raynor (eds), London: Jessica Kingsley Publishers.

McNeill, F. and B. Whyte (eds) (2007) *Reducing Reoffending*, Cullompton: Willan.

McNiff, J. and Whitehead, J. (2006) *All You Need to Know About Action Research*: London, Sage.

MacDonald, R. and Marsh, J. (2005) *Disconnected Youth? Growing Up in Britain's Poor Neighbourhoods*, Basingstoke: Palgrave Macmillan.

MacDonald, R., Shildrick, T., Webster, C. and Simpson, D. (2005) 'Growing up in poor neighbourhoods: the significance of class place in the extended transitions of "socially excluded" young adults', *Sociology*, 39(5), pp. 873–90.

MacIntyre, G. (2007) 'What Next? Opportunities for Young People with Learning Disabilities upon Leaving School', Department of Sociology, Anthropology and Applied Social Sciences, Glasgow: University of Glasgow.

MacIntyre, G. (2008) *Learning Disability and Social Inclusion*, Edinburgh, Dunedin Academic Press.

MacKay, D. and MacIntyre, G. (forthcoming) 'Personalisation and the role of the social worker', in R. Taylor, M. Hill and F. McNeill (eds) *Early Professional Development for Social Workers*, London, Venture Press.

Mackenzie, S. and Hendry, A. (2009) *Community Policing: A Review of the Evidence*, Edinburgh: Scottish Government Social Research.

Macleod, G. (2006) 'Bad, mad or sad: constructions of young people in trouble and implications for interventions', *Emotional and Behavioural Difficulties*, 11(3), pp. 155–67.

Main, M. and Solomon, J. (1986) 'Discovery of an insecure disorganized/disorientated attachment pattern', in *Affective Development in Infancy*, M. Yogman and T. B. Brazleton (eds), New Jersey: Ablex, pp. 95–124.

Malcolm, J. (2009) 'A case study investigating the ability of babies and infants to participate in the decision-making process in an early years centre', MSc in Childhood Studies dissertation, University of Edinburgh.

Malin, N. and Morrow, G. (2008) *Evaluating Sure Start*, London: Whiting and Birch.

Mann, J. J., Apter, A., Bertolote, J., Beautrais, A., Currier, D., Haas, A. et al. (2005) 'Suicide prevention strategies: a systematic review', *JAMA*, 294, pp. 2064–74.

Mansell, J. and Beadle-Brown, J. (2005) 'Person centred planning and person centred action: a critical perspective', in S. Carnaby and P. Cambridge (eds) *Intimate Care and People with Learning Disabilities*, London: Jessica Kingsley Publishers.

Maplethorpe, N., Chanfreau, J., Philo, D. and Tait, C. (2009) *Families and Children in Britain*, London: Department for Work and Pensions.

Markström, A. and Hallden, G. (2009) 'Children's strategies for agency in preschool', *Children and Society*, 23(2), pp. 113–22.

Marmot, M. (2010) *Fair Society, Healthy Lives*, London: Department of Health.

Marshall, K. (1997) *Children's Rights in the Balance*, Edinburgh: The Stationery Office, pp. 8–14.

Marshall, K. (2006) 'Human rights and children's rights in the Scottish Children's Hearings system', in M. Hill, A. Lockyer and F. Stone (eds) *Youth Justice and Child Protection*, London: Jessica Kingsley.

Marshall, T. H. (1950) *Citizenship and Social Class*, Cambridge: Cambridge University Press.

Martin, P. Y. and Jackson, S. (2002) 'Educational success for children in public care', *Child and Family Social Work*, 7, pp. 121–30.

Maruna, S. and Immarigeon, R. (eds) (2008) *After Crime and Punishment: Pathways to Offender Reintegration*, Cullompton: Willan.

Marvin, R., Cooper, G., Hoffman, K. and Powell, B. (2002) 'The Circle of Security project: attachment-based intervention with caregiver–pre-school child dyads', *Attachment and Human Development*, 4, pp. 107–124.

Matthews, H. (2001) *Children and Community Regeneration*, London: Save the Children.

Mawyer, M. (1995) *Defending the American Family*, Green Forest AR: Newleaf Press.

May, V. and Smart, C. (2004) 'Silence in court? Hearing children in residence and contact disputes', *Child and Family Law Quarterly*, 16(3), pp. 305–15.

Mayall, B. (2002) *Towards a Sociology for Childhood*, Buckingham: Open University Press.

Meadows, P. (2007) 'The costs and benefits of Sure Start local programmes' in *The National Evaluation of Sure Start – Does Area-based Intervention Work?*, J. Belsky, J. Barnes and E. Melhuish (eds) Bristol: The Policy Press.

Mediratta, K., Shah, S. and McAlister, S. (2009) *Community Organizing for Stronger Schools: Strategies and Successes*, Cambridge MA: Harvard Education Press.

Melhuish, E. and Hall. D. (2007) 'The historical and policy context', in *The National Evaluation of Sure Start – Does Area-based Intervention Work*, J. Belsky, J. Barnes and E. Melhuish (eds), Bristol: The Policy Press.

Melhuish, E., Belsky, J., Anning, A. and Ball, M. (2007) 'Variations in Sure Start local programmes: consequences for children and families', in *The National Evaluation of Sure Start – Does Area-based Intervention Work*, J. Belsky, J. Barnes and E. Melhuish (eds), Bristol: The Policy Press.

Melhuish, E., Belsky, J. and Leyland, A. (2005) *Early Impact of Sure Start Local Programmes on Children and Families. SS Report 13*, London: DfES.

Mendel, R. (2000) *Less Hype More Help. Reducing Youth Crime: What Works and What Doesn't?*, Washington DC: American Youth Policy Forum.

Menna, R. and Ruck, M. D. (2004) 'Adolescent help-seeking behavior: how can we encourage it?', *Guidance and Counseling*, 18(4), pp. 176–83.

Middleton, D. (1996) 'Talking work: argument, common knowledge, and improvisation in teamwork', in *Cognition and Communication at Work*, Y. Engeström and D. Middleton (eds) Cambridge: Cambridge University Press, pp. 233–56.

Middleton, D. (2010) 'Identifying learning in inter-professional discourse: the development of an analytic protocol', in *Activity Theory in Practice: Promoting Learning Across Boundaries and Agencies*, H. Daniels, A. Edwards, Y. Engeström and S. Ludvigsen (eds) London: Routledge, pp. 90–104.

Midgley, N. (2010) 'Improvers, adapters and rejecters: the link between "evidence-based practice" and "evidence-based practitioners"', *Clinical Child Psychology and Psychiatry*, 14(3), pp. 323–27.

Milbourne, L. (2009) 'Valuing difference or securing compliance? Working to involve young people in community settings', *Children and Society*, 23(5), pp. 347–63.

Milford, R., Kleve, L., Lea, J. and Greenwood, R. (2006) 'A pilot evaluation study of the Solihull Approach', *Community Practitioner*, 79, pp. 358–62.

Miller, J. (2009) *Never Too Young: How Young Children can Take Responsibility and Make Decisions*, London: Save the Children.

Miller, W. L. and Hussain, A. (2006) *Multicultural Nationalism: Islamophobia, Anglophobia and Devolution*, Oxford: Oxford University Press.

Modood, T. (2007) *Multiculturalism*, Cambridge: Polity.

Molcho, M., Nic Gabhainn, S. and Kelleher, C. (2007) 'Interpersonal relationships as predictors of positive health among Irish youth: the more the merrier', *Irish Medical Journal*, 100(8), pp. 33–6.

Morgan, D. (1996) *Family Connections: An Introduction to Family Studies*, Cambridge: Polity.

Morgan, D. (2006) *About Social Workers: A Children's Views Report*, London: Children's Rights Director for England.

Morgan, D. H. J. (2011) *Rethinking Family Practices*, Basingstoke: Palgrave Macmillan.

Morgan, R. (2009) 'Children and young people: criminalisation and punishment', in *Youth Offending and Youth Justice*, M. Barry and F. McNeill (eds), London: Jessica Kingsley.

Morrow, V. (1999) 'Conceptualising social capital in relation to the well-being of children and young people: a critical review', *The Sociological Review*, 47(4), pp. 744–65.

Morrow, V. (2004) 'Networks and neighbourhoods: children's accounts of friendship, family and place', in C. Phillipson, G. Allan and D. Morgan (eds) *Social Networks and Social Exclusion: Sociological and Social Policy Perspectives*, Avebury: Ashgate.

Morrow, V. (2005) 'Social capital, community cohesion and participation in England: a space for children and young people?', *Journal of Social Sciences* (special issue), 9, pp. 57–69.

Moss, D. (2008) 'The social divisions of childhood', in P. Jones, D. Moss, P. Tomlinson and S. Welch (eds) *Childhood: Services and Provision for Children*, Harlow: Pearson Education.

Moss, P. (2006) 'From children's services to children's spaces', in *Children, Young People and Social Inclusion*, K. Tisdall, J. M. Davis, M. Hill and A. Prout (eds), Bristol: Policy Press.

Moss, P. and Penn, H. (1996) *Transforming Nursery Education*, London: Paul Chapman Publishing.

Moss, P. and Petrie, P. (2002) *From Children's Services to Children's Spaces*, London: Routledge Falmer.

Muijs, D., Ainscow, M., Dyson, A., Raffo, C., Goldrick, S., Kerr, K., Lennie, C. and Miles, S. (2008) *Leading under pressure: Leadership for social inclusion*, Report for NCSL (London).

Mulcahy, A. (2006) *Policing Northern Ireland: Conflict, Legitimacy and Reform*, Portland OR: Willan Publishing.

Munn, P. (2010) 'What can active citizenship achieve for schools and through schools', in Crick and Lockyer *op. cit.*

Munro, E. (2011) *The Munro Review of Child Protection*, London: Department of Education.

Munro, E. and Calder, M. (2005) 'Where has child protection gone?', *Political Quarterly*, 76(3), pp. 439–45.

Muris, P., Merckelbach, H., Gadet, B. and Moulaert, V. (2009) 'Fears, worries and scary dreams in 4- to 12 year-old children', *Journal of Clinical Child and Adolescent Psychology*, 29(1), pp. 43–52.

Murray, C. (2009) 'Typologies of youth resisters and desisters', *Youth Justice*, 9(2), pp. 115–29.

Murray, L. and Andrews, L. (2005) '*The Social Baby*: understanding babies' communication from birth', DVD, London: NSPCC.

Murray, L., Cooper, P., Wilson, A. and Romaniuk, H. (2003) 'Controlled trial of the short- and long-term effect of psychological treatment of post-partum depression 2. Impact on the mother–child relationship and child outcome', *British Journal of Psychiatry*, 182, pp. 420–27.

Murray, L., Kempton, C., Woolgar, M. and Hooper, R. (1993) 'Depressed mothers' speech to their infants and its relation to infant gender and cognitive development', *Journal of Child Psychology and Psychiatry and Allied Disciplines*, Vol. 34, No. 7, pp. 1083–1101.

Nash, M. and Walker, L. (2009) 'Mappa – is closer collaboration really the key to effectiveness?', *Policing*, 3(2), pp. 172–80.

National Assembly for Wales (2003) *Community focused schools*. Guidance circular 34/2003, Cardiff: Department for Training and Education.

National Audit Office (NAO) (2006) *Sure Start Children's Centre*, London: The Stationery Office.

National Audit Office (NAO) (2009) *Sure Start Children's Centres*, Memorandum for the Children, Schools and Families Committee, Fifth Report of Session 2009–10, Volume II, London: House of Commons Children, Schools and Families Committee.

National Audit Office (NAO) (2010) *CAFCASS's Responses to increased demand for its services*, London: NAO.

National Institute for Health and Clinical Excellence (NICE) (2006) *Obesity: guidance on the prevention, identification, assessment and management of overweight and obesity in adults and children*, NICE clinical guideline 43, available at: http://www.nice.org.uk/nicemedia/live/11000/30365/30365.pdf.

National Scientific Council on the Developing Child (2004).

Neighbourhood Nurseries Research Team (2007) *National Evaluation of the Neighbourhood Nurseries Initiative: Integrated Report*, Research report SSU/2007/FR/024, London: HMSO.

Newman, R. S. (2000) 'Social influences on the development of children's adaptive help-seeking: The role of parents, teachers and peers', *Developmental Review*, 20, pp. 350–404.

Newman, T. (2004) *What Works in Building Resilience*, Barkingside: Barnardos.

Newman, T. and Blackburn, S. (2002) *Transition in the Lives of Children and Young People: Resilience Factors*, Edinburgh: Scottish Executive.

NHS Education Scotland (2008) A capability framework for nurses who care for children and young people who are looked after and accommodated. Access on http://www.nes.scot.nhs.uk/media/3869/lacframeworkfinallores.pdf.

NICCYP (2008) *Corporate Plan of the Northern Ireland Commissioner for Children and Young People 2008–11*, Belfast.

Nicklett, E. J. and Perron, B. E. (2010) 'Laws and policies to support the wellbeing of children: an international comparative analysis', *International Journal of Social Welfare*, 19(1), pp. 3–7.

Noell, G. H. and Witt, J. C. (1999) 'When does consultation lead to intervention implementation?', *Journal of Special Education*, 33(1), pp. 29–35.

Norman, J. (2009) 'Seen and not heard: young people's perceptions of the police', *Policing*, 3(4), pp. 364–72.

Northern Ireland Care Council (2011) *A Career in Child Care and Early Years*, http://www. niscc.info/Publications-143.aspx.

NSPCC (2010) 'The impact of abuse and neglect on the health and mental health of children and young people'. Access on www.nspcc.org.uk/inform.

Nugent, J. K. and Brazelton, T. B. (2006) 'Preventive intervention with infants and families: the NBAS model', *Infant Mental Health Journal*, 10, pp. 84–99.

Nutley, S., Morton, S., Jung, T. and Boaz, A. (2010) 'Evidence and policy in six European countries', *Evidence and Policy*, 6(2), pp. 131–44.

O'Brien, J. and Macleod, G. (2010) *The Social Agenda of the School*, Edinburgh: Dunedin Academic Press.

O'Brien, M., Bachman, M., Jones, N. R., Reading, R., Thoburn, J., Husbands, C., Shreeve, A. and Watson, J. (2009) 'Do integrated children's services improve children's outcomes?', *Children and Society*, 23(5), pp. 320–35.

O'Connor, P., Haynes, A. and Kane, C. (2004) 'Relational discourses: social ties with family and friends', *Childhood: A Global Journal of Child Research*, 11, pp. 361–82.

O'Halloran, K. (1999) *The Welfare of the Child*, Aldershot: Ashgate.

O'Neill, J. (1994) *The Missing Child in Liberal Theory; Towards a Covenant Theory of Family, Community, Welfare and the Civic State*, Toronto: University of Toronto Press.

O'Neill, J. (2000) 'So that I can more or less get them to do things they really don't want to. Capturing the "situated complexities" of the secondary school head of department', *Journal of Educational Enquiry*, 1(1), pp. 13–34.

Odegard, A. (2006) 'Exploring perceptions of interprofessional collaboration in child mental health care', *International Journal of Integrated Care*, 6(18), pp. 1–13.

OECD (1998) *Co-ordinating Services for Children and Youth at Risk: a World View*, Paris: OECD.

OECD (2010) *Obesity and the Economics of Prevention – Fit not Fat*, OECD publishing.

Office for National Statistics (2009) *Population Estimates by Ethnic Group: 2001 to 2007 Commentary*.

Ofsted (2009) *The Impact of Integrated Services on Children and their Families in Sure Start Children's Centres*, London: Ofsted.

Oldfield, A. (1990) *Citizenship and Community: Civic Republicanism and the Modern World*, London: Routledge.

Olds, D., Henderson, C. R., Cole, R., Eckenrode, J., Kitzman, H., Luckey, D., Pettitt, L., Sidora, K., Morris, P. and Powers, J. (1998) 'Long-term effects of nurse home visitation on children's criminal and antisocial behavior 15-year follow-up of a randomized controlled trial', *Journal of the American Medical Association*, 280, pp. 1238–44.

Olsson, C. A., Bond, L., Burns, J. M., Vella-Brodrick, D. A. and Sawyer, S. M. (2003) 'Adolescent resilience: a concept analysis', *Journal of Adolescence*, 26, pp. 1–11.

Onozawa, K., Glover, V., Adams, D., Modi, N. and Kumar, R. C. (2001) 'Infant massage improves mother–infant interaction for mothers with postnatal depression', *Journal of Affective Disorders*, 63, pp. 201–207.

Onyett, S. (2009) 'Working appreciatively to improve services for children and families', *Clinical Child Psychology and Psychiatry*, 14(4), pp. 495–507.

Osgood, W., Foster, M. and Courtney, M. (2010) 'Vulnerable populations and the transition to adulthood', *Future of Children*, 20(1), pp. 209–29.

Osler, A. (2010) *Students' Perspectives on Schooling*, Maidenhead: Open University Press.

Ozga, J. and Catts, R. (2004) 'Social capital concepts and implications: a discussion paper', Unpublished discussion paper. Applied Educational Research Scheme, Schools and Social Capital Network, Stirling, UK: University of Stirling.

Page, J., Whitting, G. and Mclean, C. (2007) *Engaging Effectively with Black and Ethnic Minority Parents in Children's and Parental Services*, Research Report No DCSF-RR013, London: DCSF.

Parreñas, R. (2005) 'Long distance intimacy: class, gender and intergenerational relations between mothers and children in Filipino transnational families', *Global Networks*, 5, pp. 317–36.

Parsons, M. L. and Warner-Robbins, C. (2002) 'Factors that support women's successful transition to the community following jail/prison', *Health Care for Women International*, 23(1), pp. 6–18.

Parton, N. (2004) 'From Maria Colwell to Victoria Climbié: reflections on public inquiries into child abuse a generation apart', *Child Abuse Review*, 13(2), pp. 80–94.

Penn, H. (2007) 'Childcare market management: how the United Kingdom government has reshaped its role in developing early childhood education and care', *Contemporary Issues in Early Childhood*, 8(3), pp. 192–207.

Penn, H. (2009) 'Public and private: the history of early education and care institutions in the United Kingdom', in *Child Care and Preschool Development In Europe – Institutional Perspectives*, K. Schweiwe and H. Willekens (eds), Basingstoke: Palgrave Macmillan.

Penn, H., Barreau, L., Butterworth, L., Lloyd, E., Moyles, J., Potter, S. and Sayeed, Z. (2004) 'What is the impact of out-of-home integrated care and education settings on children aged 0–6 and their parents?', in *Research Evidence in Education Library*, London: Social Science Research Unit, Institute of Education, University of London.

Percy-Smith, B. and Thomas, N. (eds) (2010) *A Handbook of Children and Young People's Participation: Perspectives from Theory and Practice*, Abingdon: Routledge.

Petch, A. (2008) *Health and Social Care: Establishing a Joint Future?*, Edinburgh, Dunedin Academic Press.

Petrie, P., Boddy, J., Cameron, C. and Wigfall, V. (2006) *Working with Children in Care: European Perspectives*, Maidenhead: Open University Press.

Petrosino, A., Turpin-Petrosino, C. and Buehler, J. (2003) '"Scared Straight" and other juvenile awareness programs for preventing juvenile delinquency. Campbell Review update', in *The Campbell Collaboration Reviews of Intervention and Policy Evaluations (C2-RIPE)*, Philadelphia, Pennsylvania: Campbell Collaboration.

Philip, K. (2008) 'Youth mentoring: a case for treatment', *Youth and Policy*, 19, pp. 17–32.

Phillips, B. and Alderson, P. (2003) 'Beyond "anti-smacking": challenging parental violence', *Child Abuse Review*, 12, pp. 282–91.

Phillips, R., Norden, O., McGinigal, S., Oseman, D. with Coleman, N. (2009) *Childcare and Early Years Providers Survey 2009*, Research Report DFE-RR012, London: Department for Education.

Pias, J. M. (2000) 'Transitions and youth cultures: forms and performances', *International Social Science Journal*, 164, pp. 219–31.

Pike, A., Coldwell, J. and Dunn, J. (2006) *Family Relationships in Middle Childhood*, York: Joseph Rowntree Foundation.

Pinkerton, J. and Dolan, P. (2007) 'Family support, social capital, resilience and adolescent coping', *Child and Family Social Work*, 12(3), pp. 219–28.

Pinkerton, J. and Katz, I. (2003) *Evaluating Family Support: Thinking Internationally, Thinking Critically*. Wiley: Chichester.

Piper, C. (2008) *Investing in Children*, Cullompton, Willan.

Platt, D. (2006) 'Investigation or initial assessment of child concerns? The impact of the refocusing initiative on social work practice', *British Journal of Social Work*, 36(2), pp. 267–81.

Plomin, R. (1995) 'Genetics and children's experiences in the family', *Journal of Child Psychology and Psychiatry*, Vol. 36, No. 1, pp. 33–68.

Pollard, A. and Triggs, P. (1997) *Reflective Teaching in Secondary Education*, London: Cassell.

Polnay, L. and Ward, H. (2000) 'Promoting the health of looked-after children', *British Medical Journal*, 320, pp. 661–62.

Pople, L. and Smith, D. J. (2010) 'Time trends in youth crime and in justice system responses', in D. J. Smith (ed.) *A New Response to Youth Crime*, Cullompton, Willan.

Porporino, F. J. (2010) 'Bringing sense and sensitivity to correction: from programmes to fix offenders to services to support desistance', in J. Brayford, F. Crowe and J. Deering (eds) *What Else Works?*, Cullompton: Willan.

Portes, A. (1998) 'Social capital: its origins and applications in modern sociology', *Annual Review of Sociology*, 24, pp. 1–24.

Poursanidou, K., Garner, P. and Watson, A. (2008) 'Hospital school liaison: perspective of health and educational professionals supporting children with renal transplants', *Journal of Health Care*, 12(4), pp. 253–67.

Power, A. (2007) *City Survivors: Bringing up Children in Disadvantaged Neighbourhoods*, Bristol: The Policy Press.

Power, S., Rees, G. and Taylor, C. (2005) 'New Labour and educational disadvantage: the limits of area-based initiatives', *London Review of Education*, 3(2), 101–16.

Pratt, J., Gordon, P. and Plamping, D. (1999) *Working Whole Systems*, London: King's Fund.

Pressler, S. J. (2010) 'Construction of childhood', in *Key Issues in Childhood and Youth Studies*, D. Kassem, L. Murphy and E. Taylor (eds), Routledge: London.

Priebe, G. and Svedin, C. G. (2008) 'Child sexual abuse is largely hidden from adult society', *Child Abuse and Neglect*, 32, pp. 1095–1108.

Prins, E., Blaire Willson Toso, B. W. and Schafft, K. (2009) '"It feels like a little family to me": social interaction and support among women in adult education and family literacy', *Adult Education Quarterly*, August 2009, 59, pp. 335–52.

Prior, D., Stewart, J. and Walsh, K. (1995) *Citizenship: Rights, Community and Participation*, London: Pitman.

Prochaska, J. O., DiClemente, C. C. and Norcross, J. (1992) 'In search of how people change: applications to addictive behaviours', *American Psychologist*, 47(9), pp. 1102–4.

Prout, A. (2005) *The Future of Childhood*, London: Sage.

Prout, A. (2011) 'Taking a step away from modernity: reconsidering the new sociology of childhood', *Global Studies of Childhood*, 1(1), pp. 4–14.

Pryor, J. (2006) 'Children and the changing families', in F. Ebtehaj, B. Lindley and M. Richards (eds), *Kinship Matters*. Oxford: Hart, pp. 99–114.

Puckering, C., McIntosh, E., Hickey, A. and Longford, J. (2010) 'Mellow babies: a group intervention for infants and mothers experiencing postnatal depression', *Counselling Psychology Review*, 25(1), pp. 28–38.

Puckering, C., Webster, J. and Wilson, P. (2011) 'Secure mother–infant attachment and the ABC programme: a case history', *Community Practitioner*, 84(1), pp. 35–7.

Pugh, G. (2006) 'The policy agenda for early childhood services', in *Contemporary Issues in the Early Years*, G. Pugh and B. Duffy (eds) London: Sage.

Puonti, A. (2004) *Learning to Work Together: Collaboration Between Authorities in Economic Crime Investigation*, Vantaa, Finland: National Bureau of Investigation.

Putnam, R. D. (1993) 'The prosperous community: Social capital and public life', *The American Prospect*, 13 (Spring), pp. 35–42.

Putnam, R. D. (1995) 'Tuning in, tuning out: the strange disappearance of social capital in America', *Political Science and Politics*, 28, pp. 1–20.

Putnam, R. D. (2000) *Bowling Alone: The collapse and revival of American Community*, New York: Simon Schuster.

Qualifications and Curriculum Authority (1998) *Education for Citizenship and the Teaching of Democracy in Schools*, (Crick Report), London: QCA.

Quinn, K. and Jackson, J. (2007) 'Of rights and roles: police interviews with young suspects in Northern Ireland', *British Journal of Criminology*, 47, pp. 234–55.

Quinton, D. (2004) *Supporting Parents*, London: Jessica Kingsley.

Qvortrup, J. (2008) 'Childhood as a structural form', in *The Palgrave Handbook of Childhood Studies*, J. Qvortrup, W. A. Corsaro and M-S. Honig (eds), Basingstoke: Palgrave Macmillan.

Raby, C. and Raby, S. (2008) 'Resilience and risk in children and young people', in K. Jackson, M. Hill and P. Lavis (eds) *Child and Adolescent Mental Health Today*, Brighton: Pavillion.

Radford, K., Hamilton, J. and Jarman, N. (2005) '"It's their word against mine": young people's attitudes to the police complaints procedure in Northern Ireland', *Children and Society*, 19, pp. 360–70.

Raffe, D. (2003) *Young people not in education, employment or training*, Centre for Educational Studies (CES) Special Briefing Paper, Edinburgh: Centre for Educational Studies.

Reder, P. and Duncan, S. (2004) 'Making the most of the Victoria Climbié inquiry report', in N. Stanley and J. Manthorpe (eds) *The Age of Inquiry: Learning and Blaming in Health and Social Care*, London, Routledge.

Rees, G., Power, S. and Taylor, C. (2007) 'The governance of educational inequalities: the limits of area-based initiatives', *Journal of Comparative Policy Analysis*, 9(3), pp. 261–74.

Rees, O. (2008) 'Devolution and the development of family law in Wales, *Child and Family Law Quarterly*, 20(1), pp. 45–63.

Rees, O. (2010) 'Dealing with individual cases – an essential role for national human rights institutions for children?', *International Journal of Children's Rights*, 18, pp. 417–36.

Rees, R., Oliver, K., Woodman, J. and Thomas, J. (2009) *Children's Views about Obesity, Body Size, Shape and Weight: a systematic review*, London: EPPI Centre, Social Science Research Unit, Institute of Education, University of London http://eppi.ioe.ac.uk/cms/Default.aspx?tabid=2463.

Reid, B. (1998) 'Panels and hearings' in A. Lockyer and F. H. Stone, *Juvenile Justice in Scotland*, Edinburgh: T. and T. Clark, pp. 184–98.

Reid, B. and Gillan, I. (2007) 'The place of lay participation in decision-making', in M. Hill, A. Lockyer and F. Stone (eds) *Youth Justice and Child Protection*, London: Jessica Kingsley.

Rhodes, J. E. and Love, S. R. (2008) 'Youth mentoring: improving programmes through research-based practice', *Youth and Policy* (19), pp. 9–16.

Ribbens McCarthy, J. (2006) *Young People's Experiences of Loss and Bereavement: Towards an Inter-disciplinary Approach*, Buckingham: Open University Press.

Richardson, G. (2004) 'Impact studies in the United Kingdom', in *Judicial Review and Bureaucratic Impact*, M. Hertogh and S. Halliday (eds) Cambridge: Cambridge University Press.

Riddell, S., Banks, P. and Thornton, P. (2003) 'Disabled people, employment and the work preparation scheme', Paper to the *Working futures: disabled people and work* seminar, University of Sunderland, 3 December 2003.

Riddell, S., Baron, S. and Wilson, A. (2001) *The Learning Society and People with Learning Difficulties*, Bristol: Policy Press.

Riddell, S. and Tett, L. (eds) (2001) *Education, Social Justice and Inter-agency Working: Joined up or Fractured Policy*, London: Routledge.

Ridge, T. (2002) *Childhood Poverty and Social Exclusion*, Bristol: Policy Press.

Rivett, M. and Street, E. (2003) *Family Therapy in Focus*, London: Sage.

Rixon, A. (2008a) 'Working with change', in P. Foley and A. Roxon (eds) *Changing Children's Services*, Bristol: Policy Press.

Rixon, A. (2008b) 'Learning together', in P. Foley and A. Roxon (eds) *Changing Children's Services*, Bristol: Policy Press.

Roberts, H., Smith, S. J. and Bryce, C. (1995) *Children at Risk: Safety as Social Value*, Buckingham: Open University Books.

Robertson, L., Campbell, A., Hill, M. and McNeill, F. (2006) 'Promoting desistance and resilience in young people who offend', *Scottish Journal of Criminal Justice Studies*, 12, pp. 56–73.

Robinson, C. and Stalker, K. (eds) (1999) *Growing up with Disability*, London: Jessica Kingsley.

Roche, J. (1999) 'Children: rights, participation and citizenship', *Childhood*, 6(4), pp. 475–93.

Roper v *Simmons*, 543 U.S. 551, 624 (J. Scalia, dissenting) in re Gault, 387 U.S. 1 (1967).

Ross, N. J., Hill, M. and Shelton, A. (2008) 'One Scotland. Many cultures', *Scottish Affairs*, 64, pp. 84–103.

Roulstone, S. (2007) *Prioritising Child Health*, London: Routledge.

Rowley, H. and Dyson, A. (2011) 'Academies in the public interest – a contradiction in terms?' in H. M. Gunter (ed.) *The State and Education Policy: The Academies Programme*, London: Continuum.

Rumgay, J. (2004) 'Scripts for safer survival: Pathways out of female crime', *The Howard Journal*, 43(4), pp. 405–19.

Rutter, M. (2006) 'Is Sure Start an effective preventive intervention?', *Child and Adolescent Mental Health*, 1(3), pp. 135–41.

Rutter, M. (2011) 'Child psychiatric diagnosis and classification: concepts, findings, challenges and potential', *Journal of Child Psychology and Psychiatry*, online version published March 2011.

Sadler, J. (2005) 'Knowledge, attitudes and beliefs of mainstream teachers of children with a preschool diagnosis of speech/language impairment', *Child Language, Teaching and Therapy*, 21(2), pp. 147–63.

Saleeby, D. (2002) *The Strengths Perspective in Social Work Practice*, Boston: Allyn and Bacon.

Sallnäs, M., Vinnerljung, B. and Kyhle Westermark, P. (2004) 'Breakdown of teenage placements in Swedish foster and residential care', *Child and Family Social Work*, 9, pp. 141–52.

Salloum, I. and Mezzich, E. (2009) *Psychiatric Diagnosis*, Chichester: Wiley.

Salmon, G. (2001) *E-Moderating*, London: Kogan Page.

Salmon, G. (2002) *E-tivities*, London: Kogan Page.

Samaritans (2008) *Media Guidelines* http://www.samaritans.org/pdf/ SamaritansMediaGuidelines-UK2008.pdf

Samaritans (2008) http://www.samaritans.org/media_centre/media_guidelines.aspx

Sammons, P., Power, S., Elliot, K., Robertson, P., Campbell, C. and Whitty, G. (2003) *New Community Schools in Scotland. Final report.* National evaluation of the pilot phase, Report for SEED (Edinburgh).

Samuel, M. (2010) 'Glasgow care partnerships scrapped over NHS–council row', *Community Care*, 1820, pp. 7–8.

Saraceno, C. (2009) 'Le polltiche della famiglia in Europa: tra convergenza e diversificazione', *Statoe Mercato*, 85, 4–30.

Sawyer, E. (2009) *Building Resilience in Families Under Stress*, London: NCB.

SCCYP (2009) Annual report of Scotland's Commissioner for Children and Young People (SCCYP) www.sccyp.org.uk.

Schofield, G. and Beek, M. (2006) *Attachment Handbook for Foster Care and Adoption*, London: BAAF.

Schofield, G. and Simmonds, J. (2009) *Handbook of Child Placement*, London: BAAF.

Schon, D. (1983) *The Reflective Practitioner*, New York: Basic Books.

Schoon, I. (2006) *Risk and Resilience*, Cambridge: Cambridge University Press.

Schor, J. (2004) *Born to Buy: the Commercialized Child and the New Consumer Culture*, New York: Scribner.

Schulz, M. (2001) 'The uncertain relevance of newness: organisational learning and knowledge flows', in *The Academy of Management Journal*, 44(4), pp. 661–81.

Scott, J. and Hill, M. (2006) *The Health of Looked-after and Accommodated Children and Young People in Scotland*, Edinburgh: SWIA.

Scott, J. and Ward, H. (2005) *Safeguarding and Promoting the Wellbeing of Children, Families and their Communities*, London: Jessica Kinsley Publishers.

Scottish Government (2008) *A Guide to Getting it Right for Every Child*, www.scotland.gov.uk/gettingitright/Publications/2008/09/22091734/1.

Scottish Executive (2001) *For Scotland's Children*, Edinburgh, Scottish Executive.

Scottish Executive (2004) *Forgotten Children*, Edinburgh: The Stationery Office.

Scottish Executive (2005a) *Getting it Right for Every Child*, Edinburgh, Scottish Executive, www.scotland.gov.uk/Topics/People/Young-People/childrensservices/girfec/

Scottish Executive (2005b) *Partnership Matters*. A guide to local authorities, NHS boards and voluntary organisations on supporting students with additional support needs, Edinburgh: The Stationery Office.

Scottish Executive (2005c) *Findings from the Scottish School Leavers Survey*, Edinburgh: Scottish Executive.

Scottish Government (2003) *Putting Our Communities First: a strategy for dealing with anti-social behaviour*, http://www.scotland.gov.uk/Publications/2003/06/17556/22908 Accessed 14 February 2011.

Scottish Government (2005) *National Care Standards: early education and childcare up to the age of 15*, revised, http://www.scotland.gov.uk/Resource/Doc/37432/0010250.pdf (27.5.10).

Scottish Government (2011) *Consulting on the common core of skills, knowledge and understanding and values that should be common to everyone working with children*, http://www.scotland.gov.uk/Publications/2011/03/14130453/2.

Scottish Statutory Instrument (SSI) Rules 2002 No. 63, The Children's Hearings (Legal Representation) (Scotland) Rules 2002.

Scottish Sun (2010) 'Fat Kid Crisis', September 29, http://www.thesun.co.uk/scotsol/homepage/news/3157459/Scotlands-fat-kids-crisis.html.

Scourfield, J., Dicks, B., Holland, S., Drakeford, M. and Andrews, A. (2006) *Children, Place and Identity*, London: Routledge.

Seckinger, M., van Santen, E. and Pluto, L. (2004) 'Comparative analyses of child and youth services in Europe', *Social Work and Society*, 2(2), pp. 199–206.

Sharp, D. and Atherton, S. (2007) 'To serve and protect?', *British Journal of Criminology*, 47, pp. 746–63.

Shaw, A. (2004) 'Immigrant families in the UK', in J. Scott, J. Tress and M. Richards (eds) *The Blackwell Companion to the Sociology of Families*, Oxford: Blackwell.

Shepperdson, B. (2000) 'Negotiating adolescence', in D. May (ed.) *Transition and Change in the Lives of People with Learning Disabilities*, London, Jessica Kingsley.

Sheridan, M. and Moller, J. (2005) 'Alleged assaults during April 2005', Paper presented to the UK College of Emergency Medicine Academic Conference.

Sherman, L. and Strang, H. (2007) *Restorative Justice: the Evidence*, London: Smith Institute.

Sims, D., Fineman, S. and Gabriel, Y. (1993) *Organising and Organisations: an Introduction*, London: Sage.

Sinclair, R. (2004) 'Participation in practice: making it meaningful, effective and sustainable', *Children and Society*, 18(2), pp. 106–18.

Sinclair, R. and Franklin, A. (2000) *A Quality Protects research briefing: young people's participation*, London: Department of Health.

Singer, P. (1973) *Democracy and Disobedience*, Oxford: Clarendon Press.

Singh, S., Paul, M., Ford, T., Kramer, T. and Weaver, T. (2008) 'Transitions of care from child and adolescent mental health services to adult mental health services (TRACK study): a study of protocols in Greater London', *BMC Health Service Research*, 8(135).

Skuse, T., Macdonald, I. and Ward, H. (1999) *Outcomes for Looked After Children: the Longitudinal Study*, Loughborough: Centre for children and family research.

Sloper, P. (2004) 'Facilitators and barriers for coordinated multi-agency services', *Child Care, Health and Development*, 30(6).

Small, M. (2006) 'Neighborhood institutions as resource brokers: childcare centers, inter-organizational ties, and resource access among the poor', *Social Problems*, 53(2), 274.

Smart, C. (2007) *Personal Life*, Cambridge: Polity.

Smith, A. B., Bjerke, H. and Taylor, N. J. (2009) 'The meaning of citizenship for children', *Children's Issues*, 13(1), pp. 43–9.

Smith, D. (2006) *Social Inclusion and Early Desistance from Crime*, Edinburgh: University of Edinburgh.

Smith, R., Smith, R., Schneider, V., Purdon, S., La Valle, I., Wollny, Y., Owen, R., Bryson, C., Mathers, S., Sylva, K. and Lloyd, E. (2009) *Early Education Pilot for Two-year-old Children – Evaluation*, Research report DCSF-RR134, London: DCSF.

Smith, T. (1996) *Family Centres and Bringing Up Young Children*, London: HMSO.

Sobotka, T. and Toulemon, L. (2008) 'Changing family and partnership behaviour: common trends and persistent diversity across Europe', *Demographic Research*, 19(6), pp. 85–138.

Social Care Institute for Excellence (2004) SCIE research briefing 9: *'Preventing teenage pregnancy in looked after children'*. Access on: http://www.scie.org.uk/publications/briefings/briefing09/index.asp.

Solomon, Y., Warin, J., Lewis, C. and Langford, W. (2002) 'Intimate talk between parents and their teenage children: democratic openness or covert control?', *Sociology*, 36(4), pp. 965–83.

Souhami, A. (2009) 'Doing youth justice: beyond boundaries?', in *Youth Offending and Youth Justice*, M. Barry and F. McNeill (eds), London: Jessica Kingsley.

Spencer, L. and Pahl, R. (2006) *Rethinking Friendship: Hidden Solidarities Today*, Princeton University Press.

Spitz, R. R. (1945) 'Hospitalism: an inquiry into the genesis of psychiatric conditions in early childhood', *Psychoanalytic Study of the Child*, Vol. 1, pp. 53–74.

Spratt, T. (2001) 'The influence of child protection orientation on child protection practice', *British Journal of Social Work*, 31(6), pp. 933–54.

Spratt, T. (2003) 'Child protection work and family support practice in five family centres', *Child Care in Practice*, 9(1), pp. 18–30.

Sroufe, L. A. (2005) 'Attachment and development: a prospective, longitudinal study from birth to adulthood', *Attachment and Human Development*, Vol. 7, No. 4, pp. 349–67.

Statham, J., Lloyd, E., Moss, P., Melhuish, E. and Owen, C. (1990) *Playgroups in a Changing World*, London: HMSO.

Stead, J., Lloyd, G. and Kendrick, A. (2004) 'Participation or practice innovation: tensions in inter-agency working to address disciplinary exclusion from school', *Children and Society*, 18, pp. 42–52.

Stephenson, M., Giller, H. and Brown, S. (2007) *Effective Practice in Youth Justice*, Cullompton: Willan.

Stevens, S. E., Sonuga-Barke, E. J. S., Kreppner, J. M., Groothues, C., Hawkins, A. and Rutter, M. (2008) 'Inattention/overactivity following early severe institutional deprivation: presentation and associations in early adolescence', *Journal of Abnormal Child Psychology*, Vol. 36, pp. 385–98.

Stewart, A., Petch, A. and Curtice, L. (2003) 'Moving towards integrated working in health and social care in Scotland: from maze to matrix', *Journal of Interprofessional Care*, 17(4), pp. 335–50.

Stone, D. (1989) 'Upside down prevention', *Health Service Journal*, 99, pp. 890–1.

Stone, D. (1993) *Costs and Benefits of Accident Prevention*, Glasgow: Public Health Research Unit.

Stone, F. H. (1995) *Report of the Committee on Children and Young Persons, Scotland (1964)* (*Kilbrandon Report*), 2nd edition with Stone's introduction, Edinburgh: HMSO.

Stovall-McClough, K. C. and Dozier, M. (2004) 'Forming attachments in foster care: infant attachment behaviors during the first 2 months of placement', *Development and Psychopathology*, Vol. 16, pp. 253–71.

Stradling, B. and MacNeil, M. M. (2007) *Delivering Integrated Services for Children in Highland*, Inverness: Highland Council and NHS Highland.

Stradling, B., MacNeil, M. M. and Berry, H. (2009) *An evaluation of the development and early implementation phases of getting it Right for every child in Highland 2006–2009*, Edinburgh: Scottish Government, www.scotland.gov.uk/gettingitright/Publications.

Stradling, B. and MacNeil, M. M. (2010) Evaluation briefing 8: *The impact on services and agencies part 2 – resource implications*, Scottish Government, www.scotland.gov.uk/gettingitright/Publications.

Strang, D. (2005) 'Policing youth in Scotland', in *Policing in Scotland*, D. Donnelly and K. Scott (eds), Cullompton, Willan.

Strang, H., Sherman, L. with Woods, D. (2010) *Effects of Restorative Justice Conferencing on Reoffending: A campbell collaboration review*, University of Pennsylvania: Jerry Lee Centre for Criminology.

Sullivan, H. and Fletcher, C. (2002) *Working Across Boundaries*, Basingstoke: Palgrave Macmillan.

Sullivan, K., Marshall, S. K. and Schonert-Reichl, K. (2002) 'Do expectancies influence choice of help-giver?', *Journal of Adolescent Research*, 17(5), pp. 509–31.

Sylva, K. and Taylor, H. (2006) 'Effective settings: evidence from research', in *Contemporary Issues in the Early Year*, G. Pugh and B. Duffy (eds), London: Sage Publications.

Tarleton, B. and Ward, L. (2005) 'Changes and choices: finding out what information young people with learning disabilities, their parents and supporters need at transition', *British Journal of Learning Disabilities*, 33, pp. 70–6.

Tarleton, B., Ward, L. and Howarth, J. (2006) *Finding the Right Support: a review of issues and positive practice to support parents with learning difficulties and their children*, London: The Baring Foundation.

TASC Agency (2003) *All I Want*, NHS Lothian/Healthy Respect, http://www.healthyrespect.co.uk/downloads-and-campaigns/resources-for-professionals.htm.

TASC Agency (2004) *Bullying: Looking to the Future*, Edinburgh: Scottish Executive Education Department.

TASC Agency (2005a) *Everyone Needs to Know Someone is There for Them*, Edinburgh: Scottish Executive.

TASC Agency (2005b) *A report on a consultation finding out more about what young people from black/minority ethnic communities need when it comes to sexual health services*, Edinburgh: NHS Health Scotland http://www.healthscotland.com/documents/1541.aspx.

TASC Agency (2006) *Confidentiality: Issues and Next Steps*, Edinburgh: NHS Health Scotland.

Taylor, C. and Dogra, N. (2002) 'Opinions to shape services', *Community Care*, 1440, pp. 42–4.

Taylor, N. J. and Smith, A. (2009) *Children as Citizens: International Voices*, Dunedin: University of Otago Press.

Taylor, R., Hill, M. and McNeill, F. (2011) *Early Professional Development for Social Workers*, Birmingham: Venture Press.

The Big Step (2001) *The Health of Young People in Care and Leaving Care in Glasgow*, Glasgow: The Big Step, Social Inclusion Project.

Theis, J. (2007) 'Performance, responsibility and political decision-making', *Children, Youth and Environments*, 17(1), pp. 1–13.

Thomas, J., Kavanagh, J., Tucker, H., Burchett, H., Tripney, J. and Oakley, A. (2007) *Accidental Injury, Risk-taking Behaviour and the Social Circumstances in which Young People Live: a systematic review*, London: EPPI-Centre, Social Science Research Unit, Institute of Education, University of London.

Thomas, N. (2000) *Children, Family and the State*, Basingstoke, Macmillan.

Thomas, N. (2007) 'Towards a theory of children's participation', *International Journal of Children's Rights*, 15, pp. 1–20.

Thomas, P. (2006) *Integrating Primary Health Care: Leading, Managing, Facilitating*, Oxford: Radcliffe.

Thorin, E., Yovanoff, P. and Irvin, L. (1996) 'Dilemmas faced by families during their young adults' transition to adulthood: a brief report', *Mental Retardation*, 34, pp. 117–20.

Tilbury, C., Buys, N. and Creed, P. (2009) 'Perspectives of young people in care about their school-to-work transition', *Australian Social Work*, 62(4), pp. 476–90.

Timms, J. (2009) 'Twenty-five years of guardians – where next?', *Seen and Heard*, 19(1), 41–53.

Tisdall, E. K. M. (2007) *School Councils and pupil participation in Scottish secondary schools* accessed at: http://www.scotconsumer.org.uk/education/SCCFinalPupilCouncilsReport.pdf.pdf (13.11.07).

Tisdall, E. K. M. and Davis, J. (2004) 'Making a Difference? Bringing children's and young people's views into policy-making', *Children and Society*, 18(2), pp. 131–42.

Tisdall, E. K. M., Davis, J. M. and Gallagher, M. (2008) 'Reflecting upon children and young people's participation in the UK', *International Journal of Children's Rights*, 16, pp. 419–29.

Tisdall, E. K. M., Davis, J. D. and Gallagher, M. (2009) *Researching with Children and Young People*, London: Sage.

Tisdall, E. K. M., Davis, J. M., Hill, M. and Prout, A. (eds) (2006) *Children, Young People and Social Inclusion: Participation for What?*, Bristol: Policy Press.

Tisdall, E. K. M. and Hill, M. (2010) 'Policy change under devolution: The prism of children's policy', *Social Policy and Society*, 10(1), 1–12.

Tizard, B., Moss, P. and Perry, J. (1976) *All Our Children*: *Pre-school Services in a Changing Society*, London: Maurice Temple Smith.

Todd, L. (2007) *Partnerships for Inclusive Education*, London: Routledge.

Tough, P. (2008) *Whatever it Takes: Geoffrey Canada's Quest to Change Harlem and America*, Boston: Houghton Mifflin Co.

Tracy, E. M. and Martin, T. C. (2007) 'Children's roles in the social networks of women in substance abuse treatment', *Journal of Substance Abuse Treatment*, 32(1), pp. 81–8.

Treasury-DfES (2007) *Policy Review of Children and Young People: a discussion paper*, London: HM Treasury.

Tremblay, R. E. (2010) 'Developmental origins of disruptive behaviour problems; the original sin hypothesis, epigenetics and their consequences for prevention', *Journal of Child Psychology and Psychiatry*, 51(1), Canada: Centre of Excellence for Early Childhood Development, pp. 333–40.

Turnell, A. and Edwards, S. (1999) *Signs of Safety: A Solution and Safety Approach to Child Protection Casework*, New York State: W. Norton and Co.

Turner, K., Hill, M., Stafford, A. and Walker, M. (2006) 'How children from disadvantaged areas keep safe', *Health Education*, 106(6), pp. 450–64.

UK Cabinet Office (2002) *Social Capital: a discussion paper*, London: UKCO.

UK Children's Commissioners (2008) *UK Children's Commissioners' Report to the UN Committee on the Rights of the Child*, London, Edinburgh, Belfast and Swansea.

UN Committee on the Rights of the Child (2008) *Concluding Observations: United Kingdom of Great Britain and Northern Ireland*, available online at http://www.unhchr.ch/tbs/doc.nsf/(Symbol)/CERD.C.63.CO.11.En?Opendocument [accessed 4 January 2011].

UNCRC (1995) UN Committee on the Rights of the Child, *Concluding Observations of the Committee on the Rights of the Child: United Kingdom of Great Britain and Northern Ireland*, CRC/C/15/Add.34, Geneva, 15 February 1995.

UNCRC (2002a) UN Committee on the Rights of the Child, *Concluding Observations: United Kingdom of Great Britain and Northern Ireland*, CRC/C/15/Add.188, Geneva, 9 October 2002.

UNCRC (2002b) UN Committee on the Rights of the Child, General Comment 2 (2002), *The Role of Independent National Human Rights Institutions in the Promotion and Protection of the Rights of the Child*, CRC/GC/2002/2, Geneva, 15 November 2002.

UNCRC (2008) UN Committee on the Rights of the Child, *Concluding Observations: United Kingdom of Great Britain and Northern Ireland*, CRC/C/GBR/CO/4, Geneva, 20 October 2008.

Ungar, M., Barter, K., McConnell, S. M., Tutty, L. and Fairholm, J. (2009) 'Patterns of abuse disclosure among youth', *Qualitative Social Work*, 8(3), pp. 341–56.

Vangen, S. and Huxham, C. (2003) 'Nurturing collaborative relationships: building trust in interorganizational collaboration', *Journal of Applied Behavioural Science*, 39(5), pp. 5–30.

VRU (2010) *The Violence Must Stop*, Glasgow: Strathclyde Police Violence Reduction Unit.

Vygotsky, L. S. (1978) *Mind in Society*, M. Cole, V. John-Steiner, S. Scribner and E. Souberman (eds), Cambridge, MA: Harvard University Press.

Vygotsky, L. S. (1986) *Thought and Language*, Cambridge, MA: MIT Press.

Vygotsky, L. S. (1987) 'Thinking and speech', in *The Collected Works of L. S. Vygotsky Volume 1: Problems of General Psychology*, Rieber, R. W. and Carton, A. S. (eds), New York: Plenum Press.

Wade, B. and Moore, M. (1998) 'An early start with books: literacy and mathematical evidence from a longitudinal study', *Educational Review*, 50, pp. 135–45.

Wade, J. (2006) 'The ties that bind: support from birth families and substitute families for young people leaving care', *British Journal of Social Work*, 38(1), pp. 39–54.

Wager, F., Hill, M., Bailey, N., Day, R., Hamilton, D. and King, C. (2009) 'The impact of poverty on children and young people's use of services', *Children and Society*, 23(5), pp. 400–12.

Wager, F., Hill, M., Bailey, N., Day, R., Hamilton, D. and King, C. (2007) *Serving Children*, Edinburgh: Save the Children.

Wajcman, J. (2008) 'Life in the fast lane? Towards a sociology of technology and time', *British Journal of Sociology*, 59, pp. 59–77.

Wallis, P. and Tudor, B. (2010) *The Pocket Guide to Restorative Justice*, London: Jessica Kingsley.

Walsh, F. (2003) 'Family resilience: strengths forged through adversity', in *Normal Family Processes*, Walsh, F. (ed.), New York: Guilford Press.

Ward, T. and Maruna, S. (2007) *Rehabilitation: Beyond the Risk Assessment Paradigm*, London: Routledge.

Warhurst, C. and Nickson, D. P. (2007) 'A new labour aristocracy? aesthetic labour and routine interactive service', *Work Employment and Society*, 21(4), pp. 785–98.

Waterman, C. and Fowler, J. (2004) *Plain Guide to the Children Act 2004*, Slough: National Foundation for Educational Research in England and Wales (NFER).

Watkins, J. (1998) *The Juvenile Justice Century: a Sociolegal Commentary on American Juvenile Courts*, Durham NC: Carolina Academic Press.

Watson, D., Abbott, D. and Townsley, R. (2006) 'Listen to me too!', *Child Care, Health and Development*, 33(1), pp. 90–5.

Weaver, B. and McNeill, F. (2010) 'Travelling hopefully: desistance theory and practice', in J. Brayford, F. Crowe and J. Deering (eds) *What Else Works?* Cullompton: Willan.

Webster, C., McDonald, R. and Simpson, M. (2006) 'Predicting criminality? Risk factors, neighbourhood influence and desistance', *Youth Justice*, 6(1), pp. 7–22.

Webster, C., Simpson, D., MacDonald, R., Abbas, A., Cieslik, M., Shilrick T. and Simpson, M. (2004) *Poor Transitions: Social Exclusion and Young Adults*, Bristol: The Policy Press.

Weller, S. (2006) '"Sticking with your mates"? Children's friendship trajectories during the transition from primary to secondary school', *Children and Society*, 21(5), pp. 339–51.

Weller, S. (2009) 'Young people's social capital: complex identities, dynamic networks', *Ethnic and Racial Studies*, 33(5), pp. 872–88.

Weller, S. and Bruegel, I. (2009) 'Children's "place" in the development of neighbourhood social capital', *Urban Studies*, 46(3), 629–43.

Wenger, E. (1998) *Communities of Practice: Learning, Meaning and Identity*, Cambridge, Cambridge University Press.

Werner, E. E. and Smith, R. S. (1992) *Overcoming the Odds*, Ithaca: Cornell University Press.

West, A., Mei, C. X., Zhou, Y., Na, Z. C. and Quiang, C. (2007) 'From performance to practice: changing the meaning of child participation in China', *Children, Youth and Environments*, 17(1), pp. 14–32.

Whitburn, S. (2003) *Education and the Human Rights Act 1998*, Slough: NFER.

White, R. and Green, A. (2011) 'Opening up or closing down opportunities?: The role of social networks and attachment to place in informing young people's attitudes and access to training and employment', *Urban Studies*, 48(1), pp. 41–60.

White, S., Wastell, D., Broadhurst, K. and Hall, C. (2010) 'When policy o'erleaps itself: The tragic tale of the integrated children's system', *Critical Social Policy*, 30, pp. 405–29.

Whitehead, J. and Clough, N. (2004) 'Pupils, the forgotten partners in education action zones' *Journal of Education Policy*, 19(2), pp. 215–27.

Whitehurst, G. J. and Croft, M. (2010) *The Harlem children's zone, promise neighborhoods, and the broader, bolder approach to education*, Report for Brown Center on Education Policy at Brookings (Washington DC).

Whitty, G. and Wisby, E. (2007) *Real decision making? School councils in action*, http://www.dfes.gov.uk/rsgateway/DB/RRP/u014805/index.shtml (accessed 18.2.08).

WHO (1948) Preamble to the Constitution of the World Health Organization as adopted by the International Health Conference, New York, 19–22 June, 1946; signed on 22 July 1946 by the representatives of 61 States (Official Records of the World Health Organization, No. 2, p. 100) and entered into force on 7 April 1948.

Whyte, B. (2008) *Youth Justice in Practice*, Bristol, Policy Press.

Widmer, E. D. and Jallinoja, R. (eds) (2008) *Beyond the Nuclear Family: Families in a Configurational Perspective*, Bern: Peter Lang.

Wierenga, A. (2009) *Young People Making a Life*, Basingstoke: Palgrave Macmillan.

Wilkin, A., Moor, H., Murfield, J., Kinder, K. and Johnson, F. (2006) *Behaviour in Scottish Schools*, Edinburgh: Scottish Executive Social Research.

Wilkinson, R. (1994) *Unfair Shares: the Effects of Widening Income Differences on the Welfare of the Young*, Ilford: Barnardos.

Wilkinson, R. and Pickett, K. (2009) *The Spirit Level: Why Equality is Better for Everyone*, London and New York: Penguin.

Williams, J. (2005) 'Effective government structures for children? The UK's four Children's Commissioners', 17, *Child and Family Law Quarterly*, pp. 37–53.

Williams, J. (2008) *Child Law for Social Work*, London: Sage.

Williams, J., Green, S., Dagle, E. and Harn's, E. (2009) *Growing Up in Ireland National Longitudinal Study of Children: the Lives of Nine-year-olds Child Cohort*, Dublin: The Stationery Office.

Williams, P. and Sullivan, H. (2010) 'Despite all we know about collaborative working, why do we still get it wrong?', *Journal of Integrated Care*, 18(4), pp. 4–15.

Willow, C., Franklin, A. and Shaw, C. (2007) *Meeting the obligations of the Convention on the Rights of the Child in England: children and young people's messages to government*, http://www.nspcc.org.uk/Inform/policyandpublicaffairs/CYP_Msg_to_Govt_wdf48658.pdf (24.10.07).

Wilson, K., Ruch, G., Lymbery, M. and Cooper, A. (2008) *Social Work*, Harlow: Pearson Longman.

Wilson, P., Barbour, R., Graham, C., Curry, M., Puckering, C. and Minnis, H. (2007) 'Health visitors' assessments of parent–child relationships: a focus group study', *International Journal of Nursing Studies*, 45, pp. 1137–47.

Wolak, J., Kimberly, J. M. and Finkelhor (2003) *'Escaping or connecting? Characteristics of youth who form close online relationships'*, *Journal of Adolescence*, 26(1), pp. 105–19.

Wood, L. J., Giles-Corti, B. and Bulsara, M. (2005) 'The pet connection: pets as a conduit for social capital?', *Social Science and Medicine*, 61(6), pp. 1159–73.

Wood, L. J., Giles-Corti, B., Bulsara, M. K. and Bosch, D. A. (2007) 'More than a furry companion: the ripple effect of companion animals on neighbourhood interactions and sense of community', *Society and Animals*, 15(1), pp. 43–56.

Woodhead, M. (2008) 'Child development and the development of childhood', in *The Palgrave Handbook of Childhood Studies*, J. Qvortrup, W. A. Corsaro and M-S. Honig (eds) Basingstoke: Palgrave Macmillan.

Woolcock, M. (1998) 'Social capital and economic development: towards a theoretical synthesis and policy framework', *Theory and Society*, 27, pp. 151–208.

World Bank (1999) *Bonds and bridges: Social capital and poverty*, http://povlibrary.worldbank.org/files/12048 Accessed 21 June 2008.

World Health Organisation (WHO) (2002) *Report on Violence and Health*, Geneva: WHO.

Worrall-Davies, A. and Cottrell, D. (2009) 'Outcome research and interagency work with children: What does it tell us about what the CAMHS contribution should look like?', *Children and Society*, 23(5), pp. 336–46.

Wu, L. and Musick, K. (2008) 'Stability of marital and cohabiting unions following a first birth', *Population Research and Policy Review*, 27, pp. 713–27.

Wylie, K. (2004) 'Citizenship, identity and social inclusion: lessons from Northern Ireland', *Journal of Educational Research*, 39(2), pp. 237–48.

Wyness, M., Harrison, L. and Buchanan, I. (2004) 'Childhood, politics and ambiguity: towards an agenda for children's political inclusion' *Sociology*, 38(1), pp. 81–99.

Yeoh, B. S. A., Huang, S. and Lama, T. (2005) 'Trans nationalizing the "Asian" family: imaginaries, intimacies and strategic intents', *Global Networks*, 5, pp. 307–15.

Young, R., Van Benumb, M., Sweeting, H. and West, P. (2007) 'Young people who self-harm', *British Journal of Psychiatry*, 191, pp. 44–9.

Ytterhus, B., Wendelborg, C. and Lundeby, H. (2008) 'Managing turning points and transitions in childhood and parenthood – insights from families with disabled children in Norway', *Disability and Society*, 23(6), pp. 625–36.

Zeanah, C. H., Larrieu, J. A., Heller, S. S. et al. (2001) 'Evaluation of a preventive intervention for maltreated infants and toddlers in foster care', *Journal of the American Academy of Child and Adolescent Psychiatry*, Vol. 40, No. 2, pp. 214–2.

Zeedyk, S. (2008) 'What's life in a baby buggy like?: The impact of buggy orientation on parent–infant interaction and infant stress', *National Literacy Trust*, http://www.literacytrust.org.uk/assets/0000/2524/Buggy_research.doc

Zelenko, M., Kraemer, H., Huffman, L., Gschwendt, M., Pageler, N. and Steiner, H. (2005) 'Heart rate correlates of attachment status in young mothers and their infants', *Journal of the American Academy of Child and Adolescent Psychiatry*, Vol. 44, No. 5, pp. 470–6.

Zigler, E. and Styfco, S. J. (1994) 'Is the HighScope Perry Preschool better than Head Start? Yes and no,' *Early Childhood Research Quarterly*, 9, pp. 269–87.

Zwozdiak-Myers, P. (2007) *Childhood and Youth Studies*, Exeter: Learning Matters.

Index